T0234895

FOR FEAR OF PAIN
BRITISH SURGERY, 1790–1850

THE WELLCOME SERIES IN THE HISTORY OF MEDICINE

The Wellcome Series in the History of Medicine series editors are
V. Nutton, M. Neve and R. Cooter.
Please send all queries regarding the series to Michael Laycock,
The Wellcome Trust Centre for the History of Medicine at UCL,
210 Euston Road, London NW1 2BE, UK.

FOR FEAR OF PAIN
BRITISH SURGERY, 1790–1850

Peter Stanley

Amsterdam – New York, NY 2003

First published in 2003
by Editions Rodopi B. V., Amsterdam – New York, NY 2002.

Stanley, Peter © 2003
Transferred to digital printing, 2006.

Design and Typesetting by Michael Laycock,
The Wellcome Trust Centre for the History of Medicine at UCL.
Printed and bound in The Netherlands by Editions Rodopi B. V.,
Amsterdam – New York, NY 2003.

British Library Cataloguing in Publication Data
A catalogue record for this book is available from the British
Library
ISBN 90-420-1024-X (Paper)
ISBN 90-420-1034-7 (Bound)

'For Fear of Pain
British Surgery, 1790–1850' –
Amsterdam – New York, NY:
Rodopi. – ill.
(Clio Medica 70 / ISSN 0045-7183;
The Wellcome Series in the History of Medicine)

Front cover:
A surgical operation to remove a malignant tumour from a man's left breast
and armpit in a Dublin drawing room, 1817.
Lettering notes: 'R Power operated on July 28th died this Augt 11th 1817.'
Image courtesy: *Wellcome Library*, London.

© Editions Rodopi B. V., Amsterdam – New York, NY 2003
Printed in The Netherlands

All titles in the Clio Medica series (from 1999 onwards) are available to
download from the CatchWord website: http://www.ingenta.com

Contents

'Who would lose, for fear of pain, this intellectual being?'

John Bell,
The Principles of Surgery, 1801

Acknowledgements

This book would not have been begun without Dr Janet McCalman of the University of Melbourne, whose example encouraged me to attempt it. At the Wellcome Institute, Dr Christopher Lawrence and the late Prof. Roy Porter gave invaluable encouragement, as did Prof. Barry Smith of the Australian National University and Prof. Jim Walvin of the University of York.

Dr John Malin, Dr Liesse Perrin and Ms Helen Hawkins of the Wellcome Trust's History of Medicine Programme provided essential support in 2000, without which the project could not have been completed. The British High Commission, Canberra, likewise provided invaluable financial support in 2000, and I am especially grateful to the then Deputy High Commissioner, Dr Andrew Pocock.

The Royal Australasian College of Surgeons has provided generous material and moral support. I am grateful to its past President, Mr Bruce Barraclough, to officers of the Section of Surgical History, notably Mr S.A. Mellick and Mr David Hardman, and members of the College's staff, notably Ms Jane Oliver. I particularly appreciate the honour of having been invited to be a Foundation Visitor of the College in 2001.

I am grateful to the librarians and archivists of the following institutions:

Australian National University; Barr-Smith Library, University of Adelaide; British Library; British Library Oriental and India Office Collections; Edinburgh Central Library; Huntington Library's Department of Manuscripts (Ms Gayle Barkley); Library of Congress, Washington; Lothian Health Services Archive, University of Edinburgh; Mitchell Library, Glasgow; Mitchell Library, Sydney; National Archives of Scotland; National Army Museum, London; National Library of Australia; National Library of Scotland; National Maritime Museum, Greenwich; National War Museum of Scotland (Mr Stephen Wood and Ms Edith Phillip); Old Operating Theatre, St Thomas's Street, London (Mr Kevin Flude, Ms Marietta Ryan and Mr Stewart Caine); Public Record Office, London; Royal Australasian College of Physicians (Ms Brenda Heagney); Royal

3

College of Surgeons of Edinburgh (Ms Marianne Smith); Royal College of Surgeons of England (Ms Claire Jackson); Royal Naval Museum (Dr Matthew Sheldon); the Royal Society of Medicine; State Library of New South Wales, Sydney; State Library of South Australia, Adelaide; State Library of Victoria, Melbourne; University of Adelaide; University College Archives, D.M.S Watson Library, University of London; University of Edinburgh Library; University of Melbourne, and its Brownless Bio-Medical Library; The State University of Ohio; Wellcome Institute for the History of Medicine.

I am grateful to colleague and participants in a number of talks and seminars presented in the course of researching and writing this book, at the Australasian College of Anaesthetists, the Australian Historical Association, the Australian National University, the Canberra Hospital, the Flinders University of South Australia, the Medical History Society of New South Wales, the Old Operating Theatre, London, the Royal Australasian College of Surgeons, the University of Melbourne and the University of Sydney.

Many individuals assisted and supported in many ways. They include Dr Richard Bailey; Dr Michael Barfoot (Lothian Health Services Archive, University of Edinburgh); Mr Gordon Cruickshank; Prof. Bruce le Quesne; Dr Bryan Egan, Prof. Bryan Gandevia, Dr Judith Godden; Dr David Hardman; Ms Rosalind Hearder; Dr Anthea Hyslop, Prof. Pat Jalland; Dr David Kinshington; Prof. David Lodge of the University of Birmingham; Ms Pamela Miller of the Osler Library of the History of Medicine, Montreal; Lt Col Clem Sargent; Dr Craig Wilcox; Rev. Robert Willson. My colleagues in the Military History Section, especially Anne-Marie Condé and Peter Londey offered welcome support.

Michael Laycock at the Wellcome Trust Centre for the History of Medicine at UCL has been a conscientious and co-operative editor. I thank him and Fred van der Zee, Marieke Schilling and their colleagues at Editions Rodopi who have produced this book handsomely.

Claire Cruickshank has been a painstaking editor without whose careful eye and judicious suggestions this book would have been much the poorer. This book brought us together and I dedicate it to her with love and gratitude.

Abbreviations

The location of contemporary works is indicated by the following abbreviations:

ANU	Australian National University, Canberra
BLUM	Brownless Bio-Medical Library, University of Melbourne
BL	British Library, London
ECL	Edinburgh Central Library
LC	Library of Congress, Washington
LHSA	Lothian Health Services Archive, University of Edinburgh
NAM	National Army Museum, London
NLA	National Library of Australia, Canberra
NLS	National Library of Scotland, Edinburgh
MLG	Mitchell Library, Glasgow
MLS	Mitchell Library, Sydney
MLSA	Mortlock Library of South Australiana, Adelaide
NMM	National Maritime Museum, London
NWMS	National War Museum of Scotland, Edinburgh
OIOC	Oriental and India Office Collections, British Library, London
PRO	Public Record Office, London
RACP	Royal Australasian College of Physicians, Sydney
RACS	Royal Australasian College of Surgeons, Melbourne
RCPE	Royal College of Physicians of Edinburgh
RCSEd	Royal College of Surgeons of Edinburgh
RCSEng	Royal College of Surgeons of England, London
RNM	Royal Naval Museum, Portsmouth
SLNSW	State Library of New South Wales, Sydney
SLSA	State Library of South Australia, Adelaide
SLV	State Library of Victoria, Melbourne
UA	Barr-Smith Library, University of Adelaide
UE	University of Edinburgh Library
UCA	University College Archives, D.M.S Watson Library, University of London
UM	University of Melbourne Library
WIHM	Wellcome Institute for the History of Medicine, London

Prologue

'Into the depths of our common nature'

John Brown qualified as a surgeon in Edinburgh in 1833. He had been apprenticed to one of the greatest of Scotland's surgeons in the first half of the century, James Syme, whom he revered. Brown practised as a physician, gaining modest fame through his literary endeavours following the publication of the story 'Rab and His Friends'.[1] Appearing in 1858 as a pamphlet, the story was often reprinted and translated in the following half century. It long outlasted its author, who died in 1882 having never equalled his first literary work in power or popularity.

Ostensibly the story of Rab, a big, scarred mongrel belonging to James, an Edinburgh carter, it is rather a deeply felt description of the death of James's wife Allie after a surgical operation. Brown later recorded how he had come to write the story while on holiday at Biggar, south of Edinburgh, in the mid-1850s. He sat down at twelve one mid-summer's night, not rising to go to bed until dawn. He recalled how the story had come on him 'at intervals, almost painfully, as if demanding to be told'.[2] Pressed later to declare it fact or fiction, he told a friend and colleague that it was 'in all essentials strictly a matter of fact'.[3]

Brown's story tells how, as a medical student late in 1830 he meets James and Allie, a devoted and seemingly childless couple in their sixties. Allie consults Brown over a growth in her right breast. He examines her and finds it 'hard as a stone, centre of horrid pain' and he muses why she should have been 'condemned by God to bear such a burden'. He calls in his senior, the taciturn Syme, who declares the growth to be malignant. Syme explains Allie's predicament succinctly: 'there could be no doubt it must kill her, and soon. It could be removed – it might never return – it would give her speedy relief – she should have it done.' Allie looks at James and asks, 'When?' 'Tomorrow', Syme replies.

Brown's description of the operation occupies a few lines. He relates how the operating room of Syme's private clinic, Minto House, is crowded with noisy students eager to secure good places to observe a 'capital operation'. 'Don't think them heartless,' he counsels. He explains that for students pity lessened as an emotion but gained power and purpose as a motive. Then, amid the clamour, Allie enters, her quiet dignity hushing the students. Behind her come James and Rab the dog. Allie climbs onto the table, still in her street clothes. She arranges her dress to expose her chest, rests on Brown and holds his hand as Syme begins cutting. She remains composed and silent all through a long operation. James sits with Rab's head between his knees, staring at the floor, restraining his growling.

At the end, Allie steps down from the table, turns to Syme and his still silent students and curtsies, begging their pardon if she has behaved ill. Brown and his fellow students weep like children. She is helped to a room where, at first, the wound appears to be healing cleanly – 'at first intention', as they said. Four days later, however, she lapses into delirium, imagining that she holds a long-dead baby to her bandaged chest, and she dies of post-operative infection. Victorian sentimentality and Presbyterian piety cannot mask the profound feeling of Brown's description of Allie's last hours, and of James's grief. Reflecting upon what he had witnessed as Syme's surgical pupil, Brown felt that his exposure to the operating room had allowed him to 'see down into the depths of our common nature'. Like Allie, he had felt 'the strong and gentle touch that we all need and never forget'. A sort of literary Landseer, Brown saw in the noble, pugnacious Rab 'the three cardinal virtues of dog or man – courage, endurance and skill'.[4] We infer that his mentor, Syme, and his patient, Allie, shared at least the first two qualities.

The popularity of John Brown's story – among a generation for which painful surgery was a recent memory – suggests how the dread of surgery had penetrated deeply into the psyche of its readers. The tale embodies many of the elements of this book. It illuminates the character and skill of surgeons; the place of students; the drama of the operating room; the limitations of contemporary medicine: above all, the plight of patients and their fortitude in undergoing an ordeal which is for us almost – but not quite – unimaginable. The story of Allie's operation brings us into this world.

This book, then, investigates the training and practice of British surgeons in the first half of the nineteenth century, between the death of John Hunter in 1793 and the acceptance of chemical anaesthesia about 1850: the final decades of painful surgery. It focuses on the relationships between surgeons, between surgeons and their pupils and between both and their patients. It is motivated by two central questions: how could surgeons like James Syme bring themselves to operate upon conscious patients, and how could patients like Allie bear to submit to surgery? Exploring these questions will, I hope, help us to gain insights into both the experience of painful surgery, and into 'the depths of our common nature'.

Notes

1. 'Rab and His Friends', in John Brown, *Horae Subsecivae* (London: Edmonston & Douglas, 1907), 265–80
2. John Brown to Miss Nancy Smith, July 1857, John Brown, *Letters of John Brown* (London: A.& C. Black, 1907), 117
3. Alexander Peddie, *Recollections of John Brown* (London: Percival & Co., 1893), 18
4. From the Preface to the first edition of *Horae Subsecivae*, quoted in *Letters of John Brown*, 5

Introduction:
'Painful, difficult, bloody, tedious and dangerous'

The operating room of pre-anaesthetic surgery remains largely closed to historians, who have permitted themselves understandably timid peeks within. As a consequence medical history has perpetrated a stereotyped view of surgery before anaesthesia. Adrian Desmond and James Moore's biography of Charles Darwin, in explaining Darwin's revulsion at the surgery he witnessed as a medical student in Edinburgh in the mid-1820s, puts the conventional view succinctly. Darwin, they wrote, would have seen 'Dirty hands clasp ... dirty saws, hacking and cutting quickly, the blood running into buckets of sawdust'.[1] Despite decades of research in medical history this view remains as dominant as ever. Here, in just sixteen words, we see painful surgery defined. It was crude, dirty, rapid, bloody, the last resort of desperate doctors, largely confined to amputation and resulted in high mortality: that it was agonising remains unstated but obvious. Much of this view is based upon fact. To defeat shock surgeons needed to operate rapidly: infection largely confined surgery to the extremities and the surface of the body. Ignorance of germ theory made infection probable and death likely. As a result hyperbole comes easily to descriptions of painful surgery. The *Encyclopaedia of Medical History*, for example, describes it as 'an explosion of agony, gouts of blood, and rapid movement'.[2] Agony and rapidity certainly – though perhaps less of either than we might imagine – but whether painful surgery was necessarily unduly gory is questionable. Certainly poor surgeons hoped that, as John Bell put it scornfully, 'the blood and cries' would conceal ignorance of anatomy or clumsiness but the conventional picture distorts, and it requires a careful re-consideration.[3] Accepting – as we will see – that surgeons, hospitals and nations operated differently through the period, the reality was significantly different.

This is a subject painful to contemplate, often disturbing to research and write as well as to read. During the first six months or so of pursuing it I found myself feeling physically uncomfortable reading the material. That the unease wore off is in itself an insight into the habituation that medical students experienced in the course of their clinical instruction. Confronting accounts of horrible suffering you might ask, as I did, why you should continue. You should persevere because contemplating painful surgery from the perspectives of both surgeon and subject, offers us insights into what has been for almost all of history one of the profound realities of the human condition: the experience of suffering.

•

In seeking to understand what surgery meant to surgeons, students and patients we must note several qualifications. This study is about one aspect of medical history. It does not deal substantially with the development of medical education, with the place of the hospital in medical thought and practice, with medical-academic politics or with relations between the medical 'colleges'. These subjects have been canvassed, often admirably, by other historians. This book constitutes a social history of the operating room.

It explores but does not try to exaggerate surgery's importance. Surgery was and remains dramatic. Even recognising what the contemporary accolades of 'heroic', 'bold' or 'daring' entailed we can still become entranced by the terrible fascination of the extreme human situation. However not even surgeons considered surgery as the most important aspect of medical practice. Robert Liston, the epitome of the heroic surgeon, reminded his students that to think so was a 'very common belief, especially among the young and inexperienced'.[4] It is possible to become preoccupied with the drama of operating room and forget that healing occurred in many other more subtle and unspectacular ways. I recognise, as did John Bell, that surgery was 'the least part' of the profession of healing.[5]

It is crucial to understand the language of evidence and interpretation. We must be sensitive to the difficulties inherent in the imperfect sources available, to the dominance of the surgeon's view, and of the difficulty of capturing the patient's voice. It is also too easy to be seduced by medical jargon, to slip into language that distances and conceals reality rather than confronts and exposes it. Finding the right 'tone' is essential. It is especially important not to sensationalise the drama of the operating room. The reality of painful surgery was always horrible. But if we are to understand the historical experience of illness and healing we must overcome the squeamishness and horror that we surely feel about painful surgery. The study of history offers one way of comprehending what humanity has encompassed and can encompass. Observing human relations in such extreme situations – in life and death, in war and revolution, on the sick bed

Figure I.1

Sir Astley Cooper (1768-1841) about 1825.
His easy manner reflects the confidence of a man regarded as the epitome
of the heroic operator but Cooper himself thought that he 'felt too much
before he began ever to make a perfect operator'.

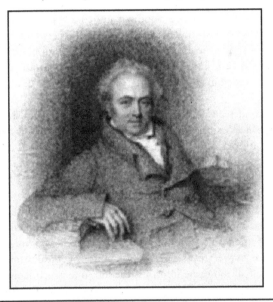

and on the operating table – offers a powerful route to understanding the limits and the possibilities of what being human can and might mean.

Surgery without pain has been a blessing for just over 150 years. Surgical operations are virtually universally performed under anaesthesia. Where they are not – in parts of the Third World and during wartime, in African conflicts and in the Balkan wars of the 1990s – the revelation of exception is regarded as shocking and newsworthy. In seeking to understand what occurred within operating rooms before the acceptance of anaesthesia then, we have to comprehend an experience entirely foreign to a modern conception of the practice of medicine. The surgeons of the pre-anaesthetic era and their students daily confronted scenes of pain, distress and suffering which are to us unimaginable without a close acquaintance with the surviving record, and then only by making a disciplined and informed leap of imagination.

In doing so we must resist the temptation to view the surgery of the early-nineteenth century through the prism of modern medicine. While implicit and individual comparison is unavoidable I have tried to avoid comparative adjectives and to avoid direct and indirect contrasts. Contemporary operative hygiene, for example, was neither 'remarkably dirty' nor 'surprisingly clean': we must seek to understand it as it was. I have therefore attempted to comprehend and express how practice appeared to contemporaries. Despite twenty years of post-modernist assault on whiggery the notion of 'progress' – and a disdain for what it supplants – still permeates our view of medicine. It is difficult but essential to avoid what E.P. Thompson called in another setting, 'the enormous condescension of posterity'.

This condescension is nowhere more apparent than in the way in which medical historians have for so long countenanced a simplistic view of surgeons and their practice. Christopher Lawrence, in an insightful and influential essay in *Medical History, Surgical Practice*, has identified the phenomenon whereby surgeons habitually boost their own era by denigrating former regimes as barbaric or inadequate. He has traced this tendency as far back as the renaissance: by the nineteenth century, with its implicit belief in the virtues of modernity and progress, the conceit was inescapable. Habituated as we are to a scientific culture of 'breakthroughs' we likewise fall all too easily into this reaction, one which hampers our ability to understand the past in its own terms. Even medical historians have displayed a reluctance to explore what painful surgery entailed or to consider the men who practised it, how they were able to inflict suffering and how they acquired the knowledge, skills and attitudes which enabled them to continue. While professional and amateur historians have long pursued medical history they have noticeably failed to enquire closely into the more challenging periods or themes. Not that the history of surgery has been neglected. Several excellent studies of surgical history are available. But they have generally adopted a technical approach, one that fails to consider surgery as an experience based on a relationship between healers and patients, or have focused unduly on the great men of surgical innovation. Historians of medicine have largely resisted the impulse to explore the subject as part of the richness of human experience.

Medicine before pain-killing has been regarded as an 'age of agony' in which the perils of shock and sepsis limited surgical treatments and condemned all those obliged to undergo them to an horrific, practically unimaginable experience. Or rather, one which,

Figure I.2

Robert Liston (1794-1847),
the greatest of the Scottish-trained operators of the first half of the century.
This bust, one of many such tributes to grace the halls of several royal
colleges of surgeons, testifies to the regard in which the great surgeons were
held. The bust, however, conceals the humanity of the man himself who
became deeply disturbed by the surgeon's responsibility.

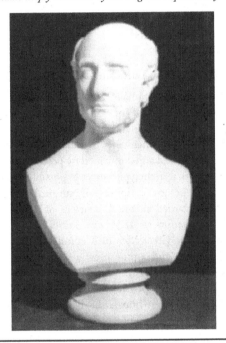

for fear of pain, we have been as a whole extremely reluctant to imagine. Abhorrence of painful surgery has arguably deterred enquiry into it. Despite the appearance of many valuable works which have vitally informed this study the practice of painful surgery has not been directly addressed.[6] Even scholars of medical history do not appear to have been interested in what it entailed or how it occurred. Roy Porter, in his *Companion Encyclopaedia of the History of Medicine and Science*, observes how pain is 'one of the more puzzling, and neglected, topics of the history of medicine' while Ghislaine Lawrence in the same work describes the state of scholarship on the history of surgery as 'undeveloped'.[7] For example, neither the Wellcome journal *Medical History* or the Johns Hopkins *Bulletin of Medical History*, the two most important journals in the field, have published much on the clinical or social history of surgical practice from the early nineteenth century over the past fifteen years. Painful surgery is a subject which, understandably, we would prefer not to contemplate: indeed the reluctance to confront it has arguably skewed the history of surgery. Otherwise useful studies dealing with medical education and practice appear to treat surgery superficially.[8] With the exception of Martin Pernick's pioneering study of American surgeons' reluctance to adopt anaesthesia universally, *A Calculus of Suffering*, no book-length study of the subject has appeared in the last two decades.[9]

'Pure surgeons': the operative surgeons of Britain, 1790-1850

Medical history has traditionally focused on great men: eminent doctors, those who named or cured conditions who became legendary as exponents or teachers of the healing art. Their formal portraits dot histories of medicine: dignified, respectable, secure in the reputations bestowed and confirmed by posterity. It is difficult to escape this traditional archetype but it is possible to subvert it: to attempt to see the great figures of surgical history as their contemporaries regarded them. A reviewer of Thomas Pettigrew's *Medical Portrait Gallery* in 1838 saw in its depictions of noted medical men not the Great Men of Medical History but men with ambitions, jealousies and animosities, a part of the robust early-Victorian medical profession.[10] Viewed in this light Sir Charles Clarke, Queen Adelaide's physician, looked to the reviewer 'like a prosperous Common Councilman'. Dr Blundell, Physician of Guy's, exuded 'the air of a smart shopman'. Sir Astley Cooper, the colossus of British surgery, appeared 'bursting with self importance like an "eminent" cheesemonger just raised to the dignity of deputy of his ward'. The great doctors of early-Victorian Britain, then, were socially much more marginal than medical professionals were to become. To their contemporaries, surgeons exhibited distinct, realistic and often uncomplimentary reputations such as a correspondent for the *Lancet* put it, 'knife-flourishing' Samuel Cooper, or 'indolent' Benjamin Travers, and 'money-scraping' William Lawrence.[11]

The surgeons of the great hospitals dominated London and Edinburgh surgery. With relatively few exceptions surgeons remained within one or two hospitals for most of their careers. They displayed a notable loyalty albeit one tinged with the self-interest inherent in a system relying on personal connection and reciprocal obligation. In virtually every hospital it is possible to ' trace a lineage of apprenticeship and promotion from generation to generation. To do so definitively would require a complex chart. For this purpose it is enough to introduce some of the protagonists and their protégés and suggest the personal and professional connections explored in greater depth in later chapters. The surgeons of Georgian and early-Victorian Britain appeared in many guises; as teachers, politicians, operators, patrons, colleagues, soldiers, scientists, charlatans and social climbers, to suggest a few. Some examples are useful.

Of the teachers John Abernethy was perhaps supreme. He dominated St Bartholomew's Hospital and, through his promotion of John Hunter's theories and robust teaching, disseminated the ideals of 'scientific surgery' far beyond it. He sought the cause of illness in the derangement of the internal organs and treated them by 'regimen' rather than surgery. Frequently commending his patients to an austere diet he was himself a notorious gourmand.

Abernethy was succeeded in 1825 by one of his pupils, William Lawrence, who inherited his standing among his pupils: his arrival in the wards was followed by the cry 'hats off'.[12] Lawrence paddled successfully in the treacherous waters of medical politics. A friend of Thomas Wakley and an early supporter of the *Lancet*, Lawrence played an ambiguous role in the struggle over medical reform, his belief in change at war with his personal ambition.[13]

Among the most long-serving of London's operators was the London Hospital's patriarch, Sir William Blizard. Known as 'Sir Billy Fretful,' Blizard became the first President of the Royal College of Surgeons at its reformation in 1800 and performed his last operation, a successful amputation at the thigh, at the age of 84.

As his papers in the Royal College of Surgeons testify, Sir Astley Cooper, 'the Wellington of British surgery' offers the example of the most successful medical patron whose connections stretched from Guy's Hospital across England. Adoring pupils 'followed him in troops'.[14] Cooper's fame generated a minor industry in itself with imposters setting up as 'associates of Dr Ashley Cooper' for years, tricking the unlettered or unwary into parting with money for bogus advice.[15] Cooper championed his nephews and relatives, precipitating the breach between Guy's and St Thomas's Hospitals early in 1825.

Success in medicine depended upon collegial diplomacy as well as on skill. Sir Anthony Carlisle succeeded as senior surgeon at the Westminster Hospital in 1793 and as a senior member of the Royal College of Surgeons defended the existing order. In 1820 his

Hunterian Oration on the ill-judged subject of 'The anatomy of an oyster' gained him notoriety as 'Sir Anthony Oyster'. (He had as many shell-fish as ... in an oyster shop', recalled Charles Bell, but broke down after 75 minutes 'amid the noise and hisses'.[16]) According to contemporaries Carlisle had only one skill, that of making friends, who remained loyal to him throughout.

As will be apparent war experience was to be crucial to the development of surgery. The surgeon who made most of his war service was George Guthrie. After serving as an army surgeon in the Peninsular war he began a civil practice in London. Once a progressive, Guthrie became a determined conservative in medical politics. 'Shrewd, quick, active and robust', although formally uneducated he possessed 'all the natural attributes of a great surgeon'.[17]

Among the greatest of clinical scientists produced by the surgical schools was Charles Bell who came to the Middlesex Hospital from Edinburgh in 1804. Bell was notable not only as a surgeon but also for his *New Anatomy of the Brain*, which established with greater certainty the function of the nerves and their relationship to the brain. An opponent of the 'philosophical anatomy' of radical colleagues at London University, he resigned in protest at its dominance.

St George's Hospital lived off the reputation of the great John Hunter. Though a capable operator its Surgeon, Everard Home, was also one of the period's great scientific charlatans. As executor of Hunter's papers and specimens he attracted suspicion for his discharge of that duty. He burned the papers, many believed after having appropriated much of their findings.

Surgeons were also alive to the material rewards of medical practice. Benjamin Brodie, a pupil of Home and a political and medical conservative, assumed much of Astley Cooper's standing after his retirement, not so much because of his skill as an operator, but because of careful diagnosis and post-operative treatment. He became immensely wealthy through surgery without displaying much of the scholarly zeal which marked his colleagues.

These men, who shared many of these characteristics, were among the most prominent of London's surgeons during the final decades of painful surgery. Acutely aware of their skill and reputation individually and collectively, they were regarded as aspiring to a particular standard of professional skill. They did not always meet that aspiration. A Scottish critic of the 'awkward and bungling' operations he witnessed at the London Hospital in October 1793 regarded the display as 'disgraceful to a Surgeon in the Metropolis of Great Britain near the end of the 18 Century'.[18] His judgement neatly introduces the London surgeons' counterparts, the surgeons of Edinburgh.

With several dozen 'pure surgeons' Edinburgh remained the kingdom's second great centre of medical and surgical practice, dominated in the final half-century of painful surgery by half-a-dozen men. Although they could rarely abide each other, collectively they and their proteges led British surgery for the best part of a century. Following the tradition of the Hunter brothers several able Scottish surgeons moved to London including Charles Bell, William Fergusson and Robert Liston. The migration of these talented men enhanced London's reputation, leading to English rivals deprecating Scottish 'clannishness'.[19] Scottish writers depicted 'the English public' as 'perfectly aware of the superiority of Scottish-educated practitioners'. This, the *Glasgow Medical Journal* soberly claimed, 'is no vain boast or hearsay'.[20]

The greatest of Scottish surgeons was James Syme, regarded (improbably in the light of his unprepossessing appearance) as the 'Napoleon of Surgery'. Barred from the Edinburgh Royal Infirmary, he opened his own surgical clinic in Minto House. A rival of Liston's (with whom he famously quarrelled and reconciled), he became Scotland's premier surgeon when Liston went to London. In the number and range of operations he devised or refined, in the number of students he taught or otherwise assisted and in his sheer longevity (practising from 1818 to 1868) Syme justifies his standing among his contemporaries.

Robert Liston arguably became the most celebrated surgeon of the period. As we will find he may also be the most enigmatic. Accused of encouraging his servant to promote him to dissatisfied patients in the Infirmary as 'the cleverest Doctor in Edinburgh' (a claim which he substantiated in a series of novel and dangerous operations), he was also barred from it, in 1822.[21] His manifest skill resulted in his reinstatement in 1828 and his elevation as 'one of the boldest and most dexterous operators' in either Scotland or England.[22] Known in Edinburgh for his bluntness, after his arrival in London in 1834 he attempted to restrain the ferocity of his address.

Perhaps the least sympathetic surgeon in either country was John Lizars. Lizars, being 'especially fond of the knife' comes closest to the popular retrospective view of the unfeeling operator.[23] His talents as an anatomist and surgeon were unquestioned but nowhere in his comprehensive *A System of Practical Surgery* does he recognise (as did his colleagues) patients' 'suffering' or 'misery' much less suggest ways of alleviating or abbreviating them. No one wrote an admiring biography of him; he attracted no followers and the only emotion apparent in his book is envy of his rivals.

These men were the 'pure surgeons' who populate this book. Physically perhaps their only common characteristic was that many possessed unusual strength and dexterity and often – notably Robert Liston, William Fergusson and Charles Aston Key – large, powerful hands. But each of them was required and prepared to perform operations which only a few hundred individuals in the kingdom could contemplate hazarding. Although disparate and often at loggerheads with each other, their careers span a period at once marked by shared assumptions and by dramatic change. They included the colleagues and students of Hunter and men who lived to see his theories overtaken by the Listerian revolution. These were the men whose lives and careers form the core of the experience of what they regarded as 'modern surgery'.

Notes

1. Adrian Desmond & James Moore, *Darwin* (Harmondsworth: Penguin, 1992), 27 .
2. Roderick McGrew & Margaret McGrew (eds), *Encyclopaedia of Medical History* (New York: McGraw-Hill, 1985), 325.
3. John Bell, *The Principles of Surgery*, 2 vols (Edinburgh: T. Cadell & W. Davies, 1801), Vol. I, 7.
4. Robert Liston, *Practical Surgery* (London: John Churchill, 1846), 15–16.
5. Bell, *op. cit.* (note 3), Vol. I, 1.
6. These works include William Bynum's *Science and the Practice of Medicine in the Nineteenth Century* (Cambridge: CUP, 1991), Susan Lawrence's *Charitable Knowledge: Hospital Pupils and Practitioners in Eighteenth-Century London* (Cambridge: CUP, 1996), Barry Smith's *The People's Health 1830–1910* (London: Croom Helm, 1979) , Alison Winter's, *Mesmerized: Powers of Mind in Victorian Britain* (Chicago: University of Chicago Press, 1998), and A.J. Youngson's *The Scientific Revolution in Victorian Medicine* (New York: Croom Helm, 1979).
7. W.F. Bynum & Roy Porter (eds), *Companion Encyclopedia of the History of Medicine and Science*, 2 vols (London: Routledge, 1993), Vol. II, 1574, 976.
8. For example, M. Jeanne Peterson's *The Medical Profession in Mid-*

Introduction

Victorian London (Berkeley: University of California Press, 1978) offers a valuable study of the composition of and changes within the profession, but virtually ignores the work of its subjects. Lisa Rosner's *Medical Education in the Age of Improvement: Edinburgh Students and Apprentices 1760–1826* (Edinburgh: Edinburgh University Press, 1991) devotes little attention to students' reactions to dissection and operations.

9. Martin S. Pernick, *A Calculus of Suffering: Pain, Professionalism and Anesthesia in Nineteenth Century America* (New York: Columbia University Press, 1985).

10. *The Times*, 13 July 1838, 5d.

11. *Lancet*, 1832–33, Vol. I, 16.

12. John Mann, *Recollections of My Early and Professional Life* (London: W. Rider & Sons, 1887), 139.

13. Forbes Winslow, *Physic and Physicians: A Medical Sketch Book*, 2 vols (London: Longman, Orme, Brown, 1839), Vol. II, 377.

14. Thomas Pettigrew, *Biographical Memoirs of the Most Celebrated Physicians, Surgeons, etc., etc.*, 3 vols (London: Fisher, Son & Co., 1839–40), 3.

15. Bransby Cooper, *The Life of Sir Astley Cooper, Bart.*, 2 vols (London: John Parker, 1843), Vol. II, 169.

16. Charles Bell to George Bell, 9 January 1826, George Jospeh Bell, (ed.), *Letters of Sir George Bell* (London: John Murray, 1870), 293 .

17. J.F. Clarke, *Autobiographical Recollections* (London: J. & A. Churchill, 1874), 258n; 293.

18. Charles Anderson, 'Memoranda during a visit to London', MS 2778, NLS.

19. *Lancet*, 1850, 136 .

20. 'The Apothecaries Hall, London, and the Medical Schools of Scotland', *Glasgow Medical Journal*, Vol. 1, (NS), No. III, 1833, 333.

21. Robert Liston, *Letter to the Right Hon. The Lord Provost ...* (Edinburgh: John Robertson, 1822), 12–13; Robert Liston, *Letter to the Honourable the Managers of the Royal Infirmary ...* (Edinburgh: J. Robertson, 1822), iii.

22. Review of *Elements of Surgery* in *Edinburgh Medical & Surgical Journal*, 1831, Vol. 31, 195.

23. Robert Paterson, *Memorials of the Life of James Syme* (Edinburgh: Edmonston & Douglas, 1874), 66

1

'Surgeons and operators':
The Surgeons' World

The characters, aspirations and achievements of the prominent
surgeons of Britain and especially their relations with their pupils and
patients form the core of this study. Before joining them in the
hospital ward, the operating room, the cockpit or the hospital tent it
is necessary to understand the medical profession of Georgian and
early-Victorian Britain.

'Surgeons' and 'subordinates': the medical profession

The medical world of the early nineteenth century was, in the words
of a contemporary, 'mixed, jumbled, brayded and blended'.[1] In the
mid-1820s nearly four thousand qualified physicians, surgeons,
apothecaries and druggists served the people of London. Compared
with Paris London boasted more than twice as many qualified
medical men per head, all rivals in an open and fiercely competitive
market. In addition to the 'regular' practitioners were 'the irregular
troops of corn-doctors, horse-doctors, tooth-doctors and quack-
doctors'.[2] Qualified practitioners disdained the irregulars living off
the sick poor: Robert Liston disgustedly described how an Edinburgh
quack had treated nasal polyps with undiluted suphuric acid which
destroyed not only the growths but also the bones of a man's nose.[3]
The expansion of formal medical education produced large
numbers of graduates. In the 1820s the Royal College of Surgeons
granted diplomas to between three and four hundred men annually,
in the early 1840s to about five hundred.[4] Positions for these
aspirants never equalled the numbers produced. The great majority
of men qualifying as 'surgeons' would in fact practise privately as
what were becoming known as 'general practitioners'. The creation of
the Apothecaries Act of 1815, by 1850 they would eclipse the earlier
'surgeon apothecary'. It was to this local doctor that all but the very
poorest or very wealthiest would resort in case of illness. The great
majority of those who entered the profession as students would never
perform a serious surgical operation except in dire emergency. Even
country practitioners would seldom operate. The journal of Gideon
Mantell who practised in rural Sussex shows that he performed nine

23

operations in the eleven years from 1819 including two operations for cataract, three trepannings and three amputations of fingers.[5] The diary of Thomas Wright discloses that as an apprentice in a Northumberland mining village he assisted at no amputations in four years in the 1820s.[6] Many general practitioners would come to resemble, as Henry Mayhew described the type, 'that bland, gentlemanly, useful humbug, the fourth-rate family doctor': and we, like Mayhew, will have little more to do with him.[7] The 'medical profession' as it was becoming known therefore encompassed at one end of the scale irregular practitioners and struggling local apothecaries and at the other the elite of the hospital surgeons.

The army and navy and the East India Company required large numbers of medical officers. These services offered situations and advancement for large numbers of young men, and not only during the French wars. The army employed just 142 surgeons in 1793 but over 950 by 1815.[8] Indian situations increased as the Company's domains grew. In 1793 the Bengal presidency directory listed 155 surgeons. By 1837 it included 379.[9] Some of the assistants of 1793 had become full surgeons by 1816 but not many. The mortality of Indian service ensured that each year the Company's directors sought replacements, and the Company's 'Cadet papers' demonstrate there was no shortage of applicants. Thomas Goldie Scott who arrived in Bengal as an assistant surgeon in the early-1840s received a discouraging letter from his father soon after. 'There is no doubt that the Indian Service offers great advantages', William Scott mused, 'but then how few live to reach that point ...'[10] Other graduates sought positions in the various colonial services and aboard emigrant or convict ships, although the merchant navy generally got by without. The acceptance of the Royal College's qualifications led to the extension of exclusive employment: the Liverpool administration decreed that surgeons to prisons needed to be members of it.[11] The cholera epidemics of the 1830s prompted a requirement that all British vessels carrying more than fifty passengers should have a qualified surgeon aboard. 'The cholera has done this good for young surgeons' the *London Medical and Surgical Journal* remarked.[12] By the late 1840s there were more emigrant ships wanting surgeons than practitioners willing to serve aboard them.[13]

For most surgeons, besides the few whose hospital positions and reputations garnered patients from distant parts, professional survival was a continuing preoccupation. Adopting hospital surgery did not represent an easy or certain route to prosperity. Hospital appointments were almost entirely honorary. Guy's paid its surgeons and physicians £40 a year.[14] They carried with them, however, two sources of income. First, appointments enabled surgeons to obtain perquisites in the fees for various services, notably their teaching duties, which allowed them to make a basic income. Second, their position, allied with their reputation and contacts, allowed them a substantial advantage in the competitive market place of the time. Ironically, this obliged them to cultivate those they called 'the subordinates', the surgeon-apothecaries in the suburbs and provinces who would refer the patients to them who paid private fees. ('I have heard my good friend BRODIE say,' a satirist claimed in the *Lancet*, 'that nothing remunerated him better than the outlay for dinner to a dozen of the subordinates'.[15]) Their official position therefore became a significant element in their capacity to attract private patients. It would be crude to suggest that pure surgeons adopted their distressing trade solely in hope of gaining a competitive advantage. At the same time, given the income those few at the head of their profession commanded, it must have been a sore temptation to some young men to contemplate embarking on a surgical career in the hope of sharing in the bloodily-won boon. The rewards of success could be considerable. The surviving receipt books of Benjamin Brodie, for example, show that he made over £8,000 a year in the late 1820s while Astley Cooper was believed at the time to have made over £15,000 a year from private practice.[16]

Obtaining situations at and promotions within hospitals demanded more than medical skill. Securing even junior appointments entailed arduous canvassing among a hospital's hundreds of contributors and governors: a man had to become an operator in another sense. Hospital positions, valuable investments, were often traded in the coinage of influence, sometimes openly. In London the aged William Lynn could be induced to retire only on the condition that his son would be made the Westminster's fourth surgeon. In Edinburgh Syme only succeeded James Russell in 1833 on condition that he pay Russell a £300 annuity.* The appointments of Assistant Surgeon and Surgeon were generally filled by elections in which hospital governors voted, in person or by proxy, in open and fiercely contested competitions. Candidates secured votes by energetic lobbying of governors and by seeking the endorsement of a powerful professional patron. Canvassing for the position of Surgeon at the Middlesex Hospital in 1814, Charles Bell described his

---

* Fortunately for Syme – though not Russell – he died only three years later.

preparations: 'dressed to a T; lists made out, and cards arranged ... a most unpleasant business'.[17] James Simpson's daughter recalled how he had been obliged to write fifty or more four-page letters, spending hours soliciting testimonials and votes only to be elected by a majority of one.[18]

Medicine was an uncertain profession in more than continuity and regularity of employment. In 1841 published figures suggested that doctors died prematurely. Based on a sample of over a thousand medical men, an actuary found that only 24 in a hundred would reach the age of 62 compared to 43 theologians, 85 clerks and 32 soldiers. 'There is not any career', he concluded, 'which so rapidly wears away the powers of life.'[19] The practice of medicine whether in the fever or surgical wards carried inherent risks of infection or contagion or overwork. A doctor commented wryly that 'it would be rather singular if many of us were left to die a natural death'.[20] Students confronted the sudden death of friends. John Mann who commenced at St Thomas's in 1813, realised one day that he had not seen about a young man named Consett who had worked at his dissecting room table. He asked the demonstrator, John South, what had become of Consett. 'He is dead,' South answered bluntly, 'he wounded one of his fingers in dissecting'.[21]

Surgery was a risky business in a more conventional sense. Many surgeons sank large amounts of money in positions, private practices and schools naturally hoping to recoup and better their investments. Buying out recalcitrant seniors John Erichsen bought a half-share in the lectureship in anatomy at the Westminster Hospital Medical School only to find that because the hospital discontinued the school for two years he could attract no students and therefore no income.[22]

'Our adversaries': apothecaries, physicians and surgeons

Surgeons strove to maintain their professional standing. After treating an opera dancer's soft corns William Lawrence entreated a friend to 'not mention to anyone that I have turned chiropodist'.[23] Physicians, surgeons and apothecaries fought to maintain a hard-won but increasingly untenable distinction between their professional spheres. Both physicians and surgeons looked askance on the apothecary, whom they tended to deprecate as 'a mere compounder of medicines'. Robert Kerrison complained that the Royal Colleges, of Physicians and Surgeons respectively, treated his own Society of Apothecaries with 'a coldness bordering on contempt'. Over the first half of the century, though, apothecaries would become 'general practitioners', the most numerous group, the first resort of most

working people and much of the middle class.[24] Most medical
students were destined to take the Licentiate of the Society of
Apothecaries and return to provincial towns.

Physicians regarded themselves as superior to surgeons, 'our
adversaries', as an Edinburgh physician put it.[25] The Royal Colleges
of Physicians in both London and Edinburgh, the oldest medical
companies (dating from the sixteenth century) retained great
influence and social standing. The surgeons' growing confidence
challenged the physicians' authority. Several London surgeons
commanded large fees as great as the formerly more prestigious
physicians. The story is often told how Astley Cooper was paid by a
wealthy patient tossing him a cheque for a thousand guineas in a
night cap: what is less well-known is that the fee was three times that
paid to the attending physicians.[26] By the 1820s many hospital
surgeons no longer sought a physician's endorsement before
operating and physicians became increasingly irrelevant in the
treatment of surgical conditions. In 1838 Charles Bell counselled his
colleagues against allowing physicians to sound for the stone before
lithotomies, 'by way of making them parties to the event'.[27] The
Royal College of Surgeons grew out of the Company of Surgeons,
which in 1750 had separated from the barbers with whom they had
been united since 1540. The surgeon's rising status was marked by
the grant in 1800 of the royal charter. The College's prestige – or at
least pretensions – was embodied in the grand building in Lincoln's
Inn Fields which was successively extended throughout the century.

The differences between physicians and surgeons could be
represented as profound. Anthony Carlisle explained the
demarcation to the 1834 Select Committee on Medical Education
using a graphic example that might have taken aback its members. If
a condition of the lower intestine were out of reach of a finger
inserted in the rectum, he explained, it belonged to the physician.
But, he continued, 'the moment it comes down and within reach of
the finger, it belongs to the surgeon': not that a physician would have
stooped to rectal, or indeed any physical examination.[28] Both,
however, sought to maintain distinctions deriving more from
professional identity than from clinical necessity. While only
surgeons operated and only physicians treated many conditions (such
as fever), in practice their spheres overlapped considerably. Both
prescribed and treated ostensibly internal conditions.

The barrier which had become inflexible through the obduracy of
the respective colleges began to erode in the face of the obvious need
to treat patients and conditions rather than restrict practitioners

arbitrarily. Benjamin Travers recalled that until the late 1820s surgeons at St Thomas's Hospital 'literally could not prescribe beyond a black draught, or a dose of opening medicine'. About 1827, however, the hospital's two professions reached a 'gentlemanlike understanding' which allowed surgeons to prescribe (though the physicians declined to cut).[29] The formation of the Medical and Chirurgical Society in 1805 which brought together physicians, surgeons and some apothecaries 'to converse upon professional subjects', suggests that the demarcation had provided a firm professional identity from which to work.[30] In his Hunterian Oration in 1834 William Lawrence quoted John Abernethy to express a working consensus. He acknowledged that because there was 'only one kind of pathology' so there must be no distinction between medical and surgical treatment.[31] By the 1850s relations had improved markedly, perhaps because each had established both their social and clinical standing beyond doubt. In 1851 *The Times* carried a curious exchange in which the physicians and surgeons involved in a delicate but successful caesarean operation referred with grave courtesy to the 'cordial co-operation' prevailing between them.[32]

The only way to make a name as a surgeon, however, was by performing operations, and young men hoped that by performing an operation first, more daringly or more spectacularly it would enhance their reputation. 'Humanitas', a correspondent in the *Lancet* in 1836, accused his colleagues of 'heartless butchery' by which they '"cut their way" to the temple of Fame'.[33] George Macilwain, having seen forty graduating classes embark upon a medical career, wearily bemoaned the ambitious country practitioner who, he claimed, knew that saving twenty limbs without surgery would not gain him the fame he could gain from a single amputation.[34]

'Title and privileges': the surgeon's social standing

The rise of a self-conscious discipline of 'modern surgery' had created since the final decade of the previous century what Benjamin Brodie called 'a new profession altogether'.[35] Unlike their continental colleagues, surgeons in Britain had long severed their ties with barbers. British surgeons serving abroad during the French wars encountered, and objected to, the echoes of the old pairing of barber-surgeon. J.G. Millingen recorded that in 1801 British assistant surgeons serving in the Swedish navy were dismissed for refusing to act as barbers. Millingen himself, while serving in the Peninsula, offended one of his Portuguese assistant surgeons when he declined an offer to be shaved, a service reflecting in Millingen's eyes a subordination that British surgeons had escaped fifty years before.[36]

To Regency and early-Victorian Britain, the term 'surgeon' covered a great diversity of character, commitment and competence. It included the operative surgeons in the great metropolitan hospitals and civil medical officers in Indian cantonments, regimental surgeons and men who were also becoming known as general practitioners. It included men who practised dissection daily, who rehearsed operations on 'the dead subject' and who operated once a week or more and also those who drew no more blood than that spilt using a lancet and avoided operating at all costs. It encompassed men who practised at the highest level of professional knowledge and those barely removed from quacks. Despite the names 'surgeon' or 'surgeon apothecary' the great majority of men graduating from these various institutions were destined to practise medicine in general rather than surgery in particular. Men nominally 'surgeons' could practise for years without cutting more than a boil or a vein. Except for isolated practitioners called out to accidents, emergencies and especially childbirth most practitioners could avoid cutting altogether if they chose to. Understandably, many did. Their practice would, of course, entail much that was demanding and unpleasant but it need not have entailed the infliction of surgical pain. Instead, as George Guthrie explained to a parliamentary committee, "if there is a great operation to be done, the patient is sent to the hospital in the county town'.[37] Consequently of the two thousand members of the Royal College of Surgeons in the mid-1830s, only some two hundred practised surgery exclusively. 'Pure' surgery, then, distinguished between those who where prepared to cut in healing, irrespective that they also prescribed, and those who declined to cut as well as prescribing. The distinction, inherited from the demarcation disputes of the previous century, remained both untenable and tenacious

The term 'pure surgeon' concealed a paradox. Their claims to being scientific practitioners relied as much as anything on men recognising the unity of medicine and surgery. As all conceded, surgery did not involve merely operative skill. Indeed, the mechanical aspects of medicine were regarded as an inferior branch of the art of healing. While proud of their status as an elite they simultaneously proclaimed that their qualifications and experience were as good as those of their rivals. Robert Liston, defending the treatment in an aneurism case, asserted that his training was 'equally full in all its branches with that of any physician or general practitioner'. He claimed to be as able to 'avert and do away with' an operation as to 'perform it when it is absolutely required'.[38] Astley Cooper admitted that 'the fact is that we are all physician-surgeons, and it is folly to say that any man is a pure surgeon': which in no way diminished their pride in their skill with the knife.[39]

While in the eighteenth century individual surgeons had attained fame performing particular operations, these tended only to distinguish men skilled in lithotomy from those willing to attempt anything else. From about 1800 the greater range of operations introduced tended to mark out surgeons willing or able to undertake certain operations in preference to others. William Fergusson, for example, favoured excisions; James Wardrop ophthalmic surgery; Joseph Carpue rhinoplasty and John Lizars ovariotomies. Frederick Salmon specialised in anal fistula operating on 3,500 successfully including Charles Dickens. Others would not undertake particular procedures; lithotomy in particular retained its reputation as an operation requiring exceptional anatomical knowledge and surgical judgement. Despite the beginnings of specialisation most surgeons appeared willing to undertake most procedures if required. Only later in the period could Arthur Farre complain that the mother of a boy he was examining protested that his eyes were under Mr A., his limbs under Mr P., and to Farre's question as to what he should inspect answered irritably 'his stomach, sir, his stomach'.[40]

Surgery at the highest level was practised in the three great cities of the kingdom, Dublin, Edinburgh and pre-eminently, London. Their provincial colleagues had to bear the condescension of London surgeons especially; a considerable impost on their patience. Although every large provincial hospital included at least one surgeon on its staff (mostly in honorary capacities like their London counterparts) surgery remained in the eyes of the colleges a metropolitan calling. While George Guthrie conceded that 'many improvements are made by surgeons in the country' he believed that 'the great advance in anatomy and surgery is due to the surgeons of the metropolitan cities'.[41] Astley Cooper exemplified the arrogance of London surgeons. William Hey of Leeds had made a point in the preface to the third edition of his *Practical Observations in Surgery* of expressing his gratitude for Astley Cooper's condescension. Since the previous edition Cooper had favoured Hey with 'a wet preparation of a strangulated Femoral Hernia' upon which Hey 'set a high value', not only for its scientific interest but because it 'afforded a repeated instance of his civility to me'.[42] Cooper's civility did not long outlive Hey. Asked by a member of the Parliamentary committee on medical education whether Hey would have been fit to examine for the

College, Cooper replied, airily patronising. 'He was a good practical surgeon' he conceded 'and an ingenious man; but he had not that foundation in anatomy, which fits a man for the highest scientific views of his profession'.[43] The London surgeons' condescension was galling and unmerited: as John Shepherd showed in tracing the history of operations for ovarian tumours it was provincial surgeons who attempted ovariotomy with growing success when London surgeons regarded them as impossible.[44]

In the 1790s the surgeon's emergence as a gentleman remained incomplete: indeed, it would not be confirmed so for a further century. Surgeons, however, were already contesting the widespread assumption that they must be marginal gentlemen. The armed services provided the acid test of gentlemanly standing: not until 1843 did the Admiralty consider surgeons worthy of commissions as naval officers.[45] 'A nobleman' had told Cooper that he had sought to place his sons in the church and the law but 'as to your profession, it is out of the question'.[46] Joseph Green of St Thomas's, in a letter to Astley Cooper, identified two courses by which surgeons had established the social standing they enjoyed; their 'intimate connexion with [the] liberal sciences' and the 'conduct and character of individual members'. These approaches he believed had secured for surgeons 'the title and privileges of GENTLEMEN'.[47] The profession's leaders supported the retention of high fees for medical education not only because a good proportion of the money went to themselves but also because if reduced, as Astley Cooper put it, 'you would have persons of all descriptions coming into the profession'. It would, he protested, become 'exceedingly degraded'. Abernethy embodied the social aspirations of surgeons. He remained as avaricious as any: one of the many Abernethy anecdotes has him searching the floor after being paid a guinea, looking pointedly 'for the other half'.[48] He sought esteem as well as wealth, once telling Astley Cooper that he intended to live seven years in the city, seven in the middle of town and seven in the fashionable west end. Sadly, as a biographer observed, 'he never advanced further west than Bedford Row'.[49] It was not, however, status that long marred surgeons' social standing but the corporeal realities of their craft and especially their dealing in dissection.

'Turning up the ground': body-snatching and the Anatomy Act

Public disquiet about 'body-snatching' remained until the 1830s one of the principal reasons for surgeons' inability to secure the esteem they craved. The growth of formal medical education, the increasing

31

numbers of students to be served and the interest of scientific surgeons in investigating and explaining the body placed a premium on the supply of cadavers. Although obliging students to acquire anatomical knowledge the law denied them the means of acquiring it. Legitimate sources of supply – the bodies of executed criminals – were, even in an age of capital punishment, inadequate to the demand. Proposals that the bodies of prostitutes, suicides and duellists be made available foundered and in any case would not have met the need.[50] In Edinburgh,.where dissection became compulsory in the mid-1820s, 300 students sought cadavers at any one time. In London the number was more than twice as great.[51] In 1831 however, just eleven bodies could have been obtained legally in London.[52] Anatomists therefore fell into an association with a clandestine criminal fraternity prepared to meet their needs for gain.

Astley Cooper's servant, Charles Osbaldston, a powerful figure in granting private patients access to Cooper's surgery, became an intermediary between Cooper and 'resurrection men'. Nor was Cooper alone. Procurers became intimate with many surgeons and the proprietors of schools of anatomy: Bransby Cooper acknowledged that resurrection men could have been seen 'flitting about' dissecting rooms 'complacently bowing to the lecturers'.[53] Notable surgeons were known to consort with resurrection men, the subjects of Thomas Hood's rightly often-quoted satirical verse, 'Mary's Ghost, a Pathetic Ballad'. Mary, whose grave has been opened and her body distributed to anatomists, addresses her fiancée thus:

> I vowed that you should have my hand,
> > But Fate gives us denial;
> You'll find it there at Mr Bell's
> > In spirits in a phial.

> I can't tell where my head has gone,
> > But Dr Carpue can;
> As for my trunk it's all packed up
> > To go by Pickford's van.

> The cock it crows, I must be gone,
> > My William we must part:
> And I'll be yours in death although
> > Sir Astley has my heart.[54]

Hood's ballad identified five well-known surgeons but it was an open secret that virtually every surgeon and anatomist was implicated in body-snatching. They included students many of whom became respected surgeons later in their careers. An anonymous memoir, 'Twenty four hours of my pupillage', describes a nerve-wracking expedition in which a London student participated in the winter of 1830. It includes a song sung by men at a reunion dinner many years later:

> Our professors sometimes look black, but then we never fear
> When fortified with Kennett, or by Barclay's strongest beer
> And now we'll drink success to our next nocturnal round
> When we hope to be employed Sir by turning up the ground.[55]

Resurrection men – often sometime dead-house porters, hospital janitors, sextons and grave-diggers – represent the dark underside of the anatomical revolution. Gangs sent bodies from the provinces to London and by the new steamboat from Ireland to Scotland and London. Procuring 'things' – the body-snatchers' cant term for corpses – involved tough dealing. Tension over the supply and price of cadavers implicated surgeons in bribery, intimidation, double-crossing and shady dealings with groups of resurrection men such as the 'Borough Gang' supplying the United Hospitals. In 1816 a gang of disgruntled body-snatchers broke into St Thomas's dissecting room, terrorised the students and hacked the corpses into useless fragments.[56]

The popular horror and anger at the resurrectionists' depredations needs to be appreciated. Bereaved families' anger at the theft of loved ones combined with a Christian culture which largely believed in the literal resurrection of the body, to arouse a deep outrage at body-snatching and those involved. The poor especially feared desecration (a resurrection man explained to a Parliamentary committee that they seldom took 'the rich ... because they were buried so deep').[57] Concern approaching moral panic coloured the popular perception of medical education and mobs often followed alleged resurrection men, attacking hospitals or private medical schools. Richard Grainger had to call constables to prevent a mob ransacking the Webb Street School. In 1831 Andrew Moir at Aberdeen had to take shelter (in a nearby cemetery) as a crowd burned the university's anatomical theatre after a dog unearthed bones in shallow soil.[58] Despite serious lobbying and a Parliamentary enquiry in 1828 many years passed before a solution could be found. The scandal of Burke and Hare in Edinburgh in 1828 – who were murderers rather than grave-robbers – precipitated a crisis. William Burke and William Hare, two Irish navvies, killed some sixteen people, mostly women, including several prostitutes and a simpleton 'Daft Jamie' in the slums of Edinburgh's West Port. They sold their bodies to, among others, the prominent anatomical teacher, Robert Knox. Students recognised Jamie, and William Fergusson cut off his head and his distinctive feet in an attempt to evade discovery. Burke and Hare's crimes were soon unmasked, however. Hare turned King's evidence to convict Burke who was hanged and duly dissected in January 1829. Robert Knox, obtuse and obstinate, continued to prepare his hitherto popular courses but was publicly disgraced. Edinburgh doggerel identified his association with the murders: 'Burke's the butcher, Hare's the thief/ Knox the boy who buys the beef.'[59] As an anatomist he must have known of the murders from the characteristic signs of strangulation. Admitting his own 'long intercourse with the Resurrectionists', John Lizars concluded that 'exhumation cannot answer'.[60]

This scandal, followed soon afterwards by the similar case of John Bishop and Thomas Williams who offered Richard Partridge of King's College bodies (and who avoided Knox's fate by sending for the police), produced an Anatomy Act legalising the supply of bodies for dissection. After it was passed in 1833 Benjamin Travers explained 'the system of body-snatching has been entirely put down', though the supply of legal corpses barely met the demand of the anatomy schools.[61] While the regulation of the supply of cadavers may have relieved the popular fear of their bodies being stolen for sale clandestinely to anatomists and their students, it did not, however, relieve the popular horror of legitimate post-mortem examination. Incidents reported periodically reinforced rather than allayed that unease. In 1831 Fanny Lawrence died in the Middlesex Hospital. When her relatives claimed her body they found that she had been 'ill-used after death'. Her body was in a 'mangled state', her hair cut off and teeth removed, disfigured by being laid open and stitched up in a 'rude and disgustful' manner. The hospital's Board of Governors was obliged to investigate. It transpired that one Enright, one of the hospitals' surgerymen, had extracted the teeth at the request of a hospital governor. The Middlesex's surgeons, on whom suspicion naturally fell, treated the investigation with 'unbecoming levity'. Enright was dismissed, the House Surgeon reprimanded and the public again persuaded that given the opportunity, surgeons would indeed cut up those whom they had allowed to die.[62]

That this fear remained a real one is suggested by an incident in 1852 – twenty years after the Anatomy Act – in which a surgeon became a victim of a distressed relative. A surgeon had been summoned to perform an autopsy on the body of Marian Jones who had apparently killed herself by swallowing oxalic acid. While dissecting her body in a locked room the surgeon was startled to hear a battering on the door and to find Mrs Jones's distraught husband bursting in. Snatching up portions of her body – including her entrails – Mr Jones rushed out into the street haranguing a growing crowd that his wife had been butchered. Flinging body parts into the street, he ran back into the house and attacked the surgeon with his own dissection knives, restrained by the surgeon's assistant. The whole time Jones's 16-year-old daughter was on her knees crying and cursing. The violent, grief-stricken (and perhaps guilt-stricken) widower was at last apprehended to be bound over to keep the peace, while the shaken surgeon was left to retrieve his instruments from the Jones's privy.[63] Even so, despite the lingering association in the popular memory the Anatomy Act enabled surgeons to 'avoid ... that very disgraceful connexion with men of desperate character' and their respectability profited accordingly.[64]

'Golden ointment': medical patronage

Like the society which sustained it, the medical profession functioned by and because of patronage. Merit became a factor only belatedly and remained subordinate to the influence deployed by mentors and the loyalty displayed by their protégés. In this, medicine resembled virtually every other sphere of public life, in which family connections and reciprocal ties of obligation bound individuals and groups in close and now often untraceable associations. While ability counted for something in attracting the support of patrons it remained a relatively minor matter in deciding many questions of selection and promotion. Brodie, in the words of his protege and biographer Charles Hawking, 'knew the value of worldly influence, of rank, of station when rightly used'.[65] Whether influence was 'rightly used' rather depended upon the benefit those concerned expected to have gained. Appointments invariably went to those allied to powerful figures, either on the medical staff or boards of governors of the great hospitals or to members of the councils of the medical corporations. To challenge the power of these bodies would have brought exclusion and ruin.

Evidence of the networks underpinning medical careers is apparent from the dedications and inscriptions in John Aitken's *A*

Probationary Essay on Stone in the Bladder and Lithotomy, published in Edinburgh in 1816. Aitken dedicated it to his master Thomas Winterbottom of South Shields, to his mentor John Barclay, the Edinburgh professor and to George Townshend Fox Esq., his local patron. He then inscribed the copy to Donald Butte Esq., 'with the Compliments of his Friend The Author': Aitken acknowledged the vertical and lateral links in the web of deference, obligation and influence that sustained his entry to the profession.[66] Even more striking is the web of patronage Astley Cooper commanded from London. His correspondence includes a letter from a former pupil recommending to Cooper 'a nephew of mine, [a] Pupil of Guy's Hospital & son of an old pupil of yours ... [whose] friend is an intimate friend & Patient of mine & Art[icle]d Pupil of my Brother-in-law ... also a student of yours'.[67]

Individual members of the College's Council between them influenced virtually every worthwhile appointment in the profession. Influence often depended upon an aspirant's medico-political orientation but, as with many other spheres of British society, medical positions commonly went to relatives, friends and the relatives of friends. 'Does nepotism prevail?' an MP asked James Wardrop in enquiring into medical education. 'No doubt of it', Wardrop replied firmly, 'very considerable'.[68] 'Notorious' nepotism is most clearly seen in the entrenchment of the Cooper dynasty at the Borough hospitals over several decades. Astley Cooper became infamous for the clutch of relatives whom he installed. Cooper himself obtained a position at Guy's because his uncle was Surgeon there. He successively manoeuvred into positions at St Thomas's his godson John Henry Green, his nephew Walter Tyrrell, his former apprentice Benjamin Travers and Edmund Cock, another relative. Having severed his connections with St Thomas's (through a schism deriving from the frustration of another family appointment) he had his nephews Aston Key and Bransby Cooper also appointed to Guy's. Cooper's 'nevies' – a cruel parody of his Norfolk burr – became a standing jest among those who resented the workings of patronage. Those who believed that the claims of family had prevailed over talent less charitably described them as his 'nevies and noodles': a resentment based in many cases not on principle, but on having missed out on the boon conferred.[69] Ironically, in the opinion of at least one contemporary, Key and Tyrrell at least would have gained situations on merit without Cooper's aid. As Wardrop made clear, though, Cooper's gladhanding was only the most celebrated example of a widespread if not universal practice. Wardrop invited 'his questioners to look over the lists of surgeons at the hospitals of London. 'You would find,' he said, 'that a considerable portion of them are, either immediately or more distantly related to some one or other of the medical officers who have preceded them'. While accepting influence as an acceptable part of promotion, Charles Bell evidently decided that the boundaries of good sense had been reached and exceeded. In a testimonial he denounced the 'shifting and discreditable manner in which so many of the medical youth are introduced into the profession'.[70] The entire system was according to *The Times* 'saturated with "golden ointment"'.[71]

'Full of rivalry and contention': rancour

The medical world – then as now – was fuelled by gossip and enlivened by intrigue, the more intense for the disproportionate rewards of patronage. Anthony Carlisle, who despite his conservatism remained refreshingly candid about the profession's shortcomings, conceded publicly that 'among ourselves, conversations about sordid subjects are more frequent than discussions upon ... science'.[72] Arguments punctuate the histories of most hospitals, many relating at some level to either matters of prestige or the material reward flowing from it. 'Quarrels in the board-room', wrote J.F. Clarke, 'were soon carried into the wards'.

The small world of metropolitan surgery remained riven by jealousy, feuds, rumours and attacks upon rivals from satirical puffs in the journals to whispering campaigns on the benches of operating theatres and over the tables of the chop houses frequented by medical men. In London animosity existed between Charles Bell and Astley Cooper, John Abernethy and William Lawrence, Frederick Skey and Lawrence, John Erichsen and Richard Quain (until Erichsen won him over), William Blizard and Astley Cooper and Samuel Cooper and Robert Liston. Edward Tuson offended all his colleagues at the Middlesex Hospital who resigned in a body to oblige him to leave. Despite his mediocrity as an operating surgeon, and his uninspired teaching, Edward Stanley's gifts as a peacemaker were greatly appreciated at St Bartholomew's.[73] Not all eruptions were as dramatic or tragic as at the Westminster in the mid-1830s when Hale Thomson fought a duel, a bitter and close-fought board-room election and, after a breach with his mentor George Guthrie, committed suicide.[74] Quarrels and jealousies found vent even in the operating room. James Latta, jealous of Charles Bell's success, once sought to upset him as he operated by imitating the croak of a raven.[75] Such dramatic gestures and emotive demeanour were, of

37

course, characteristic of the Romantic age and conversely the intensity of their collaboration generated intense friendships and strong alliances. Notable partnerships existed between Brodie and Lawrence; Erichsen and Liston, William Lynn and Charles Bell; Liston and James Miller; and William Bowman and John Simon.

Periodic and savage spats broke out in Edinburgh too, all the more diverting for the intimacy of its small surgical community. Vituperation and litigation erupted between James Syme and Robert Liston and James Syme and John Lizars, and between next-door-neighbours James Simpson and James Miller, and apparently everyone against almost everybody else at one time or another. Students and junior colleagues often inherited animosities much as they adopted their seniors' theories and remedies. The intensity of invective which these men were capable of directing at adversaries, often over seemingly trivial procedural or technical matters, was truly impressive. An anonymous author of *Remarks on a Treatise on the Rectum* directed the most vicious spleen against James Syme, sarcastically asking whether it was to the '"credit of surgery" that his ... use of the saw [was] a standing joke, amongst the profession at large?'[76] Syme's colleague at Minto House, Alexander Peddie, recalled that when Syme was at last re-admitted to operate at the Edinburgh Infirmary he encountered a hitch in his first operation. In the theatre, as the patient moaned on the table, the friends of Liston and Lizars laughed while those of Syme looked 'stern and downcast'.[77]

Much of the resultant pamphlets, broadsides and volumes of self-exculpatory correspondence is now obscure, striking only for the quality of its abuse. James Gregory, for example, vented his objection to 'that most despicable and detestable work' – Benjamin Bell's *A System of Surgery* – 'six squat, fat, vulgar-looking octavo volumes, the sight of any one of which is enough to make a man sick'.[78] In Edinburgh John Bell published at his own expense a 650-page rant, *Letters on Professional Character and Manners*, directed at Gregory and entirely concerned with pursuing obscure points of etiquette. In 1852 Samuel Dickson, under the pseudonym Jonathan Dawplunket Clearthedust (the pseudonym itself harking back to the Gregory-Bell feud of forty years before), published a pamphlet allegedly exposing *Sir Benjamin Brodie's Doings in Diseases of the Joints and Spine*. Declined for publication by the editor of the *Medical Circular* as too dangerous, Dickson accused Brodie of plagiarising his book *Unity of Disease*. Ignoring Brodie's substantial and continuing research on joints, Dickson impugned Brodie as a fraud. 'In physic, as in fermentation,' he concluded, 'the dirt and scum too often get to the top'.[79] Perhaps most tellingly over 120 items in the papers of James Simpson are described as relating to 'professional disputes'.

'The profession,' William Guy acknowledged in welcoming students to King's College in 1846, 'has been and is, too full of rivalry and contention'.[80] Some of these arguments derived from the imperfect and exploratory state of medical knowledge in which theories and explanations bounded ahead of advances in knowledge. Inevitable in the face of their contingent knowledge, their frequent controversies were all the more intense for the inadequate empirical footings and ill-founded theories on which they were based. Frederick Skey illuminated one such scholarly spat in an aside in his text *Operative Surgery* which by that time was decades old. Benjamin Brodie (Skey's teacher) recommended using a silver blade to lacerate small blood vessels thereby reducing bleeding. This idea was contested by 'the late Mr Liston' who would 'sneer at the suggestion' that the composition rather than the keenness of the blade would be relevant.[81] Liston was posthumously proved correct: the argument was only one of dozens which bubbled through the medical community.

'Self-chosen chartered jobbers': medical reform

The formal governance of the profession remained in the hands of the 'medical corporations': principally the Royal Colleges of Surgeons in London, Edinburgh and Dublin. The former military surgeon J.G. Millingen, later of the Middlesex Pauper Lunatic Asylum, spoke for the younger party of reform. 'Corporate bodies monopolising the exercise of any profession', he believed, 'will inevitably retard instruction and shackle the energies of the student'.[82] The energies of many men were therefore directed to challenging the corporations' monopoly of power. During the 1820s and '30s the politics of medical reform coincided with the science of physiological debate, as Adrian Desmond has demonstrated with dazzling scholarship in *The Politics of Evolution*. Surgeons, as the principal beneficiaries of philosophical anatomy, became among the most aggressive protagonists in the scientific-cum-political debates surrounding the reception of anatomical learning.

In the course of a century of reform the monopolies of the 'medical corporations' became identified with the abuses of 'old corruption', and the 1820s and '30s saw movements for the reform of the colleges, especially in medical education. These movements reflected and expressed the wider demand for change. A vigorous medical press became one of the principal forums for the contest: 27

new titles were launched in the 1820s and as many more in the 1830s.[83] The *Lancet*, which was to become the organ of the medical establishment, was a champion of reform in its early decades. It correspondingly became vilified by the leaders of the conservative tendency and the subject of ten actions for libel in its first decade. Its editor, Thomas Wakley (a graduate of St Thomas's who became MP for Finsbury in the reformed Parliament), jousted with the great figures over principle and with his contemporaries over circulation. Wakley's former teacher, Astley Cooper, publicly described the *Lancet* as 'a reptile press'.[84] Wakley's verbatim accounts of his lectures so incensed Abernethy that he had the lights extinguished in the theatre at Bart's. Hoping to thwart him, Abernethy was enraged to find Wakley able to transcribe the lecture from memory.[85] Late in 1824 Abernethy contested the legality of the *Lancet* transcribing and publishing accounts of his lectures on the grounds that the practice impinged on his right to publish them for gain. That *The Times* regarded the case as a matter affecting the freedom of the press in general is suggested by its publication of extracts of the *Lancet's* reports.

The College was governed by twenty one senior and in some cases elderly members of the profession constituting its Council: the 'Twenty-one self-chosen chartered jobbers of Lincoln's-inn Fields', as Wakley described them.[86] (The *Lancet* recorded with relief the resignation of Sir William Blizard from the London Hospital in 1833 aged ninety: he had qualified in the 1760s.) The College's Council enjoyed a virtual monopoly of control over entry to and advancement in the profession. Many of its members, denied a voice in its affairs, deplored their powerlessness, and in the mid-1820s Wakley's *Lancet* led a vigorous campaign to alter its constitution. A meeting of 1,200, mostly disenfranchised members of the college, met at the Freemasons' Tavern (a focus of medical public life) to be addressed by William Lawrence. Wakley's campaign may have made the College more sensitive to its members' complaints but it did not alter the essential distribution of power. Indeed, in that Lawrence soon became a member of the College's Council, it absorbed opposition rather than confronted it. Despite Wakley's campaign the proponents of reform failed to carry Parliament with them and the College retained its power. Sixteen abortive bills seeking medical reform were introduced into Parliament in seventeen years before the passing of the Medical Act in 1858 which took the regulation of the profession as a whole out of the hands of its constituent colleges.[87]

The proponents of change and the defenders of the status quo essentially split on generational lines. Students at all times, those newly qualified, those without a hospital appointment and those qualifying after the mid-1830s (significantly coinciding with the first Reform Act) challenged the existing system. Many of those who protested against the inequities of the existing system had themselves suffered from it. Thomas Hodgkin, who had missed out on a situation at St Thomas's because Astley Cooper preferred his proteges, led a meeting at Guy's in late 1827 in which students complained at the deficiencies of clinical instruction and claimed that the hospital's staff preferred to cultivate their private practices.[88] Advocates of change included James Wardrop and John Scott (surgeon to the London Hospital). They urged that merit should join (and not always supersede) connections as a means of appointment. They often recommended the French system of *concours*. The essential features of the concours were that examinations were public, based on skill, and often included among the selectors a representative of the younger faculty. In this way a talented man lacking influence could hope to prevail by skill, if not alone, then certainly much more easily than by the vote-buying and greasing which characterised the prevailing British system.

Defenders of the existing arrangements naturally included older and more influential surgeons and especially those on the College's Council. George Guthrie, a representative of the conservative faction, declared that he was 'not very favourable to any French modes of proceeding'.[89] Despite their energy the reforming faction made little headway until the 1850s. For the first half of the century, then, power in the profession remained in the hands of a relatively small number of senior, metropolitan surgeons.

'Important operations': surgeons as celebrities

Despite the understandable fear and distaste of the surgeon's bloody and painful work, early in the nineteenth century (and long before the possibility of painless surgery) the public perception of the surgeon began to change. In the 1820s, for the first time, disgust at their business began to be accompanied by a wonder at their achievements. It is perhaps no coincidence that Abernethy's *Lectures on Anatomy, Surgery and Pathology* appeared in 1828. Written in 'plain, lucid and colloquial style' the book became 'in families, a book of familiar consultation and reference'.[90] Those intrigued by Abernethy's book may have been among the 9,000 members of the public who viewed the Edinburgh college's pathological museum in 1844.[91] The London college's visitors, many members of the public,

41

almost doubled during the 1820s and in 1832 reached '2746 Persons and 3 Noblemen' including Robert Peel.[92] These were the readers of *Blackwood's Magazine* who from 1830 read Samuel Warren's memoir *Passages from the Diary of a Late Physician* including a moving and frank description of the excision of a scirrhous breast.[93]

The change in sensibility is also apparent in the reportage of important or novel operations. Before about 1820 newspapers carried very few accounts of surgical operations and those were brief. In 1799, for example, *The Times* reported a 'very extraordinary' operation performed on a 70-year-old, Mrs Flight, for a 'dreadful complaint of the bowels'. It gave no details except that the complaint was 'removed' leaving Mrs Flight in 'a fair way to recovery'.[94] Thereafter newspapers began to publish more detailed reports of operations. Booksellers commissioned and sold mezzotints, lithographs and woodcuts of surgeons – at least a dozen each of Abernethy and Astley Cooper. The effect was to turn the surgeon into a kind of hero: one also suspect and sinister but still a celebrity. Part of this admiration derived from the evident material success which the most eminent surgeons enjoyed. They could be seen getting about in carriages and attracting crowds as they arrived and left their hospitals. The *Evening Paper's* report of an address Astley Cooper delivered to medical students at the commencement of the autumn term in 1822 remarked on his prosperity. There had been a time Cooper had recalled when he had wanted a shilling more than anyone present. As a senior member of the profession, *The Times* commented in reprinting its contemporary's account, he was 'supposed to be in receipt of a larger income ... than any professional man in Europe'.[95] Cooper's wealth did not in some eyes make him a gentleman but it did not diminish his appeal in a society which admired wealth as well as breeding. When he died in 1841 he was reputedly worth £500,000. Within three years a statue had been erected to his memory in St Paul's by public subscription.[96]

By the 1830s *The Times* was carrying long articles sparing few details of 'important operations'. The front-page account of the operation performed upon Mary Cave, 'a woman in very humble station' aged about 45, illustrates contemporaries' growing willingness to confront the horror of surgery. Mrs Cave suffered from a large tumour which consumed the whole of the right side of her face. It pressed against the orbit of her eye, projected two inches out of her mouth, encompassed her tongue and approached her windpipe, giving off a fetid stench. A 'frightful object', she had 'sunk almost under the deepest humiliation' of the 'foul, dark, irregular growth'. Enduring repeated examinations by the students of Bart's, she repeatedly implored Mr James Earle to deliver her from her affliction. Professional opinion remained divided on whether Earle ought to proceed but Mrs Cave's appeals at last overcame his reluctance. He informed her that he was prepared to operate but that she might not survive. Desperate beyond endurance she consented. Earle's candour and the consideration with which he treated her confirmed her confidence in him. 'I place my life in your hands' she said 'and I hope that through you, the Almighty God will preserve it'.

Before an 'immense concourse' in Bart's theatre Mrs Cave lay on the table restrained but without any anaesthetic, neither opium nor alcohol. Earle first 'took up' her carotid artery before cutting out the mass of fungus haematodes congesting her face. The Times's correspondent (probably a student) declared that Mrs Cave's stoicism 'better deserves the name of heroism than any conduct I have ever witnessed ... in a patient under the knife'. Earle displayed the attributes of the heroic surgeon: 'self-possession, serenity and ease of manner'. Even so, he worked cautiously taking sixteen minutes to cut out the tumour. At the conclusion the spectators applauded. Several days on Mrs Cave was described as doing well, her confidence in Earle and her courage rewarded.[97] Mrs Cave's operation had captured the imagination of the nation's premier daily newspaper which had reported the event in unprecedented detail. Surgery enjoyed a popular, if prurient, interest and surgeons had become figures of renown.

These men were surgeons and operators in the accepted sense that they alone, among the thousands of surgeon-apothecaries, performed the capital operations of surgery. An American translation of an Italian surgical manual, available to English-speaking readers from 1825, imparted a new inflection to this familiar distinction. In the manner of the time, the translator, John Goodman, added his own views in footnotes contrasting the 'surgeon and a mere operator'.[98] A surgeon, he wrote, enquired into and treats the cause of a condition: an operator enquired only of his patient's willingness to submit to the knife. A surgeon sought to help the body heal: the operator amputated without further thought. A surgeon reflected on the feelings of his patient, striving to prevent pain and deformity: an operator considered the notoriety gained by operating. And so on: one operated reluctantly: the other waited only to sharpen his knife. One was noted for those he had preserved from mutilation; the other the number of cripples he had caused. One was an honour to his profession; the other rendered the profession odious. Men of both complexions could be found among the surgeons of Britain.

Notes

1. *London Medical Repository and Review*, NS (1827), p. 188, quoted in Irving Loudon, *Medical Care and the General Practitioner 1750–1850* (Clarendon, Oxford, 1986), 227.

2. *The Times*, 17 May 1826, 3c.

3. Robert Liston, *Letter to the Ladies and Gentlemen Contributors to the Royal Infirmary of Edinburgh*, (Edinburgh: Balfour & Clarke, 1821) 10.

4. PP 1833, Vol. XXXIV, 'An Account of the Number of Persons who have obtained Diplomas from the Royal College of Surgeons', 117; PP 1846, Vol. XXXIII, 'Returns from the Colleges of Physicians and Surgeons'; 474.

5. C. Cecil Curwen, (ed.), *The Journal of Gideon Mantell: Surgeon and Geologist* (Oxford: Etchells & Macdonald, OUP, 1940) .

6. Johnson, 'The Diary of Thomas Giordani Wright: Apprentice Doctor in Newcastle upon Tyne, 1824-29', *Medical History*, 1999, 43: 468–4.

7. Henry Mayhew, *London Characters* (London: Chatto & Windus, 1881), 34.

8. *A List of [All] the Officers of the Army*, 1793; 1815.

9. *Bengal or East India Calendar, The Original Calcutta Annual Directory, The Army List of the Company's Troops on the Bengal Establishment.*

10. William Scott to Thomas Goldie Scott, 20 December 1842, Acc. 9266, NLS.

11. Bransby Cooper, *The Life of Sir Astley Cooper, Bart.*, 2 vols (London: John Parker, 1843), Vol. II, 221.

12. *London Medical and Surgical Journal*, 28 March 1832 .

13. Royal College of Surgeons, Minutes of Council, November 1847, A4g, RCSEng.

14. Guy's Hospital, Table II, CHAR/2, 385, PRO.

15. 'Intercepted Letter', *Lancet*, 1833–34, Vol. I, 798.

16. Brodie receipt books, Add Ms 370, 380, 390, RCSEng; Forbes Winslow, *Physic and Physicians: A Medical Sketch Book* (London: Longman, Orme, Brown, 1839), Vol. II, 345.

17. Charles Bell to George Bell, 24 March 1814, George Jospeh Bell, (ed.), *Letters of Sir George Bell* (London: John Murray, 1870), 214.

18. Eve Blantyre Simpson, *Sir James Y. Simpson* (Edinburgh: Oliphant, Anderson & Ferrier, 1896), 37–40.

19. *The Times*, 6 July 1841, 3d.

20. *The Times*, 17 May 1826, 3c.

21. John Mann, *Recollections of My Early and Professional Life* (London: W. Rider & Sons, 1887), 119.

22. Victor Plarr, *Lives of the Fellows of the Royal College of Surgeons*, 2 vols (London: Simpkin, Marshall Ltd, 1930), Vol. I, 378.

23. Rees Gronow, *The Reminiscences and Recollections of Captain Gronow*, 2 vols (London: J.C. Nimmo, 1900), Vol. II, 231.

24. Robert Masters Kerrison, *Inquiry into the Present State of the Medical Profession in England* (London: Longman, Hurst, Rees, Orme & Brown, 1814), 27; x; 29.

25. J. Gregory, *Censorian Letter to the President and Fellows of the Royal College of Surgeons of Edinburgh* (Edinburgh: Murray & Cochrane, 1805), 35.

26. James Johnston Abraham, *Lettsom: His Life, Times, Friends and Descendants* (London: William Heinemann, 1933), 418.

27. Charles Bell, *Institutes of Surgery*, 2 vols (Edinburgh: Longmans & Co., 1838), Vol. II, 57.

28. Evidence of Anthony Carlisle to the Select Committee on Medical Education, PP 1834, Vol. XXXIV, 147.

29. Evidence of Benjamin Travers to the Select Committee on Medical Education, PP 1834, Vol. XXXIV, 126.

30. Norman Moore, & Stephen Paget, *The Royal Medical and Chirurgical Society of London, 1805-1905* (Aberdeen: Aberdeen University Press, 1905), 5.

31. William Lawrence, *The Hunterian Oration* (London: J. Churchill, 1834), 26.

32. *The Times*, 16 July 1851, 6c; 18 July, 8e; 19 July, 5d.

33. *Lancet*, 1835-36, Vol. II, 187.

34. George Macilwain, *Memoirs of John Abernethy*, 2 vols (London: Hurst & Blackett, 1854), Vol. II, 222.

35. Evidence of Benjamin Brodie to the Select Committee on Medical Education, PP 1834, Vol. XXXIV, 113.

36. John Millingen, *Curiosities of Medical Experience* (London: Richard Bentley, 1839), 288.

37. Evidence of George Guthrie to the Select Committee on Medical Education, PP 1834, Vol. XXXIV, 27.

38. *The Times*, 21 June 1845, 5b.

39. Evidence of Astley Cooper to the Select Committee on Medical Education, PP 1834, Vol. XXXIV, 104.

40. Arthur Farre, *On Some of the Circumstances which have Retarded the Progress of Medicine* (London: John Churchill, 1849), 33–34.

41. Evidence of George Guthrie to the Select Committee on Medical Education, PP 1834, Vol. XXXIV, 74.

42. William Hey, *Practical Observations in Surgery* (London: T. Cadell Jnr & W. Davies, [1803; 1814]), v.

43. Evidence of Astley Cooper to the Select Committee on Medical Education, PP 1834, Vol. XXXIV, 102.

44. John Shepherd, *Spencer Wells: the Life and Work of a Victorian Surgeon* (Edinburgh: E. & S. Livingstone, 1965), 42–50.

45. W.J. Reader, *Professional Men: The Rise of the Professional Classes in Nineteenth Century England* (London: Weidenfield & Nicolson, 1966), 65.

46. Evidence of Astley Cooper to the Select Committee on Medical Education, PP 1834, Vol. XXXIV, 105.

47. J.H. Green, *A Letter to Sir Astley Cooper, Bart ...* (London: Sherwood, 1825), xii, xiii.

48. Reader, *op. cit.* (note 45), 36.

49. Winslow, *op. cit* (note 16), Vol. I, 100.

50. James Blake Bailey, *The Diary of a Resurrectionist 1811–1812* (London: Swan Sonnenschein & Co., 1896), 31.

51. Clarendon Creswell, *The Royal College of Surgeons of Edinburgh Historical Notes from 1505 to 1905* (Edinburgh: Oliver & Boyd, 1926), 201; 203.

52. Isobel Rae, *Knox: the Anatomist* (Edinburgh: Oliver & Boyd, 1964), 61.

53. Cooper, *The Life of Sir Astley Cooper, Bart, op. cit.* (note , 11), Vol. I, 360.

54. Thomas Hood, *The Poetical Works of Thomas Hood* (London: E. Moxon, 1890), 124–25.

55. 'Twenty four hours of my pupillage', UE, DK.7.58, LHSA.

56. Hubert Cole, *Things for the Surgeon: A History of the Resurrection Men* (London: Heinemann, 1964), 38.

57. Evidence of 'F.G.', PP 1828, Vol. VII, Part 1, Report of the Select Committee on Anatomy, 119 .

58. Ella Hill Burton Rodger, *Aberdeen Doctors at Home and Abroad* (Edinburgh: W. Blackwood, 1893), 240.

59. Rae, *op. cit.* (note 52*)*, 65.

60. John Lizars to Dr Burnett, Medical Commissioner, Navy Office, London, 23 May 1829, Ms 13, Letters on Scottish Affairs, 1810–30, f. 255, NLS.

61. Extraordinary Meeting, May 1846, Royal College of Surgeons of England, Minutes of Council, 1843-49, A4g, RCSEng.

62. *The Times*, 30 May 1831, 3d; 4 June 1831, 4a.

63. *The Times*, 30 October 1852, 4a.

64. Evidence of George Guthrie to the Select Committee on Medical

Education, PP 1834, Vol. XXXIV, 40.

65. Benjamin Brodie, (C. Hawking, ed.), *Autobiography*, (London: Longmans & Co., 1865), xxi.

66. John Aitkin, *A Probationary Essay on Stone in the Bladder and Lithotomy* (Edinburgh: 1816), copy in the Gordon Craig Library of the Royal Australasian College of Surgeons.

67. Robert Elliott to Astley Cooper, 13 November 1840, Astley Cooper papers, 67.b.9, RCSEng.

68. Evidence of James Wardrop to the Select Committee on Medical Education, PP 1834, Vol. XXXIV, 173.

69. J.F. Clarke, *Autobiographical Recollections* (London: J. & A. Churchill, 1874), 26.

70. Volume of Testimonials of Dr Blyth, from the collection of the Aberdeen Medical and Chirurgical Society, nd, 2–3, WIMH.

71. *The Times*, 19 October 1827, 3a.

72. *The Times*, 8 November 1827, 3f.

73. Plarr, *op. cit.* (note 22), Vol. II, 344.

74. W.C. Spencer, *Westminster Hospital - An Outline of its History* (London: H.J. Glaisher, 1924), 103–104.

75. Amédée Pichot, *The Life and Labours of Sir Charles Bell* (London: R. Bentley, 1860), 69n.

76. Anon, *Remarks on a Treatise on the Rectum* (Edinburgh: Stevenson, [1852]), 8.

77. Alexander Peddie, *Recollections of John Brown* (London: Percival & Co., 1893), 194.

78. J. Gregory, *Additional Memorial to the Managers of the Royal Infirmary* (Edinburgh: Murray & Cochrane, 1803), 411 .

79. [Samuel Dickson?], *Sir Benjamin Brodie's Doings in Diseases of the Joints and Spine* (London: John Oliver, 1852).

80. William Augustus Guy, *On Medical Education* (London: Henry Renshaw, 1846), 23.

81. Frederic Skey, *Operative Surgery* (London: John Churchill, 1850), 34.

82. Millingen, *op. cit.* (note 36), 294.

83. Adrian Desmond, *The Politics of Evolution: Morphology, Medicine, and Reform in Radical London* (Chicago: University of Chicago Press, 1989), 14.

84. Clarke, *op. cit.* (note 69), 26.

85. Mann, *op. cit.* (note 21), 161.

86. *Lancet*, 1839–40, Vol. II, 753.

87. Noel Parry & José Parry *The Rise of the Medical Profession: A Study of Collective Mobility* (London: Croom Helm, 1976), 117–26.

88. *The Times*, 19 October 1827, 3a.

89. Evidence of George Guthrie to the Select Committee on Medical Education, PP 1834, Vol. XXXIV, 69.

90. John Abernethy, *Lectures on Anatomy, Surgery and Pathology* (London: James Bullock, 1828), np.

91. Violet Tansey & D.E.C. Meikie, *The Museum of the Royal College of Surgeons of Edinburgh* (Edinburgh: Royal College of Surgeons of Edinburgh, 1982), 22.

92. Visitors' Books, 1823-26, 1830-32, 275.g.41; 275.g.42, RCSEng.

93. *Blackwood's Magazine*, September 1830, 474–76.

94. *The Times*, 8 January 1799, 3d.

95. *The Times*, 4 October 1822, 2d.

96. *The Times*, 13 February 1841, 6c; 16 February 1841, 6a; 20 September 1844, 5a.

97. *The Times*, 6 December 1831, 1e. 'A London Hospital pupil' soon wrote to point out that Earle's operation, though impressive, was not original. Both Robert Liston and John Scott had recently removed tumours from upper jaws, in Edinburgh and London respectively; *The Times*, 8 December 1831, 6b.

98. J. Coster, *Manual of Surgical Operations* (Philadelphia: H.C. Carey & I Lea, 1825), vi–vii.

2

'Modern surgeons':
Medical Knowledge and Surgery

On the afternoon of Wednesday 16 October 1793 the board of St George's Hospital convened. Its members included five ecclesiastical or medical gentlemen and John Hunter, anatomist and Surgeon to the hospital. Relations within the board had been strained. Hunter had clashed with his colleagues recently over appointments for their proteges and the distribution of fees from students. He planned to present a memorial to the board that day arguing that two unqualified fellow Scotsmen should be allowed to enter as his pupils. That morning, despite arriving at breakfast humming a Scottish air, he had again felt the foreboding that his heart was unsound and that tension at the meeting could be dangerous. He arrived late. In the course of the meeting, one of his pupils recalled, he could not contain his anger and had 'several words' with his opponents. They may have been arguing over the appointment of his friends – opinions differed – but he abruptly ceased speaking. He stood up, staggered to an adjoining room, uttered a deep groan and collapsed into the arms of James Robertson, one of St George's physicians. The physician Dr Baillie and the surgeon Everard Home tried to revive him, relenting only after an hour. His body was carried home in a sedan chair to be buried in St Martin-in-the-Fields a week later at a modest private funeral. The meeting broke up with the matter of Hunter's Scottish students unresolved. A post-mortem examination confirmed that the cause of his death had been – as he had foreseen – heart disease.[1]

The period between John Hunter's death in 1793 and the acceptance of painless surgery around 1850 constitutes a unity, a period marked by the accumulation of anatomical and physiological knowledge and by rapid change in the techniques, range and success of surgical practice. While surgical practice in the period was anything but static and its practitioners anything but united there is about these decades a coherence, not least in the sense of excitement and adventure that surgeons shared. The period centres on a conundrum, for surgical progress did not depend upon the elimination of pain but proceeded in spite of it. At a time when surgery remained hideously painful its practitioners embarked upon bolder and more intense innovation than ever before. This tension between the human experience of surgery and its ostensible motivation gives the period its interest and power. What then was the 'modern surgery' which was John Hunter's principal legacy to his profession?

'Mr Hunter's Opinions': contemporary medical understanding

Over the preceding fifty years John Hunter had created a revolution in the understanding of human anatomy. The insights he derived and stimulated transformed surgery from a craft based on apprenticeship and received lore into a discipline professing to be 'scientific', based on research and reason. Hunter had learned surgery as an apprentice of William Cheselden in the late 1740s. As well as gaining a command in the practicalities of surgery, he had embarked upon a prolonged and devoted study of human and animal anatomy. The results of his research and the spirit in which he sought to gain and impart knowledge inspired several succeeding generations of British surgeons. His students included men who became leaders of the profession during the decades preceding the introduction of anaesthesia: such as John Abernethy, William Blizard, Anthony Carlisle, Henry Cline, Astley Cooper, William Hey and William Lynn. His discoveries – in the circulation of the blood, the treatment of wounds, the nature and management of inflammation – imparted an impetus which led to the idea that surgery had become both 'modern' and 'scientific'. The line of Milton's which Hunter's contemporary John Bell chose for the epigram to his *Principles of Surgery*, published in 1800, grew out of the humane rationalism characteristic of these enlightened men of science: 'Who would lose for fear of pain, this intellectual being?'*

Hunter's experimental methods inspired doctors to enquire into and understand the structure and functions of the human body with a determination and even a passion, hitherto unknown. Anatomy became the surgeons' touchstone: 'he must mangle the living', Astley Cooper told the Parliamentary committee enquiring into the proposed Anatomy Act, 'if he has not operated on the dead'.[2] The best surgeons continued to dissect throughout their careers. Cooper – the extreme example – barely allowed a day to pass without dissecting a human or animal cadaver. For the first time students

---

* I am grateful to Prof. David Lodge of the University of Birmingham whose novel *Thinks* enabled me to locate the source of the epigram in Milton's *Paradise Lost*.

Figure 2.1

*Joshua Reynolds's portrait of John Hunter (1728-93),
who inspired the rise of the 'modern' and 'scientific' surgeon. Hunter
taught, among others, Benjamin Bell, John Abernethy,
William Blizard, Anthony Carlisle, Henry Cline, Astley Paston
Cooper, Everard Home, William Lynn and William Hey.*

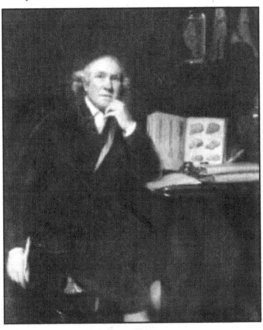

were exhorted to understand the structure and function of the body by detailed dissection. Dissection of cadavers became a mania. In 1801 Hampton Weekes, a student, told his father (an apothecary) that St Thomas's apothecary had given him a foetus ('very perfectly formed about 4 Inches long'). Weekes, himself occupied in dissecting another 'little female', passed the foetus on for three shillings to a friend 'crazey for it'.[3] Anatomy to these men meant 'surgical anatomy': the knowledge they needed in order to operate. Many surgical students became demonstrators in anatomy in hospitals or private medical schools before becoming operating surgeons, and medical journals and medical societies ceaselessly disseminated and published the results of the anatomical spirit animating the profession. Rude though their work may appear in retrospect, the surgeons of the early nineteenth century considered that they practised in an age in which greater progress was being made than at any previous time. They were excited by discoveries in anatomy and physiology, challenged by the introduction of new operations and led by men who saw themselves as practising a self-consciously scientific medicine, in which developments in surgery were among its most distinctive features. Even so, most would have agreed with William Fergusson who described himself as 'the Practical Surgeon'. While not discounting the contributions made by physiology, chemistry and pharmacy, their fundamental skill remained in the cutting of the body to effect healing.[4]

'Mr Hunter's Theory of Life', John Abernethy told fellow members of the Royal College of Surgeons in 1814, 'was verifiable'. Although not necessarily accepted or even understood by all surgeons, Hunter's views reflected the essential basis of medicine in the early nineteenth century. Hunter's insights were based on acceptance of the principle of 'universal sympathy'. 'Irritability' – general disturbances of the human system – was the product of local diseases or wounds. A sympathy existed between the parts of the human frame, if surgeons could only discern it, which provided the basis of the treatment of both illnesses and injuries. A product of the Enlightenment, Hunter's ideas, said Abernethy, 'afforded the most rational solution of the cause of irritability'. 'Even the French,' he proclaimed in the year of Waterloo, 'seem to admit the triumph of English physiology'.[5]

Understanding contemporary medical thought is complicated by the absence of uniform terminology and usage. William Hey, for example, named a condition 'fungus haematodes'. A colleague called the same phenomenon 'spongoid inflammation', John Abernethy 'medullary sarcoma' and John Hunter 'soft cancer'. They all referred to a soft caries of bone.[6] We need to enter into and accept the terminology and disputations of contemporary medicine. Retrospective and speculative diagnosis is enjoyable but hazardous, and correction encourages an unproductive condescension. It is usually enough to comprehend the explanations offered by contemporaries and salutary to avoid the temptation to show up their ignorance by correcting it. This obliges modern students to contemplate the ugly realities of contemporary medicine. Pus, for example, is understandably distasteful to the early twenty-first century sensibility. To Robert Druitt's contemporaries however, it was a vital element in diagnosis. In his *Principles and Practice of Modern Surgery* he discussed pus in detail, distinguishing half a dozen varieties – including 'healthy', 'serous', 'clotty or curdy' and putrid. It was described as 'ichorous' when thin and acrid, 'sanious' when thin and bloody and 'gruminous' when mingled with half-curdled blood.[7] This was the reality of contemporary treatment, and surgeons came to know it intimately from its appearance and smell.

Contemporaries pondered and debated three competing explanations for the sepsis that they encountered every day in their hospitals. Some favoured a recognisable 'germ theory', although it lacked empirical support and represented a minority view. A few others clung to the obsolete theory of 'spontaneous generation' although it too lacked evidence. The most popular theory was the 'atmospheric' which held that gases or miasmas generated by decomposition transmitted disease.[8] Surgeons observed the connection between inflammation and sepsis but seemed incapable of explaining it. John Bell mused that he could not explain why the sores and stumps of patients in hospital should turn gangrenous while even poor patients who had undergone the same operations, but in private, should escape.[9] Their obtuseness seems almost perverse. According to a former student John Gay, surgeon to the Royal Free Hospital, 'almost boasted' that he operated upon a frequently-used dissecting table.[10] Though bacteria had been identified microscopically, they were not to be connected to the transmission of sepsis until the 1870s, and even then many, such as James Simpson, rejected the germ theory. Sepsis was ascribed rather to the presence of 'morbid matter'. This understanding nevertheless led some to decide that cleanliness – of a rough and ready kind to our eyes – would help to deter contamination. For example, Benjamin Brodie asked in a paper in the *Lancet* in 1832 'What is it that prevents union by first intention?' – without suppuration. His answer – clots of coagulated blood and air. Brodie's analysis is ludicrous to modern eyes but his conclusion was to urge colleagues and students to cleanse wounds thoroughly.[11]

'Counter-irritation': pain in healing

Hunter's theories validated rather than initiated the therapeutic regime prevailing in the first half of the century. Essentially it held that injury disturbed the 'sympathy' inherent in the living body. 'Disturbance in one part,' explained James Syme, 'occasions disturbance in others', and the almost universal condition confronting medical practitioners was 'inflammation' or 'irritation'. So common was sepsis that many surgical texts such as those by Lizars, Erichsen, Castle, Miller and both Coopers opened not with discussions of surgical anatomy, instruments or common operations but with the varieties of inflammation that accompanied almost every wound and which followed almost every operation. Injuries – or 'irritants' – caused inflammation, a 'tendency to excited action by the parts or the patient', producing reddened, painful or swollen tissue. 'Excited actions' included 'haemorrhage, inflammation, increased nutrition, and excited secretion' (that is, the formation of pus or other discharges).[12] These actions could be induced to supplant each other because the body was believed to be unable to sustain both. Astley Cooper explained that creating a new inflammation drew blood from a neighbouring, diseased part. The surgeon's skill lay in identifying the place to excite the fresh inflammation: a blister on the nape of the neck could remedy a brain inflammation while a blister on the chest would not affect an inflamed lung.[13]

This belief became the foundation of the doctrine of 'counter-irritation'. Surgeons called on a great range of methods of displacing irritation including bleeding, fomentations and poultices, acupuncture, pressure and the application of heat, the infliction of pain and purgatives. The range of counter-irritants inflicting pain was formidable. It included the process of 'dry-cupping', the 'potential cautery' of blistering agents and the use of burning agents, notably the moxa and the 'actual cautery'. These practices offer one of the clearest illustrations of surgeons' willingness to inflict pain in the hope of healing.

Bleeding – the 'anti-phlogistic regime', the practice of 'depletion' or bleeding from veins – was based on the perception of the symptoms of inflammation. Redness, swelling and heat suggested congestion of blood ('a perverted action of the capillary system') which could be relieved or halted by taking blood from the region. Methods included venesection, usually in hospitals performed by students, the application of leeches and scarification. The usual quantity in an adult male was 16 to 20 ounces stopping short of syncope, or fainting. Depletion long remained the most common single medical procedure, regarded as useful in itself, the essential preparation for other treatments. Depletion sometimes reached heroic proportions. In 1809 *The Times* reported on an American, Captain James Niblett, who over two months had been bled of 600 ounces of blood, more than fifty instances in addition to leeches.[14] Hospitals consumed prodigious numbers of leeches: Bart's in 1822 used over 50,000; St Thomas's in the mid-1830s 23,000.[15] As a 'clerk' or dresser at the Edinburgh Royal Infirmary, James Syme had been directed to successively bleed a patient of 65, 35 and 20 ounces. Noticing that bleeding weakened patients, Syme became sceptical of the practice and contributed to its demise.[16] Opposed by influential teachers such as John Abernethy, depletion gradually fell into disrepute and by the 1840s the use of leeches marked an old-fashioned practitioner – itself a liability in a profession concerned to demonstrate its modernity. John Mann attributed the decline of the 'depletory system' to its manifest ineffectiveness during the cholera epidemics of the 1830s.[17]

Counter-irritation subjected patients to considerable suffering. A boiling water blister meant just that: a half-pint basin of boiling water wrapped in flannel and pressed against the skin. 'The effect', wrote John James ingenuously, 'is almost instantaneous'.[18] Dry-cupping entailed the use of heated vacuum glasses to raise blisters on the skin. Caustic ointments such as tartar emetic, cantharides or nitrate of silver were applied to raise blisters. Repeated applications, William Fergusson warned, could cause mortification and death especially in children. The moxa – a metal box full of burning linen impregnated with nitre – could be applied to the skin which would shrivel and brown. 'The more slowly it burns,' John Lizars advised, 'the more powerful is the effect'.[19] The cautery was a narrow iron blade, heated on a brazier black or red hot depending on the condition being treated. Robert Druitt wrote winningly that 'its effects are speedy and not attended with very much suffering'.[20] James Syme regarded the pain it caused as 'severe but almost momentary'. Of all counter-irritants, Syme felt the cautery was 'the best' because, provided it burned deeply, the lesion remained open for weeks or months. He continued to use it into the 1860s albeit in conjunction with chloroform.[21]

Notwithstanding pretensions to science and progress much of the medicine of the time smacked of the homely. Poultices – of half-dried linseed meal or even stale bread – were used to ease abscesses or joints. Mustard poultices irritated the skin and often produced 'pustular eruption'. Skey condemned them as 'one of the most remarkable relics of the barbarous surgery of the past age', but they remained popular.[22] Likewise, many surgeons placed faith in the elimination of toxins through enemas and 'opening medicines'. Ironically, the one method still used, acupuncture ('held in much esteem in eastern countries'), fell into disuse over the first quarter of the century.[23] Robert Druitt regarded acupuncture as 'very efficacious' although he was at a loss to explain how it might work.[24]

Despite the misgivings of some colleagues who deprecated

'Continental' barbarity and had abandoned all but the use of mild
caustics, most British surgeons continued to employ powerful
counter-irritants. They included a paste of potassa fusa and soap
which, smeared on the skin, produced a black slough. William
Fergusson recalled how his former colleague John Lizars used potash
extensively (and, it seems, indiscriminately). Fergusson described 'the
groans and stifled screams of agony heard in his wards a few hours
after his visit'. Fergusson pleaded 'guilty to the same kind of cruelty'
but appeared in his *System of Practical Surgery* of 1846 not to
repudiate it. Paradoxical though it seemed, counter-irritation
encompassed the use of 'setons' and other objects placed in wounds
to prevent healing and promote a suppuration that would, they
hoped, diminish another less desirable inflammation. ('Dressing
must be so managed', advised an authority on gun-shot wounds, 'so
as not to interfere with the process of suppuration'.[25]) A seton could
be inserted beneath the skin and left, or a pea replaced daily. In the
1840s James Syme was among the earliest notable surgeons to express
scepticism of their value, but he nevertheless described setons and
they remained in common use into the 1870s.

The reality of the regime is suggested by the treatment that Sir
Walter Scott received when in 1819 he was seized by a recurrence of
'stomach cramps'. Subjected again to 'profuse bleeding and liberal
blistering' he screamed without interval through the night, terrifying
his family and servants. So weak from repeated blistering he could
not bear to be shaved, his arms so mangled by lancet punctures that
he could not hold a pen, for ten days he could take nothing but toast,
water and a few teaspoons of rice. Looking back on the ordeal Scott
reflected wryly that his doctors had told him that 'mere pain cannot
kill'.[26]

Although gradually opposed, this regime remained in force for
much of the first half of the nineteenth century. Counter-irritation
came under challenge, particularly in Britain, from the 1840s but was
not supplanted by a more benign regime until long after 1850.
Younger surgeons sought to abandon older practices on the grounds
not only of ineffectiveness but also of undue cruelty. By 1840 James
Macartney was describing the custom of promoting inflammation as
having 'descended to us from ... dark ages', advocating the 'cure of
wounds without inflammation'.[27] The suffering inseparable from
treatment before or besides surgery, however, explains how the acute
pain of surgery was perhaps merely an intensification of a regime in
which prolonged pain was seen as an inevitable part of healing.

Figure 2.2

A successful Taliacotian operation, in which skin from the forehead was used to repair George Culver's nose, depicted in the <u>Lancet</u>. Culver's nose had been destroyed after a quack applied arsenic to cure 'pain, swelling and fetor' following a blow while lifting a wheelbarrow. Robert Storks gave him a new nose in a series of operations over six months from January 1843.

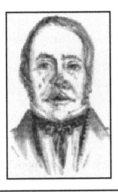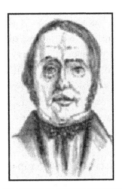

'My God, there is a nose!': innovation in scientific surgery

The drama, wonder and exhilaration of Modern Surgery was captured by an account of the ligation of the common iliac artery, published in the *Transactions of the Medical and Chirurgical Society* in 1830. The surgeon, Philip Crampton, described what he saw as he looked down at 'a more striking view' than he had ever witnessed. Unobscured by a drop of blood, 'there lay the great Iliac Artery, nearly as large as my finger, beating awfully at the rate of 120 in a minute, its yellowish white coat contrasting strongly with the dark blue of the Iliac Vein ....'[28] Crampton passed a ligature around the artery, tying it in accordance with the findings of John Hunter, and saved a patient's life. This was the triumph and the glory of 'modern', 'scientific' surgery such as had never been practised before Hunter.

The heading 'New Operation' recurs in the medical journals. They are permeated by an awareness of progress. It is an excitement easy to miss if we only notice condescendingly the mistakes and shortcomings of these men rather than the spirit in which they worked. The growth of medical knowledge and the purposes to which it could be put were matters of current moment. The title page of the *Edinburgh Medical and Surgical Journal* advertised its scope to be 'a concise view of the latest and most important discoveries'.[29] A contributor in 1828 reflected that it had only been in the previous twenty or twenty-five years that anatomical knowledge had allowed surgery of hernia and aneurism to be tackled on 'fixed rational principles'. It had been 'rather less than that' since surgeons had attempted to disarticulate the humerous and the thigh bone. Even more recently the writer acknowledged, were operations on the lower jaw and the carotid artery made possible.[30] 'Since this article was printed', Samuel Cooper added to the introduction to his dictionary, 'the aorta has again been tied': interestingly, not by a metropolitan surgeon but by Mr James, of Exeter.[31] The medical and the wider community regarded surgery as able to produce near miracles of healing. Joseph Carpue published an account of two operations in which he restored noses to two army officers. The first operation, using the 'Indian' method in which a graft was taken from the forehead and shaped to form a new nose, took 37 minutes. As the dressings were removed a bystander exclaimed 'My G__d, there *is* a nose!'[32]

Understanding contemporary surgery involves appreciating, as Christopher Lawrence has shown, the abiding tendency of surgical authors to project their own period as one of progress and enlightenment, and to cast that of preceding generations as periods of barbarism.[33] Just as representing the early-nineteenth century as a period of progress involved denigrating the eighteenth century as barbarous, so in turn surgeons after the introduction of anaesthesia and asepsis portrayed the period of painful and dirty surgery as horrific and crude. While the painful era may appear in superficial retrospect to have been static, contemporaries remarked upon the rapidity of change. New technology, terminology and techniques arose to be debated and accepted, modified or discarded. Modern surgeons distinguished their practice from what Robert Liston called 'the cruel and debased handicraft of the dark ages', and for many the dark ages of surgery ended late in the eighteenth century. Liston's contemporaries considered that the essential difference between their own surgery and that performed by their forebears was 'in limiting the expenditure of blood and pain'. The surgeon's aim, Liston declared, was to avoid operating as much as possible.[34] This logic of the 'scientific surgeon' led to the belief that truly scientific surgeons would eschew and eventually repudiate cutting altogether. This – and his revulsion at causing pain – could explain John Abernethy's aversion to operating. Abernethy decried the '*prestige* in favour of operations' because it diminished surgeons' claims to be men of science.[35]

The proliferation of surgical innovation is suggested by William Fergusson, who described fifteen methods of amputating at the hip, an operation which remained hazardous and rare, even in the 1840s justifying articles and even monographs describing particular operations.[36] The pace of the development of surgical ideas is suggested by Liston referring to 'old books' by Benjamin Bell and even Samuel Cooper.[37] 'Modern practitioners', as Samuel Cooper described them (and himself), reflected explicitly upon the changes which they had witnessed over the period. William Fergusson recalled how the French surgeon Roux had in 1814 seized the opportunity to visit London following Napoleon's first abdication. There he had witnessed a circular amputation which took twenty minutes in cutting alone. Roux 'could have seen nothing of the kind' during a second visit in 1841 Fergusson pointed out.[38] The example emphasises how in virtually every measure – speed, variety of techniques, morbidity and mortality – the intervening thirty years had seen immense changes in the conduct of operations.

For example, in 1840 British surgeons took up a new French technique intended to correct lateral curvature of the spine. The first operation attempted in Britain was performed in October by Robert Hunter, Professor of Anatomy at the Andersonian University, Glasgow. Hunter cut under the skin to divide the muscles distorting the spine, 'a formidable operation' in that it demanded dexterity and knowledge of exactly what to cut and where. His patient, 'a young delicate lady', complained of no pain, lost three drops of blood and was restrained for only thirty seconds. A month later George Childs of the Aldersgate Medical School performed the new operation for the first time in England on a seventeen-year-old boy. Dividing the muscles of the back on one side, the operation lasted less than a minute, entailed 'little pain' and a 'trifling' loss of blood and the lad walked to his bed. Ten days later Frederick Skey of Bart's performed a similar operation taking ten seconds to replicate it to a theatre 'crowded to excess' with students and colleagues.[39] The sequence suggests not only the competitive atmosphere permeating the profession but also how it was confidence rather than equipment that enabled operators to make advances.

Surgical progress brought with it much uncertainty passed off as bravado and error trumpeted as triumph. In concert with the 'regular' practitioners' continuing campaign against the 'irregulars' it is not surprising that many supposed advances were contested or exposed. In the prevailing atmosphere of experimentation, innovation and novelty many questionable procedures were accepted by some and for a time as legitimate advances. Progress was so rapid that it is now – as it must have seemed at the time – difficult to determine the merits of new procedures. Medical journals published accounts of individual operations and operators themselves distributed pamphlets promoting their procedures. Surgeons operated in a competitive market in which an account of a successful operation was as much a trade advertisement as a scientific treatise. In 1813, for example, the young James Wardrop published a pamphlet giving an *History of James Mitchell, a Boy Born Blind and Deaf, with an Account of the Operation Performed for the Recovery of His Sight*. Wardrop became a notable surgeon: many others rose to obscurity on the strength of operations of dubious efficacy. Short-sightedness, deafness and stuttering offer cases in which novel surgical treatment appeared to offer effective treatments. With newspapers increasingly ready to publish medical detail the cases became more accessible both to practitioners willing to experiment and to patients desperate for relief.

Surgeons approached innovation with a certain ambivalence. In 1823 James Syme, emulating his friend and rival Robert Liston, performed what he described as 'the greatest and bloodiest operation', the amputation at the hip. The patient, a 19-year-old man named William Fraser, had suffered from necrosis of the thigh bone for several years. Syme advised amputation but Fraser and his friends were 'much against it'. In August 1823, however, Fraser's father stopped Syme in the street and told him that William had changed his mind. Syme, assisted by Liston, performed the operation, a brave one for both the patient and the two young surgeons. Marked by alarming haemorrhage (with 'many large and crossing jets of blood'), the operation caused Syme to become, as he wrote to a London friend, 'quite a notorious character' in Edinburgh's medical community. Syme hoped and expected that William Fraser would recover although in fact he died, reportedly of liver disease, two months later. 'Whatever way the matter ends,' Syme calculated cold-bloodedly, 'it must be favourable to me'.[40]

'New and useful suggestions': surgery as an international discipline

It is too easy to represent surgery as a monolith practised uniformly over time and in various places. Rather it is apparent that while surgeons shared many similar problems and practices, their work displayed a great many variations and differences. Not only did surgery in various countries reflect marked differences but practices also differed between surgeons in the hospitals of major cities. There was, however, an international dimension in which surgical writers and journalists reported and reflected upon innovations by colleagues overseas. Surgeons seeking to promote or justify new operations typically drew on an international literature advancing cases or evidence. In the early 1850s, for instance, G.M. Jones, Surgeon to the Jersey Hospital, developed an interest in excising the knee-joint (itself a reflection of the move to conserve rather than amputate damaged limbs). In arguing his case he surveyed thirteen attempts over the preceding century drawn from French, English and Scottish surgeons.[41] Likewise, when James Wardrop tried a new method of tying aneurismal tumours, it was adopted in Britain, by Dupuytren in Paris and by Valentine Mott in New York.[42] Surgery had became an international discipline.

British medical journalists and the authors of surgical texts described and criticised foreign approaches: not always parochially. Samuel Cooper, the strength of whose monumental *Dictionary of Practical Surgery* was his diligence in reading and digesting foreign authorities, was in turn translated into French, German, Italian and Russian and appeared in American editions.[43] For all that the fellows of the Royal College of Surgeons attracted a reputation for being parochial and self-interested their library contained German, French, Italian and American periodicals. (Wakley's *Lancet* nevertheless abused the College for spending only twice as much on the library as it had on formal dinners.[44]) From its foundation in 1805 the office-bearers of the Medical and Chirurgical Society included a 'Foreign Secretary' and it continued to purchase many foreign books for its library. In 1848 of the 432 books obtained, only 57 were in English.[45] Perhaps the most telling demonstration of surgery's international character at the highest level is found in the proceedings of the Provincial Medical and Surgical Association meeting held at Worcester in August 1843. The gathering heard a Retrospective Address by William Hey, the son and namesake of the notable Yorkshire surgeon, also Surgeon to the Leeds Infirmary. Presenting a review of surgical advances during the past year Hey referred to operations conducted not only in London and Paris but also Dublin, New York, Philadelphia, Rio de Janiero, Glasgow – and Doncaster.[46] However much metropolitan colleagues might sneer, operative surgeons read, thought and corresponded internationally.

Paradoxically, however, surgery was also practised in several distinctive national styles. Many major and minor differences existed between practitioners working in different hospitals within cities, between cities and between nations. The greatest differences existed between British and European (especially French) surgeons. German innovations by Dieffenbach and Graefe were often reported in British journals, with detailed accounts of operations less developed in Britain especially gynaecological and plastic surgery. Samuel Cooper's monumental *Dictionary of Practical Surgery* documented the differing national approaches in entry after entry. The French, less impressed by Hunter's legacy (which in any case was communicated more by a series of disciples than by comprehensible texts), failed to take up the Hunterian operations for aneurism but preferred older, often less effective methods.[47] English surgeons often decried French practices as belonging to the barbaric age from which Hunterian progress had delivered them. For example, the *Lancet* published accounts of operations at La Pitié denouncing cruelties and abuses of the sort it exposed in British operating rooms: of rash operations, surgeons deferring operations because too few students attended and of students being invited in groups to handle pulsating arteries within a surgical wound.[48] 'On some parts of the continent' Liston slyly told his students 'they still, I am told, chop off toes and fingers', showing his appalled students an array of chisels and mallets which he had collected, before describing his own meticulous use of scalpel and nippers.[49]

French practice was not always rougher: in treating fractures, for example, the French were noted for their care and neatness while English surgeons were criticised as 'slovenly'. They were regarded as ingenious – the elastic gum seton, for example, praised for its 'cleanliness and convenience', the product of 'French ingenuity'. The French also tended to develop specialised instruments – such as Bichat's for tonsillectomy – where the English made scalpels serve for most purposes. French surgeons also made a particular virtue of extreme celerity in operating. English surgeons, however, had developed better post-operative treatments which promoted clean wound-healing more effectively than French methods. French surgeons appear to have remained more tenaciously attached to conservative techniques, in applying oil-soaked charpie within wounds and promoting inflammation, as well as by taking less interest in diet and general post-operative care.[50]

Although trained in their own medical schools American students had long aspired to complete their education in Edinburgh and especially Paris. American surgery inherited something of the

French tradition of boldness. Its surgeons claimed numerous firsts – the ligation of the carotid artery, the removal of a section of the lower jaw, the removal of the clavicle and ligation of the inominate artery. Ephraim McDowell's celebrated ovariotomies, though the work of a country surgeon in remote Kentucky, were in keeping with this tradition. Samuel Cooper, observing the 'still continued progress of the boldest parts of operative surgery,' looked to the United States as 'a frequent source of new and useful suggestions'.[51] The American propensity to boldness did not go unremarked or approved by British surgeons. Robert Liston, whose alleged willingness to resort to the knife has been taken as defining the heroic surgeon, condemned ovariotomy by the 'great incision'. In this he sided with conservative metropolitan surgeons against bolder provincial operators prepared to hazard this novel and risky operation.[52]

'Trials': surgical experimentation

Although the operators of the great hospitals regarded themselves (and were generally hailed) as the principal innovators, the nature of surgery enabled other innovative practitioners to contribute to the advancement of surgical knowledge. Hospital surgeons enjoyed several advantages: a ready supply of 'interesting cases', the power to generate publicity through the established medical journals and the reputation to encourage patients to place themselves in their hands. Surgery, however, required neither expensive equipment nor special facilities. A practitioner with a case of instruments, a table, an assistant – and a trusting or desperate patient – could equally venture to experiment. New operations were therefore reported from private or even rural surgeons and verified or repeated by metropolitan operators, competing with each other for the palm of having performed an operation for the first time.

Change occurred generally as individual surgeons attempted new procedures. Surgical journals and texts were punctuated by individual and often idiosyncratic instances of surgical experimentation. Speaking often 'rather in the spirit of an experimenter ... as a surgeon', Samuel Cooper described trials of the expedient of partially closing stumps, of dressing incisions 'from the bottom' and in treating spina bifida, hernia, aneurisms and gangrene.[53] Many of these trials exposed patients to danger or even death. Dr Home Blackadder experimented with the treatment of gangrenous wounds by placing three patients with 'clean' wounds between them.[54] How many patients lost their legs or their lives in the course of such tests is unknown. Surgeons acquired a habit of mind permitting individual, unsupervised experimentation. John Lizars agreed to allow his house surgeons (that is, his senior pupils) to test various methods of treating fractures of the neck of the thigh.[55] That he was not alone is revealed by his text, *A System of Practical Surgery*, in which he reported colleagues' trials of ligatures, trials which had risked or cost patients' lives. Canvassing the eight types of thread available (from fine silk through leaden thread to catgut) he described how Mr Fielding, of Hull, 'has largely employed silk-worm-gut ... but Dr Crampton lost a patient in consequence of using it'.[56] The implicit risk is apparent and no ready answers could be expected beyond collegial advice and individual responsibility. Lamentable though it may have been there was little alternative to the development of more effective techniques.

The process of informal innovation is suggested by new procedures for the treatment of wry neck in 1840. A painful and awkward condition, it attracted the attention of rural practitioners in Boston, Lincolnshire, and Hitchen in Hertfordshire. A Dr Smith of Boston devised his own treatment, passing a knife under the sternocleidomastoid muscle and cutting upwards. The patient described the resulting sound as 'like that of breaking sticks across the knee' and the excruciating pain. His head, however, immediately bobbed up 'like an automaton'. He was declared 'perfectly cured'.[57] A few days later, having read another account in *The Times* of an earlier attempt to find a surgical treatment, Edward Blackburn of Hitchen had discussed the problem with his assistant, an enterprising and persuasive but un-named young man. Without his knowledge Blackburn's assistant sought out a sufferer in the area, a sheep-farming gentlemen with three brothers known as sporting shooters. He induced the man to submit to an operation, taking him into his wool chamber. Laying the patient over a bag of wool he cut into the man's back, making incisions 'inclined to the centre like a slice of cheese'. The loss of blood was 'inconsiderable' and after ten days the man was reported to have joined his brothers in shooting over their estate, 'as straight and well formed' as them.[58]

Much of the mystique of the heroic surgeon stemmed from the willingness of individual operators to attempt the novel and the dangerous. The most celebrated exponent of new operations was surely Robert Liston, whose confidence in his ability excused the unprecedented. 'There is this difference,' he hectored the Lord Provost, 'between boldness and rashness' explaining that he 'had some experience of the steadiness of my own nerves'.[59] Liston was justifying the excision of Robert McNair's scapula in 1822, one of the most dazzling demonstrations of surgical prowess before 1850. Working in a cottage in poor light Liston excised a tumour beneath McNair's shoulder blade. His description of the operation substantiates Liston's view:

> I began by making an incision of a foot long ... I felt my finger and knife dip into the body of the tumour ... I immediately thrust my sponge into the cavity, so as to command the haemorrhagy. The patient, who had borne the operation well ... now dropped his head off the pillow, pale, cold, and almost lifeless. I then ... saw that nothing but a bold stroke of the knife could save the boy from immediate death. Pulling out the sponge, therefore, with one rapid incision I completely separated the upper edge of the tumour ... After removing the tumour, I found it necessary to saw off the ragged and spongy part of the scapula, so as to leave only a fourth part of that bone ... In this way, ten muscles were either wholly or partly divided ....[60]

Liston's patient survived the operation but died four months later reportedly from the original condition. Liston's reputation as a fearless operator prospered, although he was also accused of attempting imprudent operations for acclaim.[61]

Thomas Pettigrew warned that 'solitary instances of success' scarcely justified dangerous trials. They excited so great a dread, he wrote, that patients would not risk them.[62] So rapid did surgical innovation become that a suspicion arose that surgeons advanced their discipline by injudicious or unjustifiable experiment. A coroner holding an inquest in 1827 on Henry Loggins, a 22-year-old man who had died in an operation for hernia, heard allegations suggesting a popular mistrust of surgeons' motives. Mr Loggins's father alleged that the operation at James Wardrop's private clinic had been performed as a 'mere surgical experiment'. Testimony tendered by Wardrop's (hardly disinterested) colleagues established that the operation had begun too late to prevent mortification and no stigma attached to the operator.[63]

'Startling notions rife amongst us': surgical controversy

Willingness to innovate and experiment encouraged diversity and, inevitably, controversy. The principles of surgery, a provincial lecturer acknowledged candidly, were 'so imperfectly diffused' that he saw 'every ingenious surgeon, author and lecturer devising his own according to his 'fancy and opinion'.[64] Partisans of novel methods wrangled in the medical press and in successive editions of texts. They debated, often rancorously, the merits of new operative techniques, dressings and instruments. Arguments continued over the various methods of lithotomy, over the desirability or otherwise of suppuration, of dressing wounds 'on the table' or of waiting for incisions to 'granulate' before closing them. Operators differed over the number of 'tails' which should be left in sutures or over the type of dressings best suited to surgical wounds. The most virulent arguments concerned amputation. The controversy between proponents of the 'flap' or 'circular' amputation persisted with more passion than clarity and with partisans making directly contradictory claims. There were, Charles Bell shuddered, 'startling notions rife amongst us'.[65]

The controversy over amputation especially precluded any surgeon of any standing evading the dispute and each was called upon to declare for one or another faction every time he took up the knife. Virtually every surgeon held an opinion on the propriety of amputating a limb immediately after injury or wounding or of waiting for days before operating. Naval and military surgery gave the argument both vast additional data and the urgency of demanding treatment. In the immediate aftermath of the wars amputation sooner rather than later tended to prevail. As a generation without war experience qualified, surgeons influenced by the conservative approach began to doubt their elders' wisdom. These disputes were not simply academic or even technical. They were conducted not simply as differences of method, but as contests between personalities and the contending parties disseminated their doctrines among their subordinates and students. Their protagonists included every teacher of surgery and operative surgeon whose work was visible in hospitals. As a result hospitals and schools became captured by proponents of particular approaches. Clinical or technical disputes often became confused with the profession's vigorous personal politics: James Gregory's personal feud with John Bell infected, as it were, their professional differences over the origins and spread of gangrene.[66]

Much of this controversy smacked of fashion (a word, William Fergusson reminded his readers, 'more applicable to the practice of surgery than some imagine').[67] Lacking developed protocols in clinical trials, protagonists often elevated theories supported by anecdotal, impressionistic or otherwise inadequate evidence to the status of dogma. The Royal College of Surgeons' examiners professed to be wary of candidates who parroted their teachers' theories but the tenacity with which they held their convictions suggests that partiality entered into every facet of surgical education. Fergusson, whose lectures embody a rare common sense, decried the 'objectionable formality' by which teachers passed on their pet theories to their students through 'needlessly dogmatic statements' which he found had 'thrown difficulty in the way of the young surgeon'.[68] James Syme reflecting in maturity on fifty years of surgical progress regretted how often supposedly scientific discussions had been 'characterised by a degree of fervour that savours more of personal acrimony'.[69] The influence and example of teachers who presided over generations of students helped to propagate their particular methods widely: none more than Syme who despite mellowing with age had been notorious for his combative demeanour.

'Perfection': humility and pride in surgery

Robert Liston argued – to students who witnessed his operations – that progress since Hunter had been such that operations had been 'shorn of their horror'.[70] He was not alone. Many surgeons believed that they practised in an enlightened era, one markedly different to that of their fathers. Writing in 1839 J.G. Millingen decried his predecessors' 'barbarity' and the 'sum of misery' inflicted on their 'victims'. By contrast he reflected on the 'perfection' to which the art had been brought within the preceding decades.[71] Likewise, Samuel Cooper thought that James Veitch's short-tailed ligatures had 'brought this part of surgery as near to perfection as it is capable of being'.[72] Modern readers sharing the assumptions of the horror of painful surgery might regard these views as grotesque. W.P. Alison, in his survey of the history of medicine published in 1833, countered that there was 'nothing irrational or Utopian' in this view of surgical progress. The proponents of scientific medicine would, he predicted, gradually but surely extend their knowledge of the nature of disease and would ultimately be able to prevent or relieve 'all the sufferings of our physical constitution'.[73] The men expressing these views practised in wards which we would regard as nightmarish. We may disregard them as woefully mistaken, unconscionably callous or unduly optimistic. Or we might accept that their belief in the perfectibility of surgery reflected their practice as well as their aspirations.

The surgery of the early-nineteenth century represented such a dramatic contrast to that taught to and practised by older colleagues within memory that few 'modern surgeons' could imagine that knowledge and skill could continue to advance at the rate they had known. Indeed it has long been maintained that by the 1840s surgery had reached the limits imposed by the surgeons' speed and skill. The introduction of anaesthesia, it has been argued, removed these limits, enabling surgeons to contemplate longer and more daring operations, building upon the anatomical and physiological knowledge accumulated during the preceding half-century. Whether this is so must mercifully remain conjectural. Given the rate of change and the range of innovation still evident in the 1840s there is no reason to believe that surgeons would not have continued to at least attempt even bolder operations.

The increasing reliance on scientific investigation brought with it a feeling that surgery – a messy and distressing business at the best of times – represented a scientific failure. If surgeons truly understood the body, its functions and pathology, they reasoned, then they ought to be able to treat disease so as to render surgery unnecessary. Abernethy told his students that having to operate ought to be 'an humiliating reflection, ... a confession that our art is inadequate to the cure of disease'.[74] Since this ideal has yet to be realised Abernethy might be regarded as too hard on himself and his colleagues. It indicates, however, not only an unjustified optimism in the capacities of contemporary science but also an illuminating humility on the part of its practitioners.

Indeed, by the 1830s a new moderation had entered the surgical literature. No longer were surgeons so eager to attempt a procedure simply because it was technically possible. Charles Bell, reflecting in old age on the boundaries of the surgical revolution he had helped to engineer, mused that 'the conviction comes tardily on the surgeon's mind that there is a limit to his boldness and ingenuity'.[75] 'Surgeons of experience' like Bell began to consider the effect of unsuccessful operations on the public perception of surgeons and surgery. Sir Benjamin Brodie reflected in 1835 how as a young surgeon in the Regency he had a very high opinion of operative surgery and believed that where nothing else could be done operations could be justified on the grounds that even if ineffective, they could do no harm. In his fifties he had changed his mind. He reminded his students of a patient often encountered in the wards of London's great hospitals, a woman seeking treatment for scirrhous breast. Suppose, he said, that the woman undergoes amputation of the breast but later dies of the condition. 'You may say,' he admonished, that no harm was done: the patient was not made worse. But, Brodie suggested, not only had the woman endured pain and anxiety; so had her friends. 'Every operation which fails', he said, deters other patients from consenting to surgery; operations which may have every chance of succeeding. 'Every failure,' he counselled Brodie, 'does harm to our art and is injurious to society'.[76]

As they buried their failures and smelled the stink of cases in progress, surgeons realised the limitations of their profession. Conscious of the precarious standing of the profession into which he had recently qualified, Hampton Weekes urged his brother that 'it will not do to say to ye wor[l]d ... that Medicine were of no use ... we must keep up ye Farce'.[77] These modern surgeons could describe more than they could diagnose, could diagnose more than they could treat and could treat more than they could cure. At the same time they were proud of living in an era making rapid and unprecedented advances in anatomical and physiological knowledge and in medical and particularly operative techniques. On the eve of the acceptance of chemical anaesthesia a contributor to the *Edinburgh Medical and Surgical Journal* reviewed four surgical texts. His conclusion offers a cogent contemporary view of the ultimate state of painful surgery. Referring to James Miller's *The Practice of Surgery*, the anonymous reviewer found that Miller had vindicated 'the art of operating' from critics' charges. He had done so by advocating 'simplicity and efficiency' in operations undertaken 'in the easiest and most direct ... simplest, most gentle, and least painful way'.[78] Emboldened by their knowledge, undaunted by their ignorance and animated by their belief in progress and confidence in their own abilities, modern surgeons sought to bring into conjunction their abundant knowledge and their inadequate practice.

Notes

1. Accounts of Hunter's death differ over details. This is taken variously from those given in Drewry Ottley, *The Life of John Hunter, FRS* (London: Longman, Rees, Orme, Brown, Green & Longmans, 1835), Jesse Dobson, *John Hunter* (Edinburgh: E. & S. Livingstone, 1969) and George Qvist, *John Hunter 1728-1793* (London: W. Heinemann, 1981).

2. Evidence of Astley Cooper, PP 1828, Vol. VII, Part 1, 15.

3. Hampton Weekes to Richard Weekes, 14 December 1801, John Ford (ed.), *A Medical Student at St Thomas's Hospital, 1801–1802 The Weekes Family Letters* (London: Wellcome Institute for the History of Medicine, 1987), 98.

4. William Fergusson, *A System of Practical Surgery* (London: John

Churchill, 1846), vii–viii.

5. John Abernethy, *Introductory Lectures Exhibiting Some of Mr Hunter's Opinions Respecting Life Diseases* (London: Longman, Hurst, Rees, Orme & Brown, 1819), 66.

6. Thomas Pettigrew, *Biographical Memoirs of the Most Celebrated Physicians, Surgeons, etc., etc.*, 3 vols (London: Fisher, Son & Co., 1839–40) (RACS), Vol. II, 6.

7. Robert Druitt, *The Principles and Practice of Modern Surgery* (Philadelphia: Lea & Blanchard, 1842), 71–72.

8. Royston Lambert, *Sir John Simon 1816–1904 and English Social Administration* (London: Macgibbon & Kee, 1963), 49.

9. John Bell, *The Principles of Surgery*, 2 vols (Edinburgh: T. Cadell & W. Davies, 1801), Vol. III, 292.

10. *Transactions of the Intercolonial Medical Congress of Australasia* (Adelaide, 1887), 127.

11. Brodie, 'Clinical Remarks by Mr Brodie', *Lancet*, 1832–33, Vol. I, 168.

12. James Syme, *Principles of Surgery* (Edinburgh: Sutherland & Knox, 1842), 12–15.

13. Astley Cooper & Frederick Tyrrell, *The Lectures of Sir Astley Cooper, Bart.* … (London: Thomas Tegg, 1824), 84–85.

14. *The Times*, 25 December 1809, 3c.

15. D'Arcy Power & H.J. Waring, *A Short History of St Bartholomew's Hospital 1123–1923* (London: C. Whittingham & Griggs, 1923), 51; PP 1840, Vol. XIX, 32nd Report of the Charity Commissioners [into St Thomas's Hospital], 708.

16. Robert Paterson, *Memorials of the Life of James Syme* (Edinburgh: Edmonston & Douglas, 1874), 17.

17. John Mann, *Recollections of My Early and Professional Life* (London: W. Rider & Sons, 1887), 140.

18. J.H. James, *Chloroform versus Pain and Paracentesis of the Bladder* (London: Churchill, 1870), 21.

19. John Lizars, *System of Practical Surgery* (Edinburgh: W.H. Lizars, 1838), 20.

20. Robert Druitt, *The Surgeon's Vade Mecum* (London: Henry Renshaw, John Churchill, 1851), 572.

21. Syme, *op. cit.* (note 12), 27; James Syme, *Observations in Clinical Surgery* (Edinburgh: Edmonston & Douglas, 1861), 91.

22. Frederic Skey, *Operative Surgery* (London: John Churchill, 1850), 52.

23. Syme, *op. cit.* (note 12), 27.

24. Druitt, *op. cit.* (note 7), 485.

25. Thomas Chevalier, *A Treatise on Gun-Shot Wounds* (London: Samuel Bagster, 1806), 125.

26. Edgar Johnson, *Sir Walter Scott: the Great Unknown*, 2 vols (London: Hamilton, 1970), Vol. I, 565–72; 644–45.

27. *Lancet*, 1839–40, Vol. II, 562-64.

28. Norman Moore, & Stephen Paget, *The Royal Medical and Chirurgical Society of London, 1805-1905* (Aberdeen: Aberdeen University Press, 1905), 62.

29. *Edinburgh Medical & Surgical Journal*, Vol. II, 1806.

30. *Ibid.*, Vol. 30, 1828, 421–22.

31. Samuel Cooper, *A Dictionary of Practical Surgery* (London: Longman, Hurst, Rees, Orme & Brown, 1829), iv.

32. J.C. Carpue, *An Account of Two Successful Operations for Restoring a Lost Nose …* (London: Longman & Co., 1816), 87.

33. Lawrence, 'Democratic, divine and heroic: the history and historiography of surgery', in Christopher Lawrence, *Medical Theory: Surgical Practice – Studies in the History of Surgery* (London: Routledge, 1992) .

34. Robert Liston, *Lectures on the Operations of Surgery* (Philadeliphia: Lea & Blanchard, 1846), 16–17.

35. George Macilwain, *Memoirs of John Abernethy*, 2 vols (London: Hurst & Blackett, 1854), Vol. II, 222–23.

36. Fergusson, *op. cit.* (note 4), 395.

37. Liston, *op. cit.* (note 34), 189.

38. Fergusson, *op. cit.* (note 4), 164.

39. *The Times*, 4 November 1840, 7e; 21 November 1840, 5f; 3 December 1840, 7e; *London Medical Gazette*, 27 November 1840.

40. Paterson, *op. cit.* (note 16), 18–23.

41. G.M. Jones, *On Excision of the Knee Joint* (London: J.E. Adlard, 1854), n.p..

42. Forbes Winslow, *Physic and Physicians: A Medical Sketch Book*, 2 vols (London: Longman, Orme, Brown, 1839), Vol. II, 383.

43. Cooper, *op. cit.* (note 31), iii.

44. *Lancet*, 1835–36, Vol. II, 152.

45. Moore & Paget, op. cit. (note 28), 6;92.

46. William Hey (jun), *The Retrospective Address in Surgery* (Worcester: Deighton, 1843), 38–44.

47. Cooper, *op. cit.* (note 31), 154.

48. *Lancet*, 1845, Vol. I, 53.

49. Liston, *op. cit.* (note 34), 189.

50. Cooper, *op. cit.* (note 31), 488, 1072, 1104, 99.

51. *Ibid.*, 1072.

52. Liston, *op. cit.* (note 34), 422–23.
53. Cooper, *op. cit.* (note 31), 133.
54. H. Home Blackadder, *Observations in Phagendaena Gangrenosa* (Edinburgh: Balfour & Clarke, 1818), 46.
55. John Lizars, *On Fracture of the Neck of the Thigh Bone* (Edinburgh: 1850), 3.
56. Lizars, *op. cit.* (note 19), 98.
57. *The Times*, 3 December 1840, 7e.
58. *The Times*, 5 December 1840, 5b.
59. Robert Liston, *Letter to the Right Hon. The Lord Provost ...* (Edinburgh: John Robertson, 1822), 7.
60. Alexander Miles, *The Edinburgh School of Surgery Before Lister* (London: A. & C. Black, 1918), 156–57.
61. William Glover, *Exposure of the Unfounded Statements and Insinuations of a Paragraph in the Caledonian Mercury ...* (Edinburgh: A. Balfour, 1828).
62. Pettigrew, *op. cit.* (note 6), 7.
63. *The Times*, 14 December 1827, 4b.
64. W. Hetling, *Introductory Lectures to the Principles and Practice of Surgery* (Bristol: Bristol Infirmary, 1832), 11.
65. Charles Bell, *Institutes of Surgery*, 2 vols (Edinburgh: Longmans & Co., 1838), Vol. II, 238.
66. James Gregory, *Additional Memorial to the Managers of the Royal Infirmary* (Edinburgh: Murray & Cochrane, 1803), 330–34.
67. Fergusson, *op. cit.* (note 4), 379.
68. *Ibid.*, 170.
69. Paterson, *op. cit.* (note 16), 167.
70. Liston, *op. cit.* (note 34), 16–17.
71. John Millingen, *Curiosities of Medical Experience* (London: Richard Bentley, 1839), 285.
72. Cooper, *op. cit.* (note 31), vi.
73. W.P. Alison, *History of Medicine* (London: Blackwood, 1833), cx.
74. Abernethy, *op. cit.* (note 5), 501.
75. 'On the Powers of Life to Sustain Surgical Operations', Charles Bell, *Practical Essays* (Edinburgh: Maclachlan, Stewart & Co., 1841), 1.
76. *Lancet*, 1835-36, Vol. I, 281–82.
77. Hampton Weekes to Dick Weekes, 17 June 1802, Ford, *op. cit.* (note 3), 179.
78. *Edinburgh Medical & Surgical Journal*, Vol. 67, 1847, 305

3

'Capital operations':
Major Surgery

Surgeons confronted the great range of injuries that humans suffer through nature, accident or intention. William Lawrence defined their province in a pamphlet advertising Bart's courses in the 1830s: 'all injuries incidental to the human frame; all diseases which custom has assigned to the care of the Surgeon'.[1] It was – and remains – an awesome responsibility. An analysis of the cases treated by the Charing Cross Hospital during its first fifteen years abundantly demonstrates how dangerous was everyday life in early Victorian London. Between 1834 and 1850 the hospital treated over 66,000 emergencies. Minutely categorised, they involved falls from scaffolds or buildings (16,552), accidents involving steam engines, mill-cogs or cranes (1,308), road accidents (5,090), burns or scalds (2,088), inhalation of gases (544), cat or dog bites (145), personal violence (7,129), attempted suicide (514), epilepsy, hernia, haemorrhage and sudden illness (12,285). Almost a third (19,767) were caused by 'broken glass or porcelain, casual falls, ... lifting of weights and incautious use of spikes, hooks, knives and other domestic implements'[2]. Surgeons also saw and were expected to alleviate or cure the shocking array of growths, tumours and deformities that can beset the human body. Far more than modern practitioners, they often saw these conditions in chronic or acute forms, implored by parents to treat crying children, or importuned by patients driven to distraction by pain or fear. In judging them, we need to bear in mind their limited skill and their patients' hopes and expectations.

At the beginning of the century surgical writers recognised several major operations: trepan, amputation, hernia and lithotomy. Innovation and boldness later added others: excision and ovariotomy. The major operations represented only a few of those that surgeons were called upon to perform. The popular modern view, that surgeons were able to perform only 'a small number' of procedures before the introduction of anaesthesia, is simply wrong.[3] On the contrary, surgeons undertook many major and minor procedures and growing competence and confidence allowed them to undertake a wider range of interventions. John Lizars, a great one for listing, identified over 23 operable conditions of the rectum alone in his *System of Practical Surgery* They included abscesses, fistula, piles, warty and granular excrescences, tumours, polyps, sarcomas, the effects of 'various foreign bodies' and 'different malfunctions'.[4] Surgeons treated fractures, burns and scalds, and diseases of the eye (described by Lizars over 45 pages). Surgical solutions for the complications of childbearing and the reproductive system were increasingly suggested and attempted.* By 1820 surgeons had re-discovered operations for the restoration of noses lost in battle, accidents or to the ravages of disease, often venereal. The achievement did not impress all. Reconstructed noses, James Syme sneered, were 'almost always more disagreeable than the deficiency'.[5]

It is impossible to describe briefly the great variety of procedures that contemporary surgeons developed and attempted. Instead I will consider several of the 'great operations': aneurism, hernia, amputation and lithotomy, and fistula, a minor procedure but one that demonstrates the impact of surgical developments on the sick. The fifth of the 'great operations', trepan, will not detain us long. Perhaps the oldest surgical operation, it was performed to correct depressed fractures. It involved dissecting back the scalp and cutting a hole in the bone using a trephine, a wide circular drill. The aim was to cut cautiously through the bone allowing the injured or diseased portion to be levered out without harming the 'dura matter' protecting the brain. If the dura matter were penetrated infection and death would surely follow. With nine out of ten trepan patients unconscious, John Lizars counselled that there was 'no necessity for operating against time'.[6]

'The point of the knife': the surgeon's instruments

Most operations called upon a relatively limited range of instruments. The newly qualified surgeon's instrument case in 1800 would have been familiar to a surgeon fifty years later. The basic instruments comprised knives of various sizes, saws, forceps, probes,

---

*The emergence of obstetrics as a medical specialty and the consequent displacement or subordination of midwives is such a large part of the medical history of western childbirth that I have chosen not to make it a focus of this study. Childbirth is a subject in itself (one rather better served by modern scholarship than is surgery). I therefore follow the advice of Sir Anthony Carlisle, who told the Select Committee into Medical Education in 1834 that parturition was 'a natural operation'. 'The less surgeons have to do with it', he declared firmly, 'the better'.

hooks, needles and ligatures. Given the popularity of venesection as a counter to inflammation, the most commonly used instrument was the lancet. It was 'a general rule' that new medical students delighted to carry big lancet-cases, and for most of their training few would do much besides bleed.[7] Several different sizes of knives (variously called scalpels and bistouries) enabled cuts in proportion to their size. The smallest permitted fine dissection; the largest (known as catlins) were used for the amputation of limbs. Earlier in the period amputating knives had been heavier, curved and broad-bladed. Anthony Carlisle had advocated the thinner, lighter, straight-bladed knives more usual from about the 1820s.[8] Bone-saws, looking like hack-saws, were later complemented by bone pliers. Forceps were used to hold tissues, probes to search out bullets and foreign bodies, hooks to grasp arteries to be tied using threaded needles. While specialised instruments existed for lithotomies (later including ingenious contrivances intended to crush or drill stones in the bladder) trepan, ophthalmic and obstetrical operations, the essential components of the instruments case remained unchanged.

Samuel Cooper's charge that Robert Liston 'endeavour[ed] to show that the saw is the only necessary thing in the case of amputating instruments' was a sarcastic exaggeration but not by much.[9] Many surgeons carried a pocket set of instruments, including all but the larger amputating knives and saw, which sufficed for perhaps nine out of ten operations. Contemporary surgery was therefore not so much a matter of technology as of technique. Surgeons ensured that their blades remained sharp. 'Everything in this operation,' George Guthrie advised those contemplating the operation to remove cataract, 'depends on the point of the knife'.[10] Experienced operators often used only their own instruments, sometimes modified to their own designs. Fergusson recommended ebony handles because they were less likely to slip in bloody fingers.[11] Robert Liston, his outrage evident in the printed transcripts of a lecture, stressed the need to employ the appropriate instruments. He distastefully described the amputation at the thigh using a common scalpel. The cutting part alone took upwards of fifteen minutes, a sight which Liston regarded as 'exceedingly tedious ... exceedingly cruel and disgusting'.[12]

The knife defined the surgeon and it assumed an almost mystical place in the instructional texts (intended for students who would not wield it for several years). It was 'amusing', wrote an admirer, to note the 'care and attention' Liston paid to his instruments. He was said to have kept scalpels up his coat sleeve 'to keep them warm and comfortable'.[13]

'Bloodless and simple': aneurism

Perhaps the operation most embodying modernity was the treatment of aneurism, a pulsating tumour in the wall of an artery usually attributed to untreated syphilis. Although able to diagnose aneurism, surgeons could hitherto do little to forestall aneurismal tumours bursting and could do nothing to prevent death by haemorrhage. John Hunter's anatomical investigations, however, disclosed the phenomenon of anastomosis; that is, the process by which vessels compensated for the blocking of an artery by developing a route through minor vessels. Applying this insight to surgery he found that tying an artery leading to a vessel would eliminate the pressure of blood leading to an aneurism while the principle of anastomosis would enable the tissues formerly sustained to continue to obtain blood. The challenge therefore became to find ways of tying blood vessels to relieve patients suffering from aneurisms. Such tumours occurred more extensively in the nineteenth century than later, a consequence of the high incidence of venereal infection among men. The representative aneurism patient, John Lizars considered, was a man in his thirties. It most often attacked, as he put it, 'the irritable, the passionate, the gluttonous, the drunken, the debauched, the syphilitic, the mercurial and the rheumatic'.[14]

Operations for the cure of aneurism became feasible through the conjunction of anatomical enquiry and the boldness of surgeons who believed that the possible ought to be attempted. The quest entailed a series of progressively bolder operations, involving tying deeper and more critical vessels. New York surgeons led the way. In 1817 Wright Post succeeded in tying the subclavian artery and soon after Valentine Mott had tied the innominate artery, within a handspan of the heart. Medical periodicals and even popular newspapers reported the operations, anticipating the coverage of 'medical breakthroughs' of the following century. By the late 1820s, as Samuel Cooper put it, few external aneurisms remained 'beyond the reach of modern surgery'.[15] By the 1840s over twenty arteries could be ligated, most frequently the aorta, the popliteal (in the calf), the femoral (in the thigh), the inguinal (in the groin) the subclavian (near the collar-bone) and the carotid (in the neck). The result was not only the inflation of surgical reputations, but also the saving of lives and limbs which otherwise would have been lost. Medical journals carrying news of successful operations in one country excited the spirit of emulation in others. In 1832 in the distant colony of New South Wales William Bland, one of Sydney's most prominent surgeons, attempted to ligate a subclavian aneurism on William Mullen, a convict. Mullen, whose wife had paid Bland twenty pounds, died after eighteen days. Bland attempted a second operation in 1837, keeping the patient on the table for five-and-a-half hours.[16]

There were several distinct operations for aneurisms in various arteries each demanding different techniques. James Syme regarded locating the site of the operation as 'the principal nicety' because the artery had to be exposed 'just as in a careful dissection on the dead body'.[17] Few attempted the operation, and of them not all were justified in embarking upon it. Samuel Cooper regarded Robert Keate's ventures as 'objectionable'. Keates's aneurism operations, Cooper alleged, resembled 'a dive made with a needle ... attended with great danger of wounding and tying parts which should be left undisturbed'.[18] When planned and executed carefully though, wrote Charles Bell, it was a 'bloodless and simple operation'. Done well, students dispersed with a feeling of disappointment asking 'is this all?' Done badly, it became a tedious dissection, distressing to observe and exciting 'looks of enquiry and alarm' from onlookers.[19]

Rates of success varied depending on which artery was to be tied. John Arnott offered statistics in his 1843 Hunterian Oration, detailing 389 cases of which 277 – just over seventy per cent – had been 'cured'. Subclavian aneurisms had the highest mortality rate of 43%, while humeral the lowest at 20%.[20] If they survived the operation it was necessary to keep a patient immobile in bed for up to three months. The procedure demonstrated that surgery could prolong and enhance life without mutilating, a profound contrast to former practice.

'When the gut is mortified': hernia

The operation for hernia, like aneurism, was relatively uncommon despite the attention it received in medical journals and texts. The City of London Truss Society over the twenty years to 1830 issued trusses to almost fifty thousand out-patients, 21,000 of whom suffered from the inguinal hernia which most often became strangulated, or blocked. Only sixty-eight of these people, however, had undergone an operation.[21] Charles Bell succinctly described the operation for hernia as that recommended 'when the gut is mortified or burst'.[22] Seemingly straightforward when so robustly defined, in fact 'hernia' operations concealed a great range of conditions. The cure of hernia demanded, as Astley Cooper put it, 'a greater combination of accurate anatomical knowledge with surgical skill' than any other kind of operation.[23] To these he might have added good fortune.

Surgeons of the pre-Listerian period are reputed to have been reluctant to trespass on the abdominal cavity because of the danger of infection to which patients were exposed. Samuel Cooper regarded the abdomen as 'claim[ing] the particular notice of every practical surgeon'.[24] Paracentesis or 'tapping', although 'merely palliative', was a procedure widely employed to drain fluid from the abdomen in cases of 'dropsy'.[25] Using a 'trochar' a surgeon would make a triangular incision and 'tap' the swollen abdomen.[26] The trick was to select a site, marked with ink, which avoided the iliac artery. While abdominal wounds were regarded as usually – though not invariably – fatal, surgeons were prepared to enter the abdomen more often than has been supposed. George Guthrie, drawing on his Peninsular case notes, demonstrated in 1847 the feasibility of limited abdominal surgery in his *On Wounds and Injuries of the Abdomen and the Pelvis*.

There were as many techniques to treat hernia as there were places and types of stricture. Astley Cooper devoted an early influential text to the subject, one exemplifying his desire to combine a superb knowledge of anatomy with a difficult operation. Willingness to attempt hernia remained one of the tests of surgical boldness and skill. 'Mr Gower', in his 'Professional Reminiscences', declared that surgery in cases of hernia should be attempted only as a last resort and texts devoted much attention to preliminary alleviation.[27] Remedies to be attempted before resorting to the knife included the 'taxis' – that is, manipulating the patient to dislodge the obstruction, involving changes of posture, warm baths, massage and pressure and infusions of tobacco.[28] Small and recent blockages often proved susceptible to operating: paradoxically, precisely those most amenable to cure by the taxis. A hernia operation was no hurried matter. In essence, it involved dividing the skin and the integuments, dissecting down to the sac and opening it, removing the stricture and replacing the protruding viscera. 'Dissecting down' involved careful and often slow cutting, working through several layers of muscle, the fibres of each running in a different direction. It demanded a profound knowledge of the structures within the abdomen and a willingness to take the time to reach and deal with the internal problem. When things went well, Syme wrote, patients experienced immediate relief. 'The tormenting pain ... the sickness and the vomiting subside, the anxious expression of the countenance disappears'.[29]

The essential conundrum surrounding hernia was that such a hazardous and uncertain procedure imposed an obligation on a surgeon to attempt non-surgical remedy before venturing to cut. But leaving an operation too late could mean finding viscera slimy with gangrene. As a result, rates of mortality depended upon the timing as well as the execution of the operation. Undertaken at the right time, a surgeon might boast of a mortality rate of one in fifty. Operating after fruitlessly hoping that a stricture might come right by hot baths or injecting an infusion of tobacco water up the rectum might lead to three out of five patients dying. Unlucky surgeons with faulty judgement might lose patients in operations which – they found – they ought never have attempted. At the same time, those risking an 'immediate operation' might lose patients who might have been saved by recourse to less drastic treatments.[30] Even 'modern surgery' entailed hazard.

'Sometimes severe and fatal': amputation

In retrospect amputation remains the archetypal operation of the era of painful surgery: 'trite, though necessary', as a contributor to the *Edinburgh Medical and Surgical Journal* put it.[31] In that it was often the only recourse for many diseases and accidents, it was difficult for contemporaries to imagine a time when amputation could be entirely dispensed with.[32] In the meantime, surgeons learned the many ways in which limbs could be severed in order to save the body. Samuel Cooper observed, not entirely approvingly, that 'modern surgeons' felt 'completely fearless' about amputating 'well knowing that it mostly proves successful'.[33] It was also possible to perform an amputation badly, as the number of patients with 'sugar-loaf stumps' (with bone pressing against or protruding from the skin) testified. In amputating, Frederic Skey counselled, 'the most experienced are but students'.[34] Amputation, wrote Samuel Cooper, was an operation 'terrible to bear, dreadful to behold and sometimes severe and fatal'. [35] It was – or should have been – the surgeon's final resort.

In ill-informed retrospect these surgeons have been regarded as having been prepared to amputate if not indiscriminately at least without seeking first to save the limb. The view may be representative of the eighteenth century but it is not sustained by the evidence for the nineteenth. 'Modern surgeons' explicitly questioned this assumption. John Abernethy admonished his students that 'no surgeon has a right to lop off any part of a man's body but for the preservation of life.'[36] Indeed the conservative tendency of 'scientific surgery' is evident from the career of Benjamin Brodie. Soon after qualifying Brodie noticed in the treatment of diseases of the joints that 'different surgeons had different nostrums' which they applied 'as it happened, without any definite rules'. Over forty years of study and experiment Brodie put joint surgery upon a rational, scientific

Figure 3.1

Charles Bell's depiction of the stages in the amputation of the
arm at the shoulder from his _Illustrations of the Great Operations of Surgery_.
On the left the patient is 'determined and upright', on the right,
exhausted from the operation.

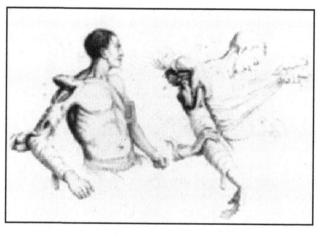

footing. The effect of the publication of 'Brodie on joints' was that,
as he proudly recalled, 'a great number of limbs are preserved which
would ... have been amputated as a matter of course'. Ironically
scientific surgery led to fewer as well as a wider range of operations
being performed.[37]

For such a common operation there was a multitude of minor
differences between surgeons and over time. In removing an arm, for
example, patients could be placed lying or sitting down. In removing
a leg the limb would usually be horizontal though Charles Bell
recommended holding it vertically. Removing an arm at the shoulder
demanded a particular facility for, as Charles Bell put it, 'the knife is
to be handled more like a sabre, than a surgeon's scalpel'.[38] Even
locating the 'place of election' for the incision was a decision
informed not only by clinical consideration (until the 1840s legs
were rarely removed at the ankle) but even by the patient's economic
circumstance. According to Everard Home 'a common man' unable
to afford an expensive artificial foot would be better off losing a leg
just below the knee.[39]

Amputation was rarely, as might be supposed (and as it often had
been earlier), a matter of making one simple cut. Although some

Figure 3.2

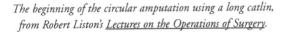

The beginning of the circular amputation using a long catlin,
from Robert Liston's Lectures on the Operations of Surgery.

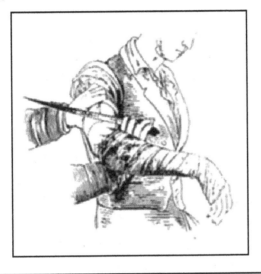

surgeons advocated making a sweeping incision around the circumference of the limb, the reality was more complex. Through the period the 'flap' operation gained ground against the 'circular' method. The essential difference between the two methods concerned the manner of making the initial incision. From the late-eighteenth century, even for the so-called circular method, surgeons had adopted the 'double' or 'triple' incision. This involved one incision through the skin, another deeper cut dividing the muscles covering the bone and often a third separating the flesh adhering to the bone. Each cut began slightly higher up the limb so that, in the case of an amputation at mid-thigh, the bone could be cut about three inches above the initial incision.

The flap operation began by 'transfixing' the limb – that is, pushing a knife through it, usually vertically downwards, before drawing the blade outwards, to pierce the skin from within. Transfixion, James Syme conceded, was 'a fearful looking and painful proceeding' and many recoiled from the idea of virtually stabbing a patient with a large amputation knife. The advocates of transfixion, however, argued that it actually subjected patients to less pain. Syme deployed evidence – unusually – from a patient. He cited a letter

Figure 3.3

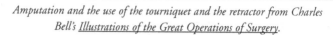

Amputation and the use of the tourniquet and the retractor from Charles Bell's <u>Illustrations of the Great Operations of Surgery</u>.

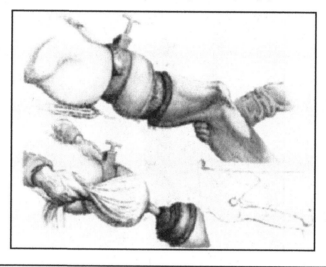

from the surgeon of a convict hospital hulk moored at Sheerness. The surgeon reported that a convict on whom he had operated using the circular method happened to see him amputate another limb using the flap method. The convict stopped the surgeon on deck and told him of his surprise. He had been 'struck with the rapidity of the process and the diminution of pain to the sufferer' and expressed regret at the 'unnecessary pain to which he had been subjected'.[40]

More than any other operation amputation required both strength and dexterity. Robert Liston advised his students to place themselves so as to 'command the limb' during the sawing.[41] The separation of the limb depended upon sawing, 'a duty of some delicacy', as Frederic Skey described it. He could saw through a femur in six double strokes of the instrument.[42] Sawing the bone required an assistant to 'draw up' the muscles, sometimes using their hands but usually by a piece of cloth called a retractor. This exposed the bone as high up the stump as possible in order to leave a large pad of muscle to form an adequate stump. Texts enjoined operators to saw cleanly; projecting fragments of bone – 'a very awkward circumstance' – would be nipped off with pliers.[43] The sawing of bone exposed the inherent tension of the act. Charles Bell gave the most succinct advice: 'saw slowly'.[44] Operators, he knew, were understandably anxious to get the sawing over with. Even those able to make 'bold, clean, and sweeping cuts', wrote William Gibson, became 'awkward and ungainly' with the saw. Nerves, undue haste or 'some booby of an assistant' could easily cause the saw to 'hitch and titter' in the groove.[45] Thomas Alcock once witnessed an amputation in which the saw became so tightly wedged in the bone that it could not be shifted.[46] Samuel Cooper believed that few surgeons did as well as would a 'plain carpenter' and William Gibson advised novices to practise sawing on wood. William Fergusson, like John Hunter, actually took up carpentry as a hobby.[47]

Having severed the limb the surgeon and his assistants would momentarily release the tourniquet to reveal the arteries to be taken up. In a mid-thigh amputation there would commonly be eleven to tie. They would be drawn out using a hook called a tenaculum, and secured by a ligature, usually by assistants. Differences over methods of closing wounds meant that some surgeons sutured the stump and bandaged it while others merely joined the flaps approximately. Dressing the wound with a piece of lint (usually wet), they closed the wound hours later after granulation had begun and the danger of haemorrhage within the stump had passed. Robert Druitt recommended waiting an hour or two: Syme perhaps six times that.

Disagreements over the efficacy of competing methods of amputation fuelled the most protracted and widespread controversy within the profession between, as James Gregory put it, 'Flappers and Anti-Flappers'. Writing in 1803, and as an accomplished disputant, he predicted accurately that the controversy 'can scarce be arrived at full maturity and violence'.[48] By the 1850s surgeons concerned with effectiveness rather than controversy resolved the issue by the adopting a hybrid operation involving amputation by flap with the circular division of muscles.[49] The controversy assumed such vehemence and prominence because experienced surgeons knew that a good proportion of amputated stumps did not in fact heal well and that it was not uncommon for amputees to require further operations to 'clean up' their stumps. Robert Liston described a man who submitted to his fourth such operation, unable to bear the pain of three badly performed operations, each of which sliced more from his arm. Liston dissected out nerves which the inept operations had imposed upon and left him more comfortable though still suffering from the pain of his 'phantom' limb. Liston (an advocate of the flap operation) argued that poor stumps were often the result of nerves being exposed and caught in ligatures (as had occurred with Nelson's arm). Correctly forming a flap which concealed the nerves deep within the wound was better, he said, than 'scooping and digging out the muscles' as surgeons were sometimes obliged to do when attempting a circular operation.[50] Liston thought it a pity that those who performed 'bungling and ill-devised operations' should not 'show a little more head'.

Encouraged by military and naval surgeons, by the 1820s bolder surgeons began to contemplate amputation at the hip. Charles Bell in 1821 could not approve of it and declined to describe it. Younger colleagues, however, embraced the challenge with several (such as James Syme) making their name by attempting it. William Sands Cox, notorious for heroic amputations, reassured his colleagues that it was 'by no means a difficult operation', although conceding that 'to the patient it is a very serious matter'.[51] Samuel Cooper, writing at the same time, disagreed, describing it as 'the most dreadful in surgery'.[52] Cox reported in 1831 that it had been ventured eighty-four times, but only successful twenty-six times. Amputation at the hip remained 'most formidable' because of the magnitude of the wound and the necessity of establishing exactly where to place and continue the incision. Nor was it a rapid procedure, requiring, as one of its pioneers wrote, 'expert and steady dissection'.[53] The claims of modernity must be balanced against reality. By the 1840s, William Fergusson claimed, it was 'frequently performed' but still only as a last resort. A survival rate of one patient in three he regarded as 'somewhat satisfactory'[54]

In a period notable for novel procedures, amputation remained a challenge for aspiring surgeons. George Guthrie by the 1840s had practised surgery for over forty years and performed or witnessed hundreds of amputations and had developed a shrewd awareness of the reality of amputation. Writing before the end of painful surgery, he wrote sarcastically that amputation had been 'deprived of all its terrors'. He found young surgeons anxious to perform the operation, the supreme test of boldness and dexterity. He compared their impetuosity to 'the fashion of the young lady pianistes, who do not consider themselves in any way advanced ... until they can play ... the Galop Chromatique of Listz [sic].[55]

'The business of taking a stone': lithotomy

Lithotomy – the removal of stones from the bladder – was an old operation, dating from the renaissance. A large number of people, from children to the aged, suffered from calcium deposits in the bladder, especially in England's eastern counties, from the chemical composition of their ground water. The great majority of lithotomy patients were male. Lithotomy in women was generally rarer and simpler (because the urethra was shorter) though 'the ingenious Dr Gooch' experimented by cutting into the bladder from the vagina.[56] Stones formed from calcium deposits in the bladder at first producing only 'uneasiness' but gradually bringing, as Benjamin Bell described it, 'the most afflicting scenes of distress'.[57] Lithotomy was such a painful and dangerous operation that it needed a powerful incentive to contemplate hazarding it. That spur was the unbearable pain imposed by bladder stones. A Gloucestershire man who submitted in 1835 had lived with constant, excruciating pain for months. Urinating was torture; he had not lain down for six weeks and could sit only with his chin on his knees. An agonising operation – in his case lasting exactly two minutes and fifteen seconds – offered a fair exchange for relief from such torment.[58] The operation to remove stones remained, as John Aitken put it, 'one of the most important' the surgeon could perform. It required not only a detailed command of anatomy but also 'a mind that never wavers, and a hand that never shakes'.[59] Samuel Cooper regarded it as the operation in which 'great awkwardness, mortifying failures, and dangerous blunders' were most clearly exposed. Surgeons who amputated, extirpated and tied aneurisms with eclat could not, he declared, 'get through the business of taking a stone'.[60]

Within each lithotomy operation, as Robert Druitt explained, 'there are an infinity of minute variations in the manner of performing it'.[61] There were, however, only two safe routes to enter the bladder; from directly above through the lower abdomen (the 'high operation') or through the perineum (the more usual 'lateral operation'). Both began by 'sounding' the stone; inserting a curved metal rod through the urethra to establish the existence and location. The sound struck the stone with a distinct 'clic'.[62]

The lateral operation – the 'English operation' – began by restraining the patient, often 'tied up' by the ankles and held by up to five assistants. John Lizars recommended securing them firmly – he had seen patients break loose more than once. The surgeon would then make an incision in the perineum, between three and five inches long in a grown man. The incision should be made, Charles Bell advised, 'slowly and deliberately'.[63] Dividing the prostate gland, the surgeon cut along the sound to enter the bladder taking great care to avoid damaging the surrounding tissues and arteries. Even so, by this stage he had encountered 'very large collections of blood'.[64] Using his fingers, a scoop or, more usually, forceps, he would extract one or

85

more stones, his actions, Astley Cooper urged, 'gradual rather than sudden'.[65] The stones could be any size but were often compared to pigeons' or hens' eggs. Some were smooth, other textured like mulberries: the rougher the texture and the larger the stone the more painful they were to extract sometimes requiring, as Benjamin Bell admitted, 'much violence'. Lying afterwards on his side, dressed with a piece of soft lint and with a drainage bristle protruding from the wound and a catheter in his penis, the patient would be exhausted by the short ordeal. A patient might sleep, 'easy and free from much pain', perhaps for the first time in months. A healthy boy's wound might heal in three weeks, that of a man in up to eight, with a protracted healing carrying the danger of sepsis and fistulous openings, leaving a patient incontinent. Though many lithotomies could be concluded within five or even three minutes even Astley Cooper and the elder Henry Cline had taken over an hour to remove large or oddly situated stones.

Lithotomy deserved its reputation. Experienced surgeons refused to perform it, some because success depended upon care – an error of a fraction of an inch could result in unstoppable haemorrhage. John Abernethy, notoriously off-hand with his patients, described it as 'a really horrible operation ... which one cannot undertake with *nonchalance*'.[66] Charles Bell usually refused to attempt it and regarded it as 'the most oppressive duty'.[67] Samuel Cooper decided that because of its 'extreme agony' and mortality it was 'a truly deplorable resource'.[68] It was possibly the most painful of all operations and involved great risks, of puncturing or severing arteries, as well as the routine dangers of shock and post-operative infection. For these reasons, lithotomies could not be hurried. Even so, it was so painful that surgeons sought to complete the operation as swiftly as possible. At worst, the neck of the bladder could be severed, one of the accidents 'most to be dreaded' advised James Syme. The patient felt incessant pain at the tip of the penis and continuous, insufferable nausea. Despite ineffectual remedies of hip baths, opiate injections and 'moderate depletion' he would inevitably die within a week.[69]

By the 1830s inventive operators had developed the techniques of lithoritry in which the stone could be ground to powder and lithotripsy which entailed crushing it. Both methods involved inserting a device into the urethra intended to break up the stone within the bladder. They entailed considerable discomfort not least in dilating the urethra to take the instrument and a danger of perforating the bladder. Few surgical authorities could resist jibes at the various lithotritic apparatus which Samuel Cooper hailed ironically as 'the greatest triumphs of modern surgery'.[70] An ingenious but complex tool, the instrument could be made to extend several arms able, with luck, to grasp the stone to allow a hand drill to bore into or crush it. Robert Druitt earnestly condemned it as responsible for 'many miserable and painful failures': witnessing a partially extended lithoritriptor dragged out of a urethra had taken the edge off his humour.[71] Those surviving the procedure – 'Sir', said one patient, 'you shall never put that three-pronged thing into me again' – were often left with fragments of stone in the bladder and sooner or later had to submit to lithotomy anyway.[72]

In many ways, except in the pain it inflicted, lithotomy contradicts many of the common assumptions about surgery. It demanded delicate rather than aggressive cutting, extracted foreign matter rather than resulted in the loss of a limb and probably was sought by rather than imposed on patients.

'A very terrible operation': excision

As surgeons developed greater anatomical knowledge and gained confidence they increasingly attempted the removal of tumours and the excision of diseased joints. The growing currency of excision is one of the clearest indications of the popular fallacy that surgeons entertained a mania for amputation. Careful surgeons, conscious of the trauma of amputation, its potential for infection and its disabling effects, sought less drastic operations. They reasoned that removing an elbow joint, say, enabled a patient to retain a limb even if the removal of the joint impeded the limb's strength and utility. By the mid-1820s excisions had become accepted and thereafter increasingly common. They appeared to be the neatest operations in a period supposedly dominated by crude operative techniques. While clearly taking longer than a 'clean' amputation they could still be completed swiftly: Syme could remove an elbow joint in fifteen minutes, including time dressing the wound.[73]

Excision became a symbol of progressive surgery. In 1829 Samuel Cooper had claimed that 'modern surgeons' would never amputate even an entire foot or hand when they saw a 'reasonable chance' of preserving a useful portion of it. Counsel such as this – carrying with it the imputation that those who amputated willy-nilly failed to live up to the ideal of modernity – itself persuaded many to reconsider their attitude to hitherto inevitable amputations.[74] This was possible because men such as Syme and Fergusson had attempted and propagated the excision of carious bone rather than countenance the amputation of limbs previously sacrificed. Conservative surgery made significant reductions in the proportion of amputations required. Frederic Skey (who became an assistant surgeon at Bart's in 1827) estimated that by 1850 they had declined there by a half.[75]

The single most common excision, however, was of tumours of the breast. This, James Latta conceded, was 'a very terrible operation, even when performed in the very best manner'.[76] The breast, James Syme wrote, was 'liable to so many diseases': 'indurations', 'Irritable Breast', milk abscesses, and half a dozen forms of tumour – vascular, sarcomatus, fibrous, cystic, carcnomatous and medullary.[77] Surgeons were well acquainted with the fact of breast diseases even if they were often perplexed as to how to treat them. Women suffering from tumours of the breast, as is apparent from John Brown's story of Allie, too often consulted a surgeon too late to have any hope of a cure. An 'improper delicacy', as Benjamin Bell wrote disapprovingly, probably cost thousands of women their lives. As with so many other conditions though surgeons could not always be certain of a growth's malignancy. 'Few questions in surgery have occasioned more discussion', Syme observed.[78] Some maintained that tumours remaining in an 'indolent, inoffensive state' could safely be left; others advocated their removal on detection for fear that by the time they were recognised as malignant surgery would be useless. Everard Home, having seen many cases end fatally, confessed that he had 'nearly lost all confidence in the operation'.[79]

The extirpation of a tumour could involve simply the dissection out of the tumour itself, or the removal of some or all of the affected breast. It entailed a long and bloody operation of 'slow and steady dissection'.[80] Careful dissection could take half an hour: Skey recalled one taking an hour and three quarters.[81] The particular horror of the amputation of a breast was that surgeons believed that they had to 'extirpate' every sign of what they believed to be malignant matter. In the course of doing so they had to take up many small arteries, making it one of the most protracted and bloody procedures: even the experienced Astley Cooper singled it out as 'a cruel operation'.[82]

Ovariotomy involved an excision performed within the abdominal cavity. Post-mortem dissection had disclosed the danger of ovarian tumours and, in the spirit of the age, surgeons resolved to try and extirpate them in order to save the lives of women afflicted. Ovariotomy long remained one of the most contentious operations. In 1832 a contributor to the *Lancet* commented on the few surgeons willing to venture such a risky procedure. He described twelve operations; three by Ephraim McDowell in Kentucky, four by John Lizars in Edinburgh and five in Germany. Of the twelve patients eight survived the operation; two because surgeons either found no tumour or decided not to remove it. The *Lancet's* reviewer decided that ovariotomy while 'dangerous' was 'not necessarily fatal'. Still, he thought that surgeons attempting it displayed 'more boldness than judgement'.[83] Liston – no stranger to daring new operations – condemned its advocates as 'belly rippers' on the grounds of the 'great incision' it demanded which he recognised as a source of sepsis.[84] Syme deprecated the operation arguing that at best 'for every life prolonged ... many must be sacrificed'.[85] On the eve of the introduction of chemical anaesthesia London surgeons still debated the propriety of the procedure (with Bransby Cooper in favour and William Lawrence cautioning prudence).[86] James Simpson, who as an obstetric physician often encountered such cases, published a pamphlet in 1846 – before the introduction of ether – in which he asked of ovariotomy *Is it - or is it not - an Operation Justifiable upon the Common Principles of Surgery?* He was in favour but only the boldest operators and the most desperate women agreed to attempt ovariotomy, a sign of the nexus between surgical possibility and the human instinct for survival.

'Clean, safe and simple': fistula

Rectal complaints were, then as now, painful and embarrassing. Some doctors, in an age when no artificial barrier could be interposed between patient and surgeon, declined to have anything to do with diseases of the rectum. Others, like Henry Smith of King's College Hospital, regarded haemorrhoids as 'a magnificent source of income'.[87] Anal surgery represented a relatively recent innovation and attracted its share of controversy and personal enmity. With characteristic lack of sympathy John Lizars considered rectal surgery 'ludicrous'. He and his rival James Syme might have agreed on this one point. Syme dismissed the operation to correct anal fistula as a 'slight incision', one that 'hardly deserves the serious title of an operation'.[88] The procedure had been a sore point between the two. In 1839 Lizars alleged that Syme had botched an operation to correct a fistula, claiming that he had 'groped about' in the patient's anus searching for a bleeding vessel. The surgeons' lawyers had enjoyed some sport claiming that medical authorities were divided into 'Pluggites' and 'Anti-Pluggites' and jesting about 'war *to the knife*' among the medical fraternity. Syme, who had sought damages of a thousand pounds, received fifty.[89]

Nevertheless, anal fistula was indeed a condition worthy of healing and some authorities regarded it as the one civil surgeons would most often face.[90] Fistulas – sinuses or passages in the rectum – imposed pain and humiliation on those afflicted. They were variously attributed to a combination of constipation and to the 'venereal virus'. Intensely painful, those afflicted dreaded defecation even going without food to avoid its pain, 'like a red hot iron in the anus' as the French surgeon Guillaume Dupuytren graphically put it. The operation for its correction was relatively straightforward. The patient stood, bending over a chair or table. The surgeon sat behind him, ready to insert an oiled finger into the rectum. After locating the sinus, he cut the tissue between it and the anus making a wound that, once healed, brought the sphincter under control again.[91] The operation exemplified the boon of modern surgery. Mr Buchanan, Surgeon to the Glasgow Royal Infirmary, extolled a new procedure among a discussion of his 'more interesting cases' for 1831. 'All is plain and open', he recorded, 'a filthy, dark, intricate and dangerous section, is at once converted into one that is clean, safe and simple'.[92]

The operation for anal fistula suggests the extent to which innovation in surgery was able to alleviate real suffering. It had not been attempted in 1790 and those afflicted were condemned to months and years of unrelieved discomfort and humiliation. Like other new operations –to correct aneurisms or to remove limbs more rapidly and safely – it was developments such as these that truly did demonstrate that surgery had developed and could relieve as well as impose suffering.

'Operating days': the incidence of surgery

Capital operations were performed relatively rarely. Once or twice a week the operating theatres of the great hospitals would be crowded with students and visitors as patients and surgeons composed themselves for the ordeal they would face together. Most large hospitals had a regular 'operating day', arranged so that students and visitors could take in operations at several hospitals each week. On these days a handful of procedures might be performed. While many surgeons undertook surgical and medical consultations privately each surgeon operated publicly infrequently. It is likely that younger surgeons were more willing to undertake more and newer operations than were their seniors. We will never know how many operations were performed not out of clinical necessity but out of a desire to establish a reputation. In 1834 Sir Anthony Carlisle decried the undue number of 'outrageously daring and hazardous operations' being performed by younger men. It is possible that the tempo of innovation had out-paced Carlisle's own surgical competence (acquired in the 1780s) but he believed that 'many violent men' were seeking 'notoriety by hazardous feats'.[93] Conversely, a review published in 1847 observed that older surgeons 'invariably become averse to operations'.[94] Liston's case books suggest that at his peak he performed two or three public capital operations a month. In the 1840s his rate declined to about one a month.[95] It is possible that he was undertaking more private consultations but also perhaps that the strain of operating had taken its toll.

Most hospitals published tables from time to time showing the operations performed by their surgical staff. The first annual report of James Syme's Edinburgh Surgical Hospital, Minto House, was published in the *Edinburgh Medical and Surgical Journal* in 1830.[96] Syme had seen 1,900 'cases' in his hospital's first year. Of these 265 were admitted and 95 had been operated upon. The operations to which they submitted included ten major amputations (all of legs) and nine minor, of fingers and toes. But Syme's list also included seven novel excisions, of elbows or knees, which obviated amputation, four excisions of scirrhous breasts (one of which could have been Allie's) and a daring excision of the upper jaw. He removed eleven tumours, performed four lithotomies, tied two aneurisms and relieved a strangulated hernia. James Syme was asserting his standing as a modern surgeon, able to conduct all the major operations at the forefront of surgical innovation. He also listed dozens of minor procedures including the relief of six cases of haemorrhoids, four anal fistulas, three nasal polyps and a cataract. At the age of just thirty, James Syme had demonstrated his competence as the complete modern surgeon.

Syme's report is both representative and exceptional. It is representative because it includes not only examples of most capital operations but also many minor procedures reflecting the variety of conditions now able to be treated. It is exceptional because it constituted a sort of advertisement to the profession of the number and range of operations undertaken by one of the foremost young Scottish surgeons. It was a manifesto of surgical prowess: a challenge to Syme's colleagues, an inspiration to his students and an incitement to his adversaries.

Notes

1. Lawrence, *St Bartholomew's Hospital Medical School, 1836-1837,* in CHAR/2, 286, PRO.

2. Benjamin Golding, *The Origin, Plan , and Operations of the Charing Cross Hospital* (London: W.H. Allen, 1867), 78.

3. David Hamilton, *The Healers: a History of Medicine in Scotland* (Edinburgh: Canongate, 1981), 147.

4. John Lizars, *A System of Practical Surgery* (Edinburgh: W.H. Lizars, 1838), 191.

5. James Syme, *Principles of Surgery* (Edinburgh: Sutherland & Knox, 1842), 496–97.

6. Lizars, *op. cit.* (note 4), 23.

7. 'The Physiology of the London Medical Student', *Punch,* 23 October 1841, 177.

8. J.G. Humble & Peter Hansell, *Westminster Hospital 1716–1966* (London: Pitman Medical, 1966), 48.

9. Samuel Cooper, *A Dictionary of Practical Surgery* (London: Longman, Hurst, Rees, Orme & Brown, 1829), 73 .

10. George Guthrie, *On the ... Operation for the Extraction of a Cataract* (London: W. Sams, 1834), 15.

11. William Fergusson, *A System of Practical Surgery* (London: John Churchill, 1846), 19.

12. Robert Liston, *Lectures on the Operations of Surgery* (Philadelphia: Lea & Blanchard, 1846), 19 .

13. Forbes Winslow, *Physic and Physicians: A Medical Sketch Book* (London: Longman, Orme, Brown, 1839), Vol. II, 362-63.

14. Lizars, *op. cit.* (note 4), 91.

15. Cooper, *op. cit.* (note 9), 125.

16. McIntosh, 'Surgery in Sydney in the 1830s', *Medical Journal of Australia,* June 1956, 998.

17. Syme, *op. cit.* (note 5), 105.

18. Cooper, *op. cit.* (note 9), 162.

19. Charles Bell, *Illustrations of the Great Operations of Surgery* (London: Longman, 1821), 79.

20. James Arnott, *The Hunterian Oration,* (London: J. Scott, 1843), 26.

21. George Macilwain, *Surgical Observations on the More Important Diseases of the Mucous Canals of the Body* (London: Longman, Rees, Orme, Brown & Longmans, 1830), table facing p. 1 .

22. Bell, *op. cit.* (note 19), 47.

23. Astley Cooper, *The Anatomy and Surgical Treatment of Abdominal Hernia* (London: Longman, Hurst, Rees, Orme & Brown, 1827),

vii.

24. Cooper, *op. cit.* (note 9), 1.

25. James Simpson, *Ovariaotomy Is It – or Is It Not – an Operation Justifiable upon the Common Principles of Surgery?* (Edinburgh: Sutherland & Knox, 1846), 4.

26. Benjamin Bell, *A System of Surgery*, 3 vols (Edinburgh: Bell & Bradfute, 1801), Vol. II, 339–48.

27. 'Mr Gower's Professional Reminiscences', *Lancet*, 1830–31, Vol. I, 39.

28. Syme, *op. cit.* (note 5), 312.

29. *Ibid.*, 318.

30. Cooper, *op. cit.* (note 9), 651.

31. 'Review of Mr Hammick's Practical Remarks on Amputation', *Edinburgh Medical & Surgical Journal*, 1830, Vol. 34, 186.

32. Fergusson, *op. cit.* (note 11), 161.

33. Cooper, *op. cit.* (note 9), 49.

34. Frederic Skey, *Operative Surgery* (London: John Churchill, 1850), 304.

35. Cooper, *op. cit.* (note 9), 49.

36. John Abernethy, *Lectures on Anatomy, Surgery and Pathology* (London: James Bullock, 1828), 307.

37. Benjamin Brodie, (C. Hawking, ed.), *Autobiography*, (London:. Longmans & Co., 1865), 98; 100.

38. Bell, *op.cit.* (note 19), 74.

39. 'Sir Everard Home's lectures', c. 1811, 'On Amputation', 1f.334, RCSEng.

40. 'Surgical observations', *Edinburgh Medical & Surgical Journal*, Vol. 27, 1827, 49.

41. *Lancet*, 1835–36, Vol. II, 135.

42. Skey, *op. cit.* (note 34), 318–19.

43. Robert Druitt, *The Principles and Practice of Modern Surgery* (Philadelphia: Lea & Blanchard, 1842, 500.

44. Bell, *op. cit.* (note 19), 62.

45. William Gibson, *Institutes and Practice of Surgery* (Philadelphia: J. Kay, Jnr & Brother, 1841), 504.

46. Thomas Alcock, 'An Essay on the Education and Duties of the General Practitioner in Medicine and Surgery' in *Transcations of the Associated Apothecaries and Surgeon Apothecaries of England and Wales* (London: the Society, 1823), 53.

47. Victor Plarr, *Lives of the Fellows of the Royal College of Surgeons*, 2 vols (London: Simpkin, Marshall Ltd, 1930), Vol. I, 399.

48. J. Gregory, *Additional Memorial to the Managers of the Royal*

Infirmary (Edinburgh: Murray & Cochrane, 1803), 414–15.

49. Skey, *op. cit.* (note 34), 317.

50. *Lancet,* 1835-36, Vol. II, 134–5.

51. William Sands Cox, *Maingault's Illustrations of the Different Amputations Performed on the Human Body* (London: Barlow, 1831), np.

52. Cooper, *op. cit.* (note 9), 1071.

53. James Veitch, *Observations on the Ligature of the Arteries* (London, 1824), 30.

54. Fergusson, *op. cit.* (note 11), 394.

55. George Guthrie, *Commentaries on the Surgery of the War in Portugal, Spain, France, and the Netherlands* (London: Renshaw, 1853), 70; 74.

56. Bell, *op. cit.* (note 26), Vol. II, 128–30.

57. *Ibid.,* Vol. II, 17.

58. *The Times,* 16 October 1835, 6b.

59. John Aitkin, *A Probationary Essay on Stone in the Bladder and Lithotomy* (Edinburgh: 1816), 2.

60. Cooper, *op. cit.* (note 9), 838.

61. Robert Druitt, *The Surgeon's Vade Mecum* (London: Henry Renshaw, John Churchill, 1851), 534.

62. Lizars, *op. cit.* (note 4), 224.

63. Charles Bell, *Institutes of Surgery,* 2 vols (Edinburgh: Longmans & Co., 1838) , Vol. II, 59.

64. Bell, *op. cit.* (note 26), Vol. II, 120.

65. Astley Cooper & Frederick Tyrrell, *The Lectures of Sir Astley Cooper, Bart.* ... (London: Thomas Tegg, 1824), Vol. II, 255.

66. Abernethy, *op. cit.* (note 36), 559–60 .

67. Bell, *op. cit.* (note 19), 116.

68. Cooper, *op. cit.* (note 9), ix.

69. Syme, *op. cit.* (note 5), 377–78.

70. Cooper, *op. cit.* (note 9), 819.

71. Druitt, *op. cit.* (note 43), 455–56.

72. *Lancet,* 1850, Vol. I, 734.

73. *Edinburgh Medical & Surgical Journal,* 1829, Vol. 31, 264–65.

74. Cooper, *op. cit.* (note 9), 105.

75. Skey, *op. cit.* (note 34), 304.

76. James Latta, *A Practical System of Surgery,* 3 vols (Edinburgh: G. Mudie, A. Guthrie & J. Fairbairn, 1795), 511.

77. Syme, *op. cit.* (note 5), 286.

78. *Ibid.,* 295.

79. 'Sir Everard Home's lectures', c. 1811, 1f.334, RCSEng.

80. Bell, *op. cit.* (note 26), Vol. II, 447.
81. Skey, *op. cit.* (note 34), 410.
82. *Lancet,* 1833–34, Vol., I, 137.
83. Review of John MacFarlane's *Clinical Reports of the Surgical Practice of the Glasgow Royal Infirmary, Lancet,* 1832-33, Vol. I, 17 .
84. Liston, *op. cit.* (note 12), 422–23.
85. Syme, *op. cit.* (note 5), 418–19.
86. *Lancet,* 1843–44, Vol. I, 549.
87. Plarr, *op. cit.* (note 47), Vol. II, 315.
88. Anon., *Remarks on a Treatise on the Rectum* (Edinburgh: Stevenson, [1852]), 2.
89. Macgregor, *A Full Report of the Jury Cause, Syme vs Lizars,* 3;15;23.
90. Thomas Castle (ed.), *A Manual of Modern Surgery* ... (London: E. Cox & Son, 1828), 128.
91. Bell, *op. cit.* (note 26), Vol. II, 297–98.
92. 'Report of a few of the more interesting cases treated in the Surgical Wards of the Glasgow Royal Infirmary', *Glasgow Medical Journal,* Vol. IV, No. XVI, 1831, 437.
93. Evidence of Anthony Carlisle to the Select Committee on Medical Education, PP 1834, Vol. XXXIV, 144.
94. *Edinburgh Medical & Surgical Journal,* 1847, Vol. 67, 305.
95. Liston's case books, University College Hospital, 1839-47, UCH/MR/1/25, /31, /39, /44, /61, UCA.
96. *Edinburgh Medical & Surgical Journal,* 1830, Vol. 34, 1–124.

4

'A hard set of butchers'?:
Wartime Surgery, 1793-1815

The death of John Hunter coincided with the outbreak of the great wars in 1793. Bransby Cooper, who himself became an army surgeon, reflected that the succeeding twenty-three years of more-or-less continual conflict had given surgeons 'ample opportunity' to investigate every kind of wound and injury and to devise and test new treatments.[1] Samuel Cooper, in a *Dictionary of Practical Surgery* replete with examples drawn from the wars, approvingly quoted Napoleon's surgeon, Dominique Larrey, who argued that the war had carried surgery to 'the highest pitch of perfection'.[2] While 'perfection' hardly seems a likely word to apply to the shambles of field hospitals and ships' cockpits in which Larrey and his counterparts operated, the connections between surgical innovation and war were substantial.

Surgeons were appointed to the military and naval forces of every combatant nation: more than had ever served before. The expansion of armies and navies itself stimulated the training of young men as surgeons and contributed, once the wars ended, to the 'overcrowding' of the profession which medical men so lamented. They included many men who were to become prominent in surgical practice and innovation in following decades: Samuel Cooper, Bransby Cooper, George Guthrie, Robert Knox and John Lizars. Even if they had not served in uniform, the arrival in Britain of large numbers of casualties after naval actions and of ship-loads of convalescent wounded soldiers gave civilian surgeons ample opportunities of developing their expertise. Charles Bell, establishing his position in London, made the most of the arrival of wounded evacuated from Corunna early in 1809. 'I am doing myself much good', he told his brother, George: 'being so much among the army surgeons', he was 'always in at the death'.[3]

'To stand forward with zeal': naval surgeons·

Britain's war against revolutionary France and then the Napoleonic empire at first pitted Britain's seapower against French dominance on land. The first decade of the struggle, the Revolutionary war, saw

97

Britain establish maritime superiority over France, a contest punctuated by a series of naval battles, all victorious. By 1814 Britain's was the largest and most powerful navy the world would see for a century. In 1814 it included over 90 ships of the line, 124 frigates and 76 sloops.[4] A qualified surgeon and perhaps several assistant surgeons were supposed to have been posted to each of these ships: smaller vessels did without, relying on cognate skills of the carpenter or sail-maker. In 1793 the Royal Navy included 500 surgeons, by 1814, 850.[5] Hundreds of young men, often imbued with notions of scientific surgery, joined during the wars. In 1808 two recently-qualified assistant surgeons aboard HMS *Gibraltar*, James Napper and Richard Speely, attracted odium when they dissected 'the *Hearts* of two Seamen lately deceased', keeping the organs in a bucket. 'The crew', their superior reported, 'is reported to be greatly exasperated', and the two young men were hastily transferred.[6]

Ships' surgeons shared cramped wardrooms with the lieutenants, Marine officers, the master, the purser and chaplain. John Lane, surgeon to HMS *Eagle*, described his quarters in verses written in Cork Harbour in 1797: 'A Cavern ... ne'er pierced by solar ray/ When Glimmering tapers only lend the day ....'[7] The surgeon, exercising a professional responsibility, was described as 'the most independent officer in the ship' but, like their fellows, they reacted against the tensions of close living and the demands of an exacting service.[8] Living in crowded proximity for months at a time imposed strains within wardrooms. Naval surgeons acquired a reputation as quarrelsome. Cases reported in *The Times* suggest something of their temper. William Kelly of the *Sparkler* was convicted of mutiny for striking the ship's clerk, saying that 'he did not care a d__n for the Lieutenant or his orders'. Mr Palmer of the sloop *Savage* was court-martialled for drunkeness and neglect of duty. Dismissed, he was allowed to serve as a surgeon's mate.[9] Surgeons were also regarded as drunken. James Gardner, who served as a lieutenant throughout the war, described 22 surgeons in his memoir. He approved of about half. His comments on some of the other half suggest the sources of shipboard strain: 'fractious little fellow'; 'drinks like a fish'; 'mad with drink'.[10] The statistics of actual courts martial, however, suggest a different conclusion. Despite the hundreds of men serving, between 1803-15 only 79 surgeons or assistant surgeons were convicted, only 16 for drunkenness and 13 for neglect of duty. The remainder breached conventions of 'gentlemanlike conduct' or the conventions of the service.[11]

The naval war involved both the constant patrolling of frigates and ships of the line in blockade and the occasional clash of great fleets. Each confronted the navy's surgeons with clinical challenges. Simply keeping a ship's company healthy demanded considerable vigilance and skill. For most of the time this was a medical rather than a surgical problem: battle only caused about one death in twenty.[12] Poor food, bad water, crowded mess-decks, damp and unremitting labour in all weathers made heavy demands on a surgeon. Just working the ship injured men routinely: one seaman in fifteen suffered from hernia.[13] Besides the accidents from slips and falls, hauling wet canvas whenever sail had to be made or taken in caused serious strains. 'Wounds and Hurts' certificates disclose the range of injuries seamen suffered: 'injury to the right testicle caused by a fall down a hatchway'; 'wound to the face sustained in a fall from the booms'; 'injury to the left leg caused when a rope broke on the main topgallant mast'.[14] Overwhelmingly, however, it was fevers, 'flux', ulcers and accidents which filled the sick bay.[15] Compared to army surgeons, naval surgeons confronted a wider range of surgical cases (including wounds and cuts but also burns and fractures) as well as a broader range of medical cases from tropical fever to frostbite.

The variety of naval practice gave its surgeons ample opportunity to ponder the effectiveness of established methods and to devise new techniques. It was a naval surgeon, James Veitch, who in 1804 introduced the small, fine gut ligatures which replaced the coarser threads hitherto used to stitch wounds.[16] David Fleming, surgeon of HMS *Tonnant*, performed the first successful ligation of the carotid artery in 1803. He saved the life of a rating named Mark Jackson who had attempted suicide by cutting his throat. Fleming acted without preparation as Jackson lay bleeding. Even more adventurous was the operation performed by Ralph Cuming at Antigua in 1808, when he amputated the entire arm, shoulderblade and collar-bone of a sailor smashed by a cannon ball. This daring and dangerous operation, attempted in tropical heat in the absence of a full set of instruments, represented a surgical triumph.[17]

The surgeon's duties were usually more prosaic, however. John Lane described the range of ailments and remedies he was called upon to treat aboard HMS *Eagle*:

> Pox, itch, scurvy and hot distempers vile
> Death's Grim Militia stand in rank and file

Unawed young Galen stands the hostile brunt
Pills in the rear and Cullen in the front[18]

Ordinary duty still demanded surgical skill. The case of Daniel
Leary of the frigate HMS *Circe* suggests something of the qualities
required. In 1797 Leary had been re-loading a gun during a drill. The
barrel exploded and Leary was thrown onto the deck with both arms
shattered and his head, face and chest shockingly scorched. 'So
hideous a spectacle' did Leary appear that all secretly hoped that
death would quickly end his suffering. The ship's surgeon, Robert
Dunn, then arrived. Undismayed he saw in Leary's plight 'something
... which induces the surgeon to stand forward with zeal'. Acting
swiftly while Leary lay in a swoon – and presumably on the open
deck – he removed the left hand. During this operation Leary
became conscious. His right arm, Dunn recorded, with the
ambivalence characteristic of the ambitious surgeon 'presented a
most awful prospect, and interested me much'. Dunn decided that
Leary must lose the arm at the shoulder, a rare and serious operation.
Leary, however, reacted with 'all the violence and obstinacy which
seamen exhibit' and refused to consent, declaring that he was
'content to die in the way he was'. At last, after appealing to the ship's
captain, the two compromised on an amputation at the forearm.
Throughout, Leary remained 'rational in his conversation',
maintaining a healthy interest in his well-being in opposition to the
surgeon's desire for professional renown. Two months after the
accident he was discharged from the naval hospital at Spithead
declared completely healed. The £20 pension he was granted would
not ensure his independence, however, and he obtained a job as a
'slopman' or storekeeper, able even without hands to move bundles
of clothing. 'Unsubdued' Leary declared that he would 'still receive
King's pay' and was 'thank God, hearty and well'.[19]

Battle remained the most severe test of a surgeon's skill. On
hearing the Marine drummers commanding the ship to 'clear for
action' the surgeon, his mates and the 'loblolly boys' who assisted
them in the cockpit, immediately began their own preparations.
They cleared the cockpit (in a ship of the line or frigate usually the
midshipmen's quarters) of unwanted furniture, setting up one or two
canvas-covered operating tables on some of the midshipmen's trunks.
In some ships surgeons distributed temporary tourniquets so that
wounded men might not bleed to death awaiting treatment. The
cockpit was located on the orlop deck, usually below the waterline. It
was dark – both because the gloom was relieved only by lanterns, and

Figure 4.1

This drawing, made in the 1820s, gives a good impression of the cramped and dark state of a warship's cockpit in battle. A 'loblolly boy' restrains the patient as a surgeon amputates. Like other artists reluctant to observe the operation too closely he has given the amputating knife a serrated blade.

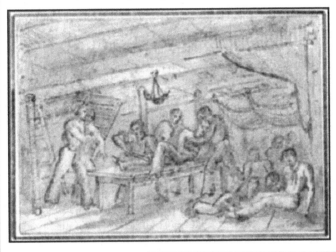

because the bulkheads and deck were often painted a dark red – for obvious reasons. Having readied their instruments, lanterns, and tubs to hold severed limbs, they stood and 'awaited the awful moment in anxious solicitude'.[20] John Bell, who did not serve at sea, imagined the feelings of naval surgeon as his ship sailed into battle cleared for action. Such a man he saw 'stands for a moment in his place alone, fixed and motionless, with folded hands, in horror and deep astonishment at the situation in which he finds himself'.[21]

One naval officer, George Jackson, recalled Evan Evans, the surgeon of his frigate HMS *Junon* as he appeared during a fight with French frigates in the West Indies in 1809: 'besmeared up to his shoulders with blood, ... plying his instruments with untiring energy and encouraging the sufferers with kind words'.[22] Jackson conjures up the nightmare of the orlop in battle, a sight we might prefer to turn from, except that the surgeon's work deserves a closer investigation.

The journals of several surgeons who saw action in sea battles suggest insights into the experience. Robert Young of HMS *Ardent* left a detailed account of the cases he treated during and after the battle of Camperdown, off the Dutch coast in October 1797.[23] Young had no qualified mate to assist him, only his loblolly boys. 'I was employed in operating and dressing till near four in the morning' he wrote, the action having opened at one the previous afternoon. He treated ninety wounded, who before long lay upon each other at the foot of the ladder, at least six with traumatic amputations from cannon balls carrying away limbs. At one point fifteen 'wretches' tumbled into the cockpit shockingly burned from an explosion. Young described the 'melancholy cries for assistance' he heard. He was obliged, he recalled, 'to preserve myself firm and collected' directing his attention to 'where the greatest and most essential services could be performed'. He reproved those who complained of painful but less pressing wounds and 'cheered and commended the patient fortitude of others'. Perhaps the greatest trial for Young was his inability to help some men. He described Joseph Broken who had his right leg taken off by a ball close to his pelvis, leaving 'a large and dreadful surface of mangled flesh'. Young was unable to apply a tourniquet, but Broken lived 'near two hours, perfectly sensible and incessantly calling out in a strong voice to me to assist him'. Sixteen died of their wounds including the *Ardent's* captain.

Likewise, George McGrath left a detailed record of the same action in HMS *Russel*.[24] Like most surgeons McGrath began his 'Physical and Surgical Journal' on that day with the most serious case, that of Henry Spence, who lost both legs to a ball striking his ankles. McGrath was obliged to amputate both of Spence's legs below the knee. Spence exhibited 'a trembling so sudden, so violent' that McGrath feared that he could not proceed. He at first thought it derived from fear as Spence stuttered, was 'much oppressed' and fainted. This alarm, McGrath wrote, 'attacks every Man ... wounded ... the brave as well as the cowardly'. Spence gathered his resolve and did not require an assistant to hold him as McGrath began operating. As he finished one leg a ball crashed through the bulkhead spraying splinters off the beams and rolling about the cockpit, injuring the 'women who formed the chief of my assistance'. Of his ship's 23 wounded, six were soon transferred to the naval hospital at Yarmouth and the rest were returned to duty within a couple of months.

The nightmare of sight and sound of the cockpits in which Robert Young and George McGrath worked cannot be diminished. At the same time, we must be careful not to exaggerate it. Surgeons' journals suggest a paradoxical conclusion. A ship's cockpit in battle was indeed a hideous place, crammed with bleeding and moaning men, buffeted by the sounds of the guns firing and recoiling overhead, with a surgeon working desperately in a feeble lantern light. But the surgical consequences of even a big sea battle were not necessarily as severe as the casualty returns might suggest. The surgeon's journal of the most famous ship in the most famous battle, the *Victory* at Trafalgar, suggests an intriguing interpretation.[25] William Beatty recorded 102 wounded aboard the *Victory* (a figure immediately suspect because it does not in fact include the ship's most famous casualty, Admiral Lord Nelson). Five men besides Nelson died of their wounds. Eleven of Beatty's patients underwent amputation, nine of the leg, two of the arm. But of the men crowding *Victory's* cockpit, 76 were 'cured on board', 59 within five weeks of the action. While *Victory's* cockpit was a horrible place to be, and while many men suffered wounds and burns, relatively few underwent amputation and most were relatively lightly wounded. Indeed, seven wounded with compound fractures did not undergo amputation, still regarded as the standard treatment.

The example of one brief but fierce single-ship action is illuminating. On 1 June 1813 the British frigate HMS *Shannon* defeated the United States frigate *Chesapeake* off Boston. The battle became one of the most celebrated of the war (notable because in most other frigate actions against the larger and more powerful American ships, British frigates did poorly). The journal of the *Shannon's* surgeon, Alexander Jack, names all those wounded and briefly describes their treatment. During the eleven-minute cannonade preceding the ships' collision about 160 projectiles struck the *Shannon* – one every four seconds. Sixty of the *Shannon's* men were wounded, two of whom died on board. Eighteen were discharged on board and forty went to hospital at Halifax. Jack amputated several limbs but mainly he applied simple dressings to wounds, allowed incised wounds to heal by first intention, poulticed splinter wounds and treated contusions with blood-letting and purging.

Perhaps because the fight ended with a chaotic boarding action, musket balls hit many of the wounded. The boatswain, Mr Stevens, sustained a grapeshot wound on the left forearm and a musket ball on the left side of the pelvis. Jack amputated his arm but Stevens died later in hospital. Splinters wounded fourteen men. Grapeshot – small balls fired by cannons in 'bunches', as the name suggests, at close range wounded ten men, most of them seriously. Blades – cutlasses or bayonets – wounded five men including the *Shannon's* captain, who lay dangerously wounded with a fractured skull. Men were also contused by flying wads (the fabric padding at the base of a cannon ball) and by objects, such as a gun-laying tool being driven into a man's body by the force of a ball. Some of these wounds presented Jack with serious and often insuperable surgical problems. Able Seaman John Robins, for instance, received a musket ball through the abdomen for which Jack could do nothing and he died two days later. Others taxed his skill, such as Corporal William Driscoll who had both knees fractured and cut down to the bone and both forearms contused and fractured. Jack brought the integuments above the knee together, reduced and splinted Driscoll's arms and administered opium. It is no surprise that surgeons complained of fatigue in the aftermath of action.[26]

Though casualties might be overlooked in the noise, smoke, darkness and confusion of the gun decks, men might reach the surgeon soon after being wounded. Men often reached the cockpit in what a naval surgeon described as 'the highest state of excitement'. 'Doctor,' a wounded midshipman exclaimed as he was carried down to have stump of his right arm dressed, 'I have lost one of my flippers'.[27] Alexander Hutchinson, surgeon of HMS *Terror* recalled an incident during a night action. A quartermaster (one of the warrant officers responsible for the ship's wheel) came crawling into the cockpit. 'Sir,' he said, 'I believe I am wounded'. He had been re-hoisting the ship's colours, which had been shot away when he felt 'something smartly strike the calf of my leg; and I felt my trowsers wet, which I suspect to be with blood'. In fact his thigh had been struck by a 24-pound ball, fracturing his leg.[28] The prevailing practice of attending to the wounded 'in rotation as they are brought down' meant that men sometimes bled to death awaiting their turn at the table.[29] Evan Evans of the *Junon* addressed the forty wounded he treated with 'N'am of goodness … bear with it a bit … I'll serve you in yer turn'.[30]

Hutchison had observed the reactions of sailors wounded in battle. 'The most severe wound,' he explained, 'is hardly felt at first'. He urged surgeons to operate before the 'smart terminating in agony'. This 'excitement of mind continues for some time,' he wrote, recalling the 'patriotic exultation' of men who 'under the knife, have joined in the shouts of victory'.[31] At Trafalgar Thomas Main of the *Leviathan* sang 'Rule Britannia' as his arm was amputated at the shoulder 'with great composure, smiling and with a steady clear voice'.[32] Characteristically John Lizars considered that men displayed a 'false courage' in the hope of deterring necessary surgery.[33] Those whom the surgeon reached after this initial numbness could become less compliant. John Adamson, surgeon of the *Raisonable* in 1805, recalled a sailor, Richard Beamsley, who had had his arm shot off at the elbow. Three hours later, when Beamsley at last reached the surgeon's table Adamson wanted to amputate to form a proper stump. Beamsley resisted 'with such determined obstinacy' that Adamson gave up and moved on to attend to other wounded.[34]

Perhaps the most telling evidence of the medical aftermath of a naval action comes from one of the most bloody but also paradoxically one of the least known; 'the memorable cannonading of Algiers' in August 1817, part of the navy's suppression of piratical threats to European commerce.[35] A British and Dutch fleet, under Admiral Lord Exmouth, bombarded the defences of the Dey of Algiers's capital, resolutely defended by gunboats and batteries protected by stone fortifications. While British casualties at Trafalgar were nine per cent of the ships' companies and eleven per cent at the Nile, at Algiers they amounted to sixteen per cent.[36] The casualties in the five ships of the line averaged about eighty, from fifteen in the *Albion* to 163 in the *Impregnable*. In the five frigates casualties ranged from fifteen in the *Hebrus* to 122 in the *Leander*, averaging fifty. The wounded reacted as they had throughout the long war at sea. In the frigate *Severn* one man, after losing a leg to a cannon ball, coolly removed his neckerchief and wrapped it about the stump before being carried to the cockpit. A witness described the scene in the cockpit of the *Leander* in a paper read to the Medical and Chirurgical Society. His stream-of-consciousness memoir carries an edge of post-traumatic shock: 'crowded to excess: without air; panting for breath; bathed in a most profuse perspiration ...' the surgeon 'unable to stand upright ... water! water! was the constant cry ....'[37] Characteristically, the ships' surgeons used their reports of their operations at Algiers to engage in the protracted debates animating the profession, arguing about the propriety of immediate or delayed amputation.

Naval surgeons clearly represented a range of age, temperament, experience, diligence and skill. The best of them matched the standard of civil and hospital surgery. Their contribution in maintaining sailors' health and in treating the effects of battle, disease, accidents and the hazards of the sea was at last recognised in a material form. In 1793 surgeons had been paid £5 a month, less than a lieutenant. By 1815 those of over ten years' service received £20, a little below the pay of a ship's captain.[38] The sailors' regard remained ambivalent. Though grateful for the surgeon's solicitude and skill, they also feared the exercise of that skill. 'You are a hard set of butchers' said Richard Dunn of the British frigate *Guerriere* after his leg had been amputated aboard the USS *Constitution* in 1812.[39]

'Active, humane, sensible and diligent': army surgeons

John Bell regarded the situation of a military surgeon as 'more important than any other'. Usually young men – nine out of ten army surgeons in 1798 had qualified after 1793 – they were responsible for the health of a regiment several hundred strong.[40] He cared for these men 'in the most perilous situations, in unhealthy climates, and in the midst of danger'.[41] The standing of the surgeon of a regiment depended upon the impression he made upon his commanding officer and fellow officers. As a novice he 'wanders about, acknowledged by none, ... not wanted by any until the time of actual battle'.[42] Then, provided he made good, he could have been 'caressed, flattered, and almost idolised'.[43] A good surgeon – 'active, humane, sensible and diligent' – could save or ease many lives.[44]

The army's expansion from 1793 drew into it a large number of men of all degrees of skill and experience. Some, like James M'Grigor who became Wellington's senior medical officer, obtained an appointment although formally unqualified. Others had gained the Licentiate of the Society of Apothecaries or were members of the Company (from 1800 the Royal College) of Surgeons. Vacancies were filled speedily. 'Placards were posted on the college gates', James M'Grigor recalled, 'offering commissions to such as could pass some kind of examination'.[45] Military service, John Bell wrote, attracted 'the young, the needy, the adventurous', drawn by 'pay, and perquisites, and pensions'.[46]

Wartime expansion brought into the army men who would otherwise never have donned the King's uniform – both in the ranks and among officers, honorary and otherwise. Many were evidently neither gentlemen nor equal to their professional responsibilities. George Guthrie disgustedly claimed that of thirty hospital mates – assistant surgeons – he had met twenty 'fit only to dispense Medicines'.[47] John Bell, observing the young men hastily appointed at the height of the struggle against Revolutionary France, described them as 'yet boys of fifteen or seventeen'.[48] Imperfectly integrated into the army's disciplinary mechanism – surgeons were honorary officers only – they were often regarded as unruly. Like their naval counterparts army surgeons also appeared before courts martial but the incidence appears to have been less, probably because they were not cooped so closely together. Still, assistant surgeons were regarded as 'puppies', 'idle and ignorant'.[49] Surgeons were, however, also part of the apparatus of discipline. Both naval and military surgeons were obliged to oversee floggings and treat those punished, confronting many with a professional and ethical dilemma. Their complicity in the system is suggested by an anecdote of George Ballingall's. He recalled a colonel known as a notorious flogger who had often asked Ballingall to find a medical reason to halt a flogging, something he could not do himself for fear of diminishing his authority. Whether they approved or not, surgeons treated flogged men. Ballingall recommended that men's backs be washed with a solution of lead acetate, while in India and the West Indies the leaf of the plantain tree soothed the gashes of the cat.[50]

Although British troops saw action from Buenos Aires to Java and from the Baltic to Mauritius, from 1808 the focus of Britain's war became Portugal and Spain – the Peninsula. An ill-advised novice might arrive in Portugal with little more than a small case of instruments and his valise. A well-provided man, by contrast, came equipped with the wherewithal to operate independently of an often rudimentary army medical system. John Hennen, a surgeon in the Peninsula and at Waterloo, described in his *Principles of Military Surgery* the 'field panniers' – wooden or wicker boxes containing instruments, dressings and drugs, and carried on horses or mules. As well as the instruments surgeons would ordinarily buy themselves, he reminded them to bring a 'good strop to touch them when blunted'. Travelling and often working in all weathers, he advised wrapping them in lint or bibulous paper, to dust them with absorbent powder and smear with oil to maintain an edge. In case of encountering men in need when separated from his panniers, Hennen recommended carrying a pocket case of basic instruments – scalpels, probes, scissors and needles – and a canteen of wine. Thus equipped an army surgeon would be prepared – physically at least – for the work he would do in the aftermath of battle.[51]

'Worthy friends': the army medical system

The Military Adventures of Johnny Newcome, a sprawling verse tragi-comic epic of the British army in the Peninsular war, offers a sustained analogy of Wellington's army as a vast estate, the workers and chattels of 'Farmer George' the King. In this clumsy pastoral the generals become 'shepherds', the soldiers their 'flock', the cavalry the farmer's 'stud' and, of course, the surgeons the 'butchers'.[52] Johnny Newcome's regard for the surgeons remained ambivalent, 'skilful as they extract, and Bleed and Cup,/ I hope my worthy friends won't cut me up.'

By the time the Peninsular campaigns began Johnny Newcome's 'worthy friends' had learned their business in a hard school. During the war's early campaigns, in the Netherlands and in the West Indies, the system broke down as often as not. These early campaigns disastrously demonstrated the 'striking ... want of system' that cost men's lives and broke their health and hearts.[53] 'We had little knowledge of hospital economy' James Fergusson, an army surgeon, admitted.[54] Almost exactly half of the 100,000 British soldiers or sailors who served in the West Indies died of illness there; many before they had seen a Frenchman, some before they disembarked from the transports.[55] Despite John Hunter's exertions (he had been an army surgeon in the Seven Years' War and became Surgeon General for the last three years of his life) the system was cumbersome and ineffective. The Army Medical Board was constrained, unable to control regimental hospitals, unable to appoint hospital staff, beholden to the Purveyor General for bedding and to the Apothecary General for medicines and dressings.[56] Not until the first several years of the Peninsular war was it made to work, much of the credit for which belongs to James M'Grigor.

The core of the army medical system was the surgeon and assistant surgeons nominally part of every regiment (that is, the fundamental fighting unit, in practice about 500 men strong). As in the navy regimental surgeons attended to their men's health, treating many more for disease than wounds. They treated the sick and the lightly wounded themselves but passed serious cases to intermediate 'marching' or field hospitals and 'general' hospitals, each staffed by surgeons of the Medical Department. Regimental hospitals were often 'brigaded' with those of adjoining units because capital operations required several surgeons. The system depended heavily upon the energy, skill and commitment of individual medical officers. Non-combatants, and poorly regarded by a society valuing the martial over its medical consequences, surgeons were rarely able to influence commanders' plans or actions. When M'Grigor once presumed to change the route of a column for the convenience of his wounded, Wellington rounded upon him with an enraged 'Who is to command the army? I or You?'[57]

Casualties often overwhelmed hospitals and surgeons. Commissariat and transport officers regarded medical supplies and comforts as less important and bureaucratic muddle and lethargy were never eliminated. Although confusion, waste and indifference continued and contributed to great and often needless suffering, it would be misleading to represent the army medical system after 1812 as the same as that prevailing in the war's early years. Wellington, who was persuaded that medical efficiency contributed to the strength of the army, supported M'Grigor's changes and reforms in the medical care provided to his men. M'Grigor weeded out the irresponsible and ineffective, exhorted the lazy, and inspired a body of surgeons who by 1814 included Europe's most experienced: William Jones of the 95th Rifles served in thirteen battles; John Gunning in eleven.[58] M'Grigor described them as 'a body of operators such as never were excelled'.[59] He established and inspected hospitals and convalescent depots. He compelled surgeons to carry a 'field Pharmacopiae' in panniers containing a month's worth of drugs. He ensured that medical depots conformed to the standards of cleanliness and regularity that existing manuals stressed but that the realities of war had so often confounded. By the time Wellington advanced across the French frontier in 1814 the army's medical system had reached, so Guthrie said, according to the expectations of the time, a 'peak of perfection'.[60]

M'Grigor made an unpromising arrangement work as the saga of the carts suggests. Divisions were supposed to be supplied with 'spring wagons' in which to evacuate wounded but there were never enough and many were transported in primitive ox carts, the jolting of which grated bones and caused many to wish themselves dead. Wellington denied M'Grigor ambulances like the French and would have 'no vehicles ... but for the conveyance of guns' but regimental surgeons and even colonels, abetted by M'Grigor, covertly subverted this intention by obtaining ox carts and even spring wagons.[61] Dependant upon the good grace of the commissariat officers in charge of wagons, arrangements for the carriage of wounded remained 'deficient and cruel' and many wounded made their own way to the surgeons, but M'Grigor's initiative and the energy of his subordinate surgeons made the system workable.[62] Late in 1812 the spring wagons of the Royal Waggon Train were detailed exclusively to the carriage of sick and wounded.[63] On the 'commissariat line' which Wellington insisted the army follow, they carried casualties along the evacuation route slowly and painfully but still more efficiently than any other army hitherto.

The French medical system has been regarded as superior in some respects. Its *Service de Santé* provided permanent orderlies for military hospitals while the 'flying ambulances' introduced by Dominique Larrey encouraged soldiers that they would be transported swiftly and reasonably comfortably to medical aid.[64] On the whole, however, French medical services were in fact inferior. There were few ambulances; the *compagnies d'infirmiers d'hôpitaux* were as untrained and uncommitted as British orderlies; the rudimentary supply system was rarely coordinated with the medical and in distant theatres – such as Spain – medical arrangements often broke down.[65] In a country in which guerrillas ruled all but the immediate vicinity of a French army, wounded often suffered at their hands. In spite of Larrey's individual genius French surgeons were generally less skilful than their British counterparts: the demand was so great that some young men treated casualties with only a few months' training.* A British surgeon was appalled at the condition of French wounded after Orthes finding their condition 'deplorable', with small wounds 'foul and sloughing' and 'sugar loaf' stumps requiring re-amputation.[66] A hospital mate described the French method of amputation as disgraceful: 'they cut them like a round of beef' he complained.[67]

The modest scale of the Peninsular war and the secure maritime base Wellington's army enjoyed gave British forces an advantage denied their enemies. The great campaigns of central Europe which decided French defeat presented not only the largest battles Europe was to see for a century but also the most horrific casualties. Apart from battles such as Albuhera when the 26-year-old George Guthrie became responsible for three thousand wounded, British surgeons were spared casualties on this scale. One consequence was that Britain was able to create a military system more economical and effective than that of any other combatant power.[68] Although surgeons were at times reduced to tearing their own shirts for bandages and tearing their hair in frustration at the laborious workings of the commissariat system, by the war's last years they were providing better medical care than any army had ever seen. Under M'Grigor's urging and example the Peninsular surgeons, experienced, purged of ineffective men and confident of their abilities, were able

---

* Larrey served in sixty battles, from Egypt to Waterloo (where he was saved from execution by the intercession of a Prussian surgeon) but his achievements should not be unduly magnified. It is often said that he amputated two hundred limbs in twenty-four hours after Borodino. The claim derives from a careless reading of his memoirs. This comes out at an average of one every eight minutes, including time for selecting, diagnosing and operating, with no allowance for refreshment, rest, or for difficult cases. In fact, he claimed no more than that the operations were performed 'under his own observation, and even under his own direction', presumably by an unknown number of subordinates. Charles Bell - who at least might have conceded Larrey's record of operating under fire - sniffed that his cases 'do not go to the point' and that his operations were 'ill-performed'.

110

Figure 4.2

George James Guthrie (1785-1856), depicted about 1840,
who founded a civil career on the knowledge and skills gained in
surgery on the battlefields of the Peninsula.
Guthrie's pose suggests something of the self-possession that
enabled him to meet the challenges of surgery.

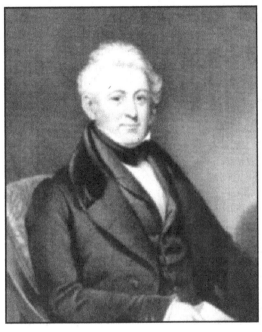

to keep Wellington's army in a condition for victory. During the final
Pyreneean campaign Wellington's army marched and fought for
twenty days and at the end, George Ballingall proudly wrote,
'mustered within thirty men as strong as before the action'.[69]
Acknowledging this achievement is not to deny the inherent horror
of the medical treatment necessarily available.

'Essential things only': treating war casualties

The most significant difference between service and civilian surgery
was, of course, that as well as having to deal with accidents and
disease, war surgeons periodically confronted large numbers of
wounded. On land and sea men were struck by musket balls and

roundshot fired from cannon. At sea men were burned and gashed by splinters sprayed when balls struck ships' timbers. All three types of projectile left ghastly wounds. Balls crushed and mutilated when they did not kill and concussed or killed even when passing close by. Roundshot striking the wood of ships sent long splinters flying. Splinter wounds, some long, large and deep, presented naval surgeons with an operating problem peculiar to themselves and one barely addressed by conventional texts. Usually formed along the grain of the wood, the individual fibres acted as barbs, making a splinter almost impossible to extract from the direction of entry and obliging the surgeon to cut it out often by a long incision. A peculiarity of ships made of mahogany in India (as were many ships on the East Indian station) was that splinter wounds inflicted by them invariably suppurated.[70] Naval surgeons also faced flash burns more often than their military counterparts.

Land warfare also inflicted its own peculiar wounds. Musket wounds were more common and wounds from cannon or grapeshot less so. Even so, grapeshot caused gashes and fractures. Wellington decried the newly-introduced shrapnel shells, complaining that they caused 'trifling' wounds and 'kill nobody'.[71] Wounds from swords and especially bayonets were, contrary to popular belief, infrequent: men facing charging opponents wielding sharp steel more often broke and ran than face them and fight hand-to-hand. Musket balls, made of soft lead travelling at low velocity, ripped flesh and shattered bone. Reports of the sensation of their impact varied. Some described the feeling as 'inconsiderable'; others as a 'dead, heavy, painful blow'.[72] Still others described the feeling as resembling 'a smart blow from a supple cane' or having a red hot wire pass through.[73]

Surgeons confronted the need to treat dozens – perhaps hundreds – of serious wounds within a short time. The response, as Charles Bell put it, was that in the field 'essential things only can be attended to'.[74] War experience taught surgeons who were able to last to distinguish the important from the unimportant. While individual army surgeons adopted their own procedures, treatment was generally a matter of 'first come, first served'.[75] As at sea, men with more serious wounds could die awaiting their turn.

The improvised hospitals of the war on land conjure up the most harrowing scenes of military surgery. Lieutenant William Grattan of the 88th Connaught Rangers offered the most frank description.[76] In May 1811, two days after the battle of Fuentes d'Onoro, he made his way to the village of Villa Formosa looking for a fellow officer. He found his friend wounded through the chest by a musket ball. The divisional surgeons had bled him copiously, three and four times a day despite which, miraculously, he recovered. Leaving the house Grattan noticed 'bustle' and 'half-stifled moaning' in the yard of a nearby house. Peering through the gate, he saw in the yard some two hundred wounded waiting to be treated. Wounded two days before, their drawn sun-burned faces were marked with dried blood which, with their fixed expressions, gave them a glazed, copper-coloured hue resembling bronzed statues. Some resigned and patient, others feebly asking for water, they awaited their turn to be carried to the surgeons. Curious rather than repelled, Grattan found the surgeons at their improvised tables. Stripped to the waist and bloody, they worked on men placed on doors wrenched off hinges and laid over barrels. The arms and legs they had removed earlier lay in heaps about the courtyard, and the ground around the tables was dyed red. Grattan arrived just as John Bell was about to amputate at the thigh the leg of a soldier of the 50th Foot. The surgeon asked Grattan to assist by holding the man down. As Grattan moved to comply, Bell pulled almonds from his pocket and offered to share them with Grattan. Though 'one of the best-hearted men' Grattan had met Bell seemed 'insensible' to the horror about him. The operation, 'the most shocking sight I ever witnessed', lasted nearly half an hour. Grattan made his excuses and left. 'This was my first and last visit to an amputating hospital' he declared. It is worth recalling that in terms of the ratio of wounded-to-surgeons Fuentes d'Onoro comes out as one of the lowest in the league table of Peninsular battles.

The surgeon's first duty, Robert Druitt advised, was to 'comfort' the patient, to 'explain to him the nature of his loss [and] to assure him of his safety'.[77] This was vital because, as Thomas Chevalier explained in a text carried by many army surgeons through the Peninsular war, 'the state of a patient's mind, and often of his body, at the moment a Gun-shot wound is inflicted, are generally the very worst that could possibly exist'.[78] We might imagine that just as soldiers entered battle under military discipline to face wounds and death, they remained under military discipline after being wounded. George Macleod claimed that the military surgeon's advantages included a freedom from the 'ill-judged kindness of relatives' and the 'headstrong wilfulness' of his patients.[79] But the surgeon's authority over their patients' treatment was more medical than military. Soldiers – who would rarely have had the reasons for procedures explained to them – understandably viewed medical treatment as 'experiments upon his fortitude'. They believed that surgeons would habitually "lop off" limbs in cart-loads.[80] It was commonly believed around camp-fires that surgeons were paid a bonus of £5 for each limb they amputated 'whether the patient lived or died'.[81]

Military patients did not meekly submit. Though there is no question that surgeons remained the more powerful half of the relationship it was possible for patients to take control of their treatment, or at least negotiate it, in ways that helped them to retain a measure of autonomy. In 1810 Lieutenant Harry Smith haggled with his surgeons before agreeing to have them cut a ball from his Achilles tendon. Having accepted the need, he 'cocked up' his leg saying 'There it is; slash away'. The jagged ball was 'half dissected and half torn out' after five minutes.[82] As an officer, Harry Smith might have been be expected to be assertive. The experience of a bugler, William Green of the 95th Rifles, illustrates the negotiation possible among all but badly wounded men.[83] Green had been wounded in the night-time storming of the fortress of Badajoz in April 1812. A ball passed through his thigh and lodged in his wrist. Bandsmen carried him on a stretcher to the surgeons' tents where a doctor treated him 'with his coat off, a pair of blue sleeves on, and a blue apron'. The tent was full of men more seriously wounded, 'an awful sight to see', and Green was hastily passed to the rear. A few days later the ball was extracted looking 'more like a soldier's three-cocked hat than a musket ball'. Green, with a swollen, painful wrist, begged for amputation: 'Do, sir, if you please, take my hand off'. This the surgeon undertook to do. While a nurse was dressing the wrist, however, a piece of bone came away relieving the pain and swelling. Overnight some fellow patients urged him 'Have it cut off' while others advised 'Let it be on'. Green decided to keep the hand, to the surgeon's annoyance because he had arranged for assistants to be present. A further 29 fragments of bone were taken out over the following eighteen months before the wound finally healed.

Surgeons became increasingly reluctant to amputate, so much so that they found themselves at odds with their patients. Alexander Hutchison, who had served at the naval hospital at Deal, observed that men were not only 'anxious to undergo an operation when they find it inevitable' but found that men 'frequently press it before the proper time'.[84] The trend is reflected in Corporal Wheeler's account of his treatment after being wounded in both ankles during the battle of Nivelle. After lying in general hospitals for nearly six months surgeons found one of his wounds to be 'sluffed' and he was moved into the 'incurable ward' of the General Hospital at Fuentarrabia. Surrounded by 'dreadful sufferings ... beyond description' he 'joyfully agreed' to lose his leg and was twice carried to the operating room.

Each time, though, surgeons deferred operating to try yet another remedy. Finally a 'little Spanish Doctor' sprinkled 'some thing like pepper and salt mixed' on the wound. It changed from 'a nasty sickly whitebrown' to a healthy red. Wheeler lived to serve again but he did not forget 'the agony of the dying, their prayers, their despair and the horrid oaths' he had heard in 'this house of misery'.[85]

The decision to operate, and especially whether to amputate, was not always taken as a matter of course. Rutherford Alcock, who served as a surgeon with the British Legion in the Carlist war fifteen years later, reflected on the reactions of soldiers under his care. Their reluctance to consent to amputation was not grounded in fear of the operation itself but on the fear that they would not receive a pension for the resultant disability. Alcock had seen men move through several emotions as they awaited the outcome of treatment and especially those whose septic or otherwise intractable wounds required surgery. Men resisted the suggestion that they should undergo amputation; 'What, lose my leg, Sir?' men had asked, 'Oh, no – no. .... What is to become of my wife and children? ... I can't – I won't ....' Alcock saw how 'a feeling of despondency, near akin to despair' could overwhelm a man. He would express 'regret and anger', anticipating a 'long vista of misery ... ending at best in a workhouse'. Then, accepting the reality of his situation, he might say 'Oh I know, Sir, my leg cannot be saved ... I wish it had been off at first ... the sooner the better.'[86]

By 1814 military surgeons had developed and advocated many notions that were to influence surgery generally. Perhaps the most striking illustration of the change through which British military medicine passed in the course of the war is that the rate of amputation declined drastically. After Toulouse, the final battle in 1814, fewer than one in twelve of the 1,200 British wounded underwent amputation and not one was lost to gangrene in hospital.[87] It is nevertheless important to remember, as an officer recalled, the 'agony and torment and shrieks' of the thousands of wounded 'scattered over miles of ground' and that 'hundreds' died before reaching the surgeons.[88] Still, the British wounded at Toulouse arguably fared better than any battle in history hitherto. As a scientific surgeon George Guthrie naturally sought verification by repetition, by experiment. The war's end dismayed him and he foolishly expressed in print his 'regret that we had not another battle ... to enable me to decide on two or three points in surgery which were doubtful'. Packing up his instruments and his voluminous case notes he returned to England and his beloved family, embarking on

Figure 4.3

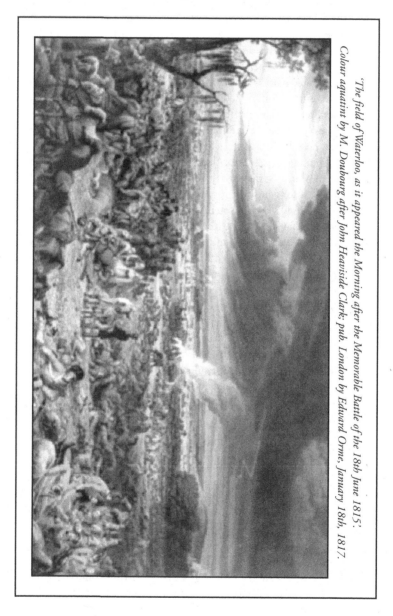

'The field of Waterloo, as it appeared the Morning after the Memorable Battle of the 18th June 1815'. Colour aquatint by M. Dubourg after John Heaviside Clark; pub. London by Edward Orme, January 18th, 1817.

a civil career in surgery. His less fervent colleagues called him an 'enthusiast' and laughed at him. In the summer of 1815, however, the battle of Waterloo afforded the desired opportunity'.[89]

'Bloody and desperate': surgeons at Waterloo

When news of the victory at Waterloo reached London four days after the battle an excited Charles Bell wrote to his brother-in-law, also a surgeon: 'Johnnie! how can we let this pass?' The wounded of Waterloo represented 'an occasion of seeing gun-shot wounds come to our very door'.[90] Bell was not alone in his enthusiasm. A dozen or more civilian surgeons and students travelled to Brussels including George Guthrie, now a civilian, arriving as 'an amateur'.[91]

If the British army of the Peninsula had learned and applied hard lessons under M'Grigor those achievements had swiftly come undone without his presence. Virtually unqualified despite his rise, he had gone on half-pay to study at the Windmill Street School to become a member of the Royal College of Surgeons, albeit belatedly. Although Wellington's army in Belgium inherited some of the legacies of the Peninsula, including some veteran senior medical officers, it was in other ways deficient. The most experienced of Wellington's Peninsular army had been transported across the Atlantic to conclude the war against the United States. Many of the troops who fought at Waterloo were inexperienced, as were many of their 270 surgeons.

A participant described the 'terrible sameness' of Waterloo, a battle of 'fierce and incessant onsets'.[92] During a long summer afternoon on 18 June 1815 Napoleon launched a succession of assaults at Wellington's British, German, Dutch and Belgian force occupying a low ridge astride the road to Brussels. Lieutenant Edward Wheatley recorded his impression of the battle in his journal. It was a kaleidoscope of 'charge after charge'. Wheatley described 'the clashing of swords, the clattering of musketry, the hissing of balls and shouts and clamours'. The noise, 'jarring and confounding the senses, [sounded] as if hell and the devil were in evil contention.'[93] Each French attack was narrowly held, with the dead marking the squares in which the British infantry stood. The victory was to become a defining moment for Britons for a century, 'an event sufficiently unique to mark the age we live in' George Ballingall later told students too young to remember the wars.[94] Those who survived took a more jaundiced view: 'are you not tired of battles?' asked a Scots officer in a letter home.[95]

The task confronting the surgeons of the British and allied forces on the field was massive and mournful. Nearly 40,000 men lay dead or wounded in an area little larger than a couple of square miles. Many remained there without aid for days – some accounts claimed up to a fortnight.[96] Some of the moribund, expected to die, John Thomson was told, 'were left to their wretched fate to die where they fell'.[97] Thousands of corpses and the carcasses of horses festered in the heat before being respectively buried in huge pits or burned. A former soldier who set out to see the battlefield four days later turned back 'sick in the stomach'.[98] For days many wounded lay in cottages and barns about the field in 'hideously bad' accommodation.[99] Eventually, the British, their allies and finally the French were brought into Brussels. Its people, including 'prodigious crowds of females' turned out to assist those arriving in the city's streets and squares.[100] Gradually they were dispersed to houses, convents, barns and fortresses around Brussels and even as far as Antwerp.

The surgeons' work was, as John James wrote, 'grim in the extreme'.[101] Isaac James wrote to his brother Richard eleven days after the battle, telling how the fighting had been 'bloody and desperate' and James had been 'extremely fatigued' with so many wounded to attend. Like other surgeons he had not slept for the three nights after the battle: 'We have had lots of legs and arms to lop off'.[102] James Elkington recorded that by 9 on the morning of the 21st he had sent every wounded man of his regiment to Brussels.[103] Most of Wellington's surgeons followed his army on its victorious advance into France: it was a mercy that surgeons and medical students arrived from Britain within a week. Charles Bell's letters had so excited him that Sir Walter Scott determined to see the field for himself and almost a month after the battle Scott wrote to encourage a medical friend to volunteer: 'I understand surgical assistance is much wanted in the hospitals at Brussels'.[104]

It was indeed badly needed. Even on the second Sunday after the battle many French wounded had still not been treated. They lay in barns and out-buildings all over Brussels, calling out piteously to passers-by 'Pansez, monsieur docteur, pansez ma cuisse. Ah! je souffre ...' ('dress my wounds ... I am suffering'). For eight days Charles Bell rose before dawn and worked late into the night.[105] 'All the decencies' of operating, he told a friend, 'were soon neglected'. While he operated on one, a dozen more lay nearby beseeching to be taken next. Though a surgeon for twenty years Bell had not previously served in war but quickly adopted the psychic armour of the military surgeon, seeing his patients as cases rather than men. 'To give one of these objects access to your feelings', he confessed, 'was to allow

Figure 4.4

*Charles Bell's watercolour of Private James Ellard of the
18th Hussars based on Bell's drawing of Ellard made
about a week after the battle of Waterloo.
Ellard had been wounded by a musket ball in the shoulder which
shattered the head of the humerus. Though losing his arm, after three
weeks he was walking about the ward. Bell's notes end 'Successful'.*

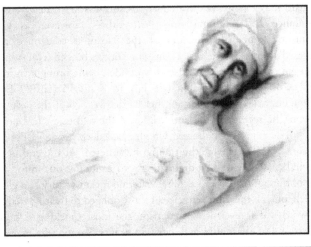

yourself to be unmanned for the performance of a duty'. Used to
weekly operating sessions at the Westminster Hospital he found it
'strange to feel my clothes stiff with blood and my arms powerless
with the exertion of using my knife'. It was not only the fighting at
Waterloo that was 'bloody and desperate': for weeks the military
surgeons and the civilian volunteers felt likewise. John Thomson who
arrived in Brussels on 8 July recalled that several surgeons felt
overwhelmed by the sight of such misery and which 'rendered them
indifferent to life'.[106]

While all British witnesses praised their soldiers' fortitude
opinions varied over French capacity to bear physical pain as well as
the burden of defeat. Edward Costello, who lost a finger at Quatre
Bras, watched a British dragoon chew a plug of tobacco while his
forearm was amputated. Irritated by an adjacent French soldier's cries
as a surgeon probed his wound, the dragoon picked up his
amputated arm and struck the Frenchman, shouting at him to 'stop
your damned bellowing'.[107] The incident hints at the psychological
wounds afflicting many of the survivors. John Scott, a journalist who

watched the convoys of carts carry the wounded into Brussels, saw in their faces 'an extravagance of wretchedness' compounded of 'pain, intoxication, and the recollections of battle'.[108] His observation hints at a condition akin to the 'shell-shock', 'combat exhaustion' or 'post-traumatic stress disorder' of later wars suffered by both surgeons and their patients.

The hospitals into which wounded went – usually segregated by their nationality and nature of wounds – varied greatly. Some, an English lady wrote, exhibited a 'cleanliness and neatness of appearance ... truly gratifying'.[109] In others, however, as John Thomson wrote, 'the horrors of the Hospital continued and increased'.[110] Some were 'very clean' while others buzzed with swarms of flies in the summer heat. He saw wounded being brought in from cottages on the battlefield in late July in 'a putrid state'.[111] Even George Guthrie, so keen for another battle, wearied of the task. 'By the end', he recorded, 'the enthusiasm of the enthusiast had oozed out'.[112] The experience affected Charles Bell deeply, one of the few surgeons to acknowledge the trauma he suffered. At the end of his time in Brussels he was left drained, prey to 'a gloomy, uncomfortable view of human nature'. To Britain Waterloo meant victory and glory. To Bell, one of the most sensitive of those obliged to treat its victims, the word was forever associated with 'the most shocking sights ... expressions of the dying and *noisome smells*.' Six months after his return he still found himself 'easily moved, easily distempered and cast down'.

Waterloo's significance is that it brought together civilian and military surgeons to treat the wounded of the final – if not the largest – battle of a twenty-year war. During, and often as a result of, that war surgeons had learned more than in any comparable period in history. It offers an opportunity to evaluate not only the experience but also the significance of military surgery and to suggest the close connection between military and civil surgery of the period. Despite the slaughter the conservative treatments pioneered by M'Grigor and Guthrie in the Peninsula were again evident. By April 1816 returns disclosed a final accounting. Though redolent of terrible suffering they demonstrated the surgeons' claims of proficiency. Of nearly 7,000 cases 5,068 – just under three-quarters – had rejoined their units. Just over five hundred had been discharged, presumably as maimed. Over 850 were still in hospital nine months after the battle and almost the same number had died of their wounds in hospital. Although the figures are ambiguous, on the most conservative estimate no more than one in ten of the British wounded lost a limb.[113] The proportion of men dying of their wounds was kept as low as the Peninsular surgeons had achieved: of 373 Gordon Highlanders wounded just 19 died in hospital.[114] Charles Bell, John Thomson and William Somerville were sufficiently proud of the conservative surgery they performed to make extensive pictorial records of interesting or important cases exemplifying their contribution to modern surgery.[115]

'An excellent school': war as catalyst of surgical progress

Although all would have expressed regret at the cost in blood and suffering, surgeons regarded the experience of wartime surgery ambivalently. As John Thomson wrote after Waterloo the battle offered 'the greatest opportunity' he could have had to learn military surgery.[116] James Veitch went further, revelling in how the naval surgeon could 'enjoy in full force, the triumph of his art'.[117] War experience shaped the generation that dominated surgery in the ensuing decades reinforcing their confidence in the healing power of their profession. The best surgeons learned in military hospitals which under M'Grigor became almost experimental establishments, emblematic of the scientific ethos with which the profession was imbued. M'Grigor believed that a military hospital was 'best for trying the effects of all new remedies' because its patients were 'more under control and observation'.[118] George Ballingall, later Professor of Military Surgery at Edinburgh, demonstrated the effects of this regime. He described how at Feversham in 1806 the wards were full of men with gangrenous ulcers. It was discovered – 'at last' – that the patients' sores were washed using the same sponge, possibly day after day. 'The sponge was destroyed', and the epidemic of gangrene ceased. Ballingall used the instance in his lectures at Edinburgh for twenty years to illustrate the idea that 'sickness is not always the necessary consequence of a military life'.[119]

The most energetic proponent of the lessons of war, however, remained George Guthrie whose commentaries on war surgery bore the subtitle 'showing the improvements made during and since that period in the great art and science of surgery'. M'Grigor saw 'a new spirit of emulation' in the army, one which brought 'much credit with our brethren in civil life'.[120] He encouraged his colleagues to publish their findings on adhesive straps, bandaging, fever and ulcers: they needed little encouragement to engage in the long-running controversy over the propriety, timing and methods of amputation. Amputation at the shoulder Guthrie argued was 'a very simple operation' after 1815, 'for which simplicity English surgery is indebted to the Peninsular war'. He claimed credit for the use of incisions in treating erysipelas, 'an improvement for which all mankind should be grateful'.[121] He even contested John Hunter's advice to defer amputation albeit with 'the greatest deference and respect'.[122]

Surgeons who had served in war argued (in Guthrie's case unremittingly) that it was war that allowed them to develop their skills and to draw conclusions from their experiences. Through treating great numbers of wounded surgeons learned and passed on many lessons. While in the eighteenth century, surgeons would dilate wounds to search for balls or foreign matter, long experience taught that, as the former naval surgeon John Lizars wrote, 'no torturing search should be made' and that 'uncalled for dilation' should be abandoned.[123] Even John Hennen, an advocate for immediate amputation ('no lacerated joint' he believed 'should ever leave the field unamputated') did not urge indiscriminate operating. Surgeons, he wrote, would betray 'a miserable want of science' if they operated on the 'weak, the terrified, the sinking and the determined'.[124] Hennen's insight suggests that even in the midst of what might appear to be blood-soaked butchery surgeons were not only making clinical judgements based on more than a desire to amputate but were also reaching understandings of the psychological dimensions of their patients' predicament.

One of the most lasting legacies of the wars lay not in clinical advances, substantial though they were. Rather, it lay in a decisive change in the minds of surgeons. War service broke the demarcation between physicians, surgeons and the prescribing apothecary and demonstrated the value of a unified approach to health. The surgeon responsible for the wellbeing of a ship or a regiment found it as George Ballingall said, 'impossible to adopt ... a minute division of professional labour'.[125] Responsible for the care of several hundred men, often relying upon his own resources, a surgeon found that he did not need a physician's advice or permission to operate and could find his own medicines in his field pannier. By the war's end thousands of surgeons had worked as medical practitioners, gaining a new confidence in their skills and capacity to heal. Few now accepted the validity of the rigid divisions which had previously obtained.

Despite the regard of medical colleagues, military and naval surgeons resented their failure to win the honours and rewards conferred on their fighting colleagues. Thirty years after Waterloo they continued to express their dismay. In vain did Guthrie point out that it would have been impossible for regimental and even staff surgeons to have been out of range of French cannon. 'No storming party' he said 'ever ascended the breach without its surgeon in company'.[126] A satirical contributor to the *Lancet*, poking fun at Guthrie's lecturing style suggested that a generation of young men who had been in petticoats during the war became restive at the recitative of their seniors' surgical triumphs:

> All the world knows that I have been the ... surgical hero of the Peninsular war ... I learned to do without a tourniquet ... I finally abandoned it at Albuhera ... Bye-the-bye, gentlemen, I hope you will always spell Albuhera ... with an h. You may as well write ... Guthrie without "baronet" (great cheering).[127]

Surgeons like Guthrie were able to observe the conduct of their fellows in some of the most extreme ordeals which humans have been obliged to endure. Few experiences can compare with the obligation to stand to a gun in a great naval battle under sail or in a line facing death within fifty yards. Military and naval surgeons saw in the reactions of their patients the full range of human emotions: how fear of wounds or death depressed the spirit, how men summoned the fortitude to endure pain or succumbed to misery. Though the evidence is ambiguous or lacking, the trauma surely marked many for life. Many of those men undoubtedly conformed to, and fuelled, the stereotypical view of incompetence and drunkenness. But many others met the challenge with a skill and courage even more admirable for the paucity of their material resources. They gained insights, many uncongenial and unwelcome, into the human condition unavailable to those who were not there. The best retained their humanity in circumstances in which it would be all too easy to give way to brutality, indifference, hopelessness or despair.

Notes

1. Cooper, 'On Amputation', *Guy's Hospital Reports*, 1839, 301.
2. Samuel Cooper, *A Dictionary of Practical Surgery* (London: Longman, Hurst, Rees, Orme & Brown, 1829), 573 .
3. Charles Bell to George Bell, 30 June 1809, George Jospeh Bell, (ed.), *Letters of Sir George Bell* (London: John Murray, 1870), 152.
4. D. Arnold & A.D. Harvey, *Collision of Empires: Britain in Three World Wars* (London: Phoenix, 1994), 125.
5. Steel's *Original and Correct List of the Royal Navy, 1793*, 1814.
6. Orders and Letters of Sir William Beattie [sic], Document 1988/

417(2) RNM .

7. 'Verses written on board His Majesty's Ship Eagle', Commonplace book of Andrew and John Johnston, 1797–1817, Acc. 5811, No. IIa, NLS.

8. William Burney, *A New Universal Dictionary of the Marine* (London: T. Cadell & W. Davies, 1815), 513.

9. *The Times*, 2 Jul 1800, 3b; 15 Sep 1801, 3b.

10. Michael Lewis, *A Social History of the Navy* (London: George Allen & Unwin, 1960), 244 .

11. *Ledger of Royal Navy Officers' Courts Martial, 1803-56*, ADM 13/103, PRO .

12. Christopher Lloyd, *The British Seaman 1200–1860: A Social Survey* (London: Paladin, 1970), 239.

13. William Turnbull, *The Naval Surgeon, Comprising the Entire Duties of Professional Men at Sea* (London: R. Phillips, 1806), 360.

14. Wounds and Hurts certificates, 1797–1815, Document 1986/537, RNM.

15. The term 'sick bay' itself exemplifies the changes in naval medicine which occurred during the French wars. While battle casualties were treated in the cockpit, below decks, the more numerous and frequent sick were treated in a more healthy area of the upper deck near the foc'sle.

16. Cooper, *op. cit.* (note 2), vi.

17. Christopher Lloyd & Jack Coulter, *Medicine and the Navy 1200–1900* (Edinburgh: E. & S. Livingstone, 1961), 365-66.

18. Verses written on board His Majesty's Ship Eagle', Acc. 5811, No. IIa, NLS. Professor William Cullen, the Edinburgh physician, wrote an influential text, *First Lines on the Practice of Physic.*

19. Thomas Trotter, *Medicina Nautica: An Essay on the Diseases of Seamen* (London: Longman, Hurst, Rees & Orme, 1804), Vol. II, 248–50.

20. A. Copland Hutchison, *Some Farther Observations on the Subject of the Proper Period for Amputating in Gunshot Wounds* (London: J. Callow, 1817), 2.

21. John Bell, *Memorial Concerning the Present State of Military and Naval Surgery* (Edinburgh: Mundell & Son, 1800), 11–12.

22. George Jackson, *The Perilous Adventures and Vicissitudes of a Naval Officer 1801–1812* (Edinburgh: Blackwood & Sons, 1927), 144.

23. 'Journal of His Majesty's Ship Ardent', 29 March 1797–3 April 1798', ADM 101/85/7, PRO.

24. 'Physical & Surgical Journal' 30 May 1797–30 May 1798', ADM

101/118/1, PRO.

25. 'Surgeon's Journal Victory 1805', ADM 101/125/1, PRO.

26. 'Journal of His Majesty's Frigate Shannon 30 July 1812–29 July 1813', ADM 101/120/3, PRO; J.G. Brighton, *Sir P.B.V. Broke Bart ...* (London: Sampson Lowe & Co., 1866), 204–08; William James, *A Full and Correct Account of the Chief Naval Occurrences of the Late War between Great Britain and the United States of America* (London: Black, Kingsbury, Parbury & Allen, 1817), 211–51.

27. 'Mr Leah's cases of tetanus', *Edinburgh Medical & Surgical Journal,* 1828, Vol. 30, 21–29.

28. Hutchison, *op. cit.* (note 20), 5.

29. William Robinson, (ed.), *Jack Nastyface: Memoirs of a Seaman* (London: Wayland, 1973), 50.

30. Jackson, *op. cit.* (note 22), 144.

31. Hutchison, *op. cit.* (note 20), 9, 8.

32. Stuart Legg, (ed.), *Trafalgar: An Eye-Witness Account of a Great Battle* (London: Hart Davis, 1966), 100 .

33. John Lizars, *A System of Practical Surgery* (Edinburgh: W.H. Lizars, 1838), 196.

34. Hutchison, *op. cit.* (note 20), 37.

35. Lizars, *op. cit.* (note 33), 194.

36. C. Northcote Parkinson, *Britannia Rules: the Classic Age of Naval History, 1793–1815* (London: Weidenfield & Nicolson, 1977), 183.

37. Norman Moore & Stephen Paget, *The Royal Medical and Chirurgical Society of London, 1805-1905* (Aberdeen: Aberdeen University Press, 1905), 65.

38. Lewis, *op. cit.* (note 10), 303 .

39. Harold D. Langley, *A History of Medicine in the Early US Navy* (Baltimore: Johns Hopkins, University Press, 1995), 177.

40. *A List of the Officers of the Army, 1798.*

41. John Bell, *The Principles of Surgery*, 2 vols (Edinburgh: T. Cadell & W. Davies, 1801), Vol. I, 2.

42. James Fergusson (ed.), *Notes and Recollections of a Professional Life* (London: Longman, Brown, Green & Longmans, 1846), 65.

43. James M'Grigor, *The Autobiography and Services of James McGrigor* (London: Longman, Green, Longmans & Roberts, 1861), 279.

44. Bell, *op. cit.* (note 21), 4.

45. M'Grigor, *op. cit.* (note 43), 93.

46. Bell, *op. cit.* (note 21), 21 .

47. Letter, 11 September 1811, M 1996.11.13, NWMS.

48. Bell, *op. cit.* (note 21), 16 .

49. W.C.E. Napier, (ed.), *The Early Military Life of General Sir George Napier* (London: John Murray, 1886), 134.

50. George Ballingall, *Outlines of Military Surgery* (Edinburgh: A.&C. Black, 1844, 1846), 479; 482.

51. John Hennen, *Principles of Military Surgery* (London: John Wilson, 1829), 27.

52. 'An Officer', [David Roberts], *The Military Adventures of Johnny Newcome* [1816] (London: Methuen & Co., 1904), 184–86.

53. M'Grigor, *op. cit.* (note 43), 32.

54. Fergusson, *op. cit.* (note 42), 56.

55. Roger Buckley, *The British Army in the West Indies: Society and the Military in the Revolutionary Age* (Gainesville: University Press of Florida, 1998), 272; 276.

56. Neil Cantlie, *A History of the Army Medical Department,* 2 vols (Edinburgh: Churchill Livingstone, 1974), Vol. I, 178.

57. M'Grigor, *op. cit.* (note 43), 303.

58. Papers of William Jones, 9109–86, NAM; Mullen, *The Military General Service Roll* (London: London Stamp Exchange, 1990), 665.

59. M'Grigor, *op. cit.* (note 43), 375.

60. Richard Blanco, *Wellington's Surgeon General: Sir James McGrigor* (Durham: Duke University Press, 1974), 139–41.

61. M'Grigor, *op. cit.* (note 43), 265.

62. Fergusson, *op. cit.* (note 42), 62.

63. S.G.P. Ward, *Wellington's Headquarters: A Study in the Administrative Problems in the Peninsula, 1809–1814* (Oxford: OUP, 1957), 89; 161.

64. Cooper, *op. cit.* (note 2), 581.

65. John Elting, *Swords Around a Throne: Napoleon's Grande Armée* (New York: Free Press, 1988), 283-95. Though Elting argues that the *Service de Santé* 'performed as well as any other medical service of its day', on the evidence he provides it manifestly did worse than M'Grigor's.

66. Pat Hayward (ed.), *Surgeon Henry's Trifles* (London: Chatto & Windus, 1970), 95.

67. Longmore, 'Description of a series of watercolour drawings', p. 5, RAMC 96, WIHM.

68. Arnold & Harvey, *op. cit.* (note 4), 145–47 .

69. Ballingall, *op. cit.* (note 50), 66.

70. James Henderson, *Sloops and Brigs* (London: Coles, 1972), 17.

71. Arnold & Harvey, *op. cit.* (note 4), 50.

72. Robert Druitt, *The Principles and Practice of Modern Surgery*

(Philadelphia: Lea & Blanchard, 1842), 138.

73. George Macleod, *Notes on the Surgery of the War in the Crimea* (London: John Churchill, 1858), 102. Russian troops used a musket essentially the same as those used in the Napoleonic wars..

74. Charles Bell, *Illustrations of the Great Operations of Surgery* (London: Longman, 1821), 56.

75. Hayward, *op. cit.* (note 66), 82.

76. William Grattan, *Adventures with the Connaught Rangers, 1809–1814* (London: Edward Arnold, 1902), 75–78. Bell was no relation to the great John Bell of Edinburgh.

77. Druitt, *op. cit.* (note 73), 149.

78. Thomas Chevalier, *A Treatise on Gun-Shot Wounds* (London: Samuel Bagster, 1806), 107–108.

79. Macleod, *op. cit.* (note 73), 89.

80. Hennen, *op. cit.* (note 51), 62–63, 75, 46–47.

81. John & Dorothea Teague, (eds), *Where Duty Calls Me: The Experiences of William Green of Lutterworth in the Napoleonic Wars* (West Wickham: 1975), 40.

82. G.C. Moore Smith (ed.), *The Autobiography of Lieutenant General Sir Harry Smith* (London: Constable, 1903), 39.

83. Teague, *op. cit.* (note 81), 36–40;44.

84. Alexander Hutchison, *Practical Observations in Surgery* (London: 1816), 4.

85. Letter, 14 June 1814, B.H. Liddell Hart, (ed.), *The Letters of Private Wheeler 1809–1828* (London: Michael Joseph, 1951), 152–53.

86. Rutherford Alcock, *Notes on the Medical History and Statistics of the British Legion of Spain* (London: John Churchill, 1838), 97.

87. Cantlie, *op. cit.* (note 56), Vol. I, 511; 345.

88. Brian Stuart, (ed.), *Soldier's Glory, being, Rough Notes of an Old Soldier by Sir George Bell* (London: G. Bell & Sons, 1956), 136.

89. George Guthrie, *Commentaries on the Surgery of the War in Portugal, Spain, France, and the Netherlands* (London: Renshaw, 1853), v .

90. Charles Bell to John Shaw, 22 June 1815, Bell, *op. cit.* (note 3), 24.

91. Bransby Cooper, *The Life of Sir Astley Cooper*, Bart., 2 vols (London: John Parker, 1843), Vol. II, 195.

92. Anon [possibly an officer of the 28th Foot], *Stories of Waterloo* (London: 1847), 291.

93. Christopher Hibbert, (ed.), *The Wheatley Diary: A Journal and Sketch-book kept during the Peninsular War and the Waterloo Campaign* (London: Longman, 1964), 67.

94. Ballingall, *op. cit.* (note 50), 20.

95. Edward Sabine, (ed.), *Letters of Colonel Sir Augustus Simon Frazer* (London: 1859), 553.

96. James M'Queen, *A Narrative of the Political and Military Events of 1815* (Glasgow: [1816?]), 346.

97. John Thomson to Mrs J. Davey, 26 July 1815, Ms 9236, NLS.

98. W.E. Frye, *After Waterloo: Reminiscences of European Travel 1815–1819* (London: William Heinemann, 1908), np.

99. R.D. Gibney, (ed.), *Eighty Years Ago, or the Recollections of an Old Army Doctor* (London: Bellairs & Co., 1896), 206.

100. 'Extracts from the Journal of a Gentleman', George Jones, *The Battle of Waterloo*, 3 vols (London: John Booth, T. Edgerton, 1817), Vol. III, 121.

101. Jane Vansittart, (ed.), *Surgeon James's Journal* (London: Cassell, 1964), 35.

102. Isaac James to Richard James, 29 June 1815, RAMC 394–396, WIHM.

103. Elkington papers, RAMC 484/2, WIHM.

104. Sir Walter Scott to Thomas Wilkie, 14 July 1815, Ms 23118, NLS; H.J.C. Grierson, (ed.) *The Letters of Sir Walter Scott 1815–1817* (London: Constable, 1933), 74.

105. Bell, *op. cit.* (note 3), 243–54 .

106. John Thomson, *Report on Observations made in the British Military Hospitals in Belgium after the Battle of Waterloo* (Edinburgh: William Blackwood, 1816), 8.

107. Anthony Brett-James, (ed.), *Edward Costello: The Peninsular and Waterloo Campaigns* (London: Longmans, 1967), 156.

108. John Scott, *Paris Revisited in 1815* (London: Longman & Co., 1817), 166.

109. [Charlotte Eaton], *Narrative of a Residence in Belgium During the Campaign of 1815 …* (London: John Murray, 1817), 210.

110. John Thomson to Mrs J. Davey, 26 July 1815, Ms 9236, NLS.

111. Jones, *op. cit.* (note 100), Vol. III, 121.

112. Guthrie, *op. cit.* (note 89), viii.

113. Cantlie, *op. cit.* (note 56), Vol. I, 391. The figures can only be approximate. Figures for 18 June generally do not include the 2300 wounded at Quatre Bras who must also have been treated at the time.

114. J.M. Bulloch, *Gordon Highlanders Wounded at Waterloo* (Aberdeen: 1916), 4.

115. Thomson & Somerville, 'Sketches of the Wounded at Waterloo', Gen 594, EUL. Charles Bell's Waterloo sketches are in the

collections of the Wellcome Institute and Royal College of Surgeons of England.

116. John Thomson to his wife Margaret, 12 July 1815, Ms 9236, NLS.

117. James Veitch, *Observations on the Ligature of the Arteries* (London, 1824), 6.

118. M'Grigor, *op. cit.* (note 43), 183.

119. Ballingall, *op. cit.* (note 50), 169; 65.

120. M'Grigor, *op. cit.* (note 43), 96.

121. Guthrie, *op. cit.* (note 89), 118; 10.

122. George Guthrie, *On Gunshot Wounds of the Extremities* (London: Longman, Hurst, Rees, Orme & Brown, 1815), viii.

123. Lizars, *op. cit.* (note 33), 193.

124. Hennen, *op. cit.* (note 51), 41, 46.

125. Ballingall, *op. cit.* (note 50), 2.

126. *The Times*, 11 July 1846, 8f.

127. *Lancet*, 1835–36, Vol. II , 567–68.

5

'In process of cure':
Hospitals and Surgical Healing

Modern surgeons practised capital operations in their consulting rooms, in the houses of their patients but, especially in hospitals. The unreformed, pre-anaesthetic, pre-Listerian, pre-Nightingale hospital has been represented as a place of horror, as a 'gateway to death'. This stereotype has been challenged.[1] Like the received beliefs about surgeons and surgery, however, it retains an obstinate popular longevity. The view of the dirty, crowded, dangerous hospital is also a product of changing standards, following swiftly on the introduction of recognisably modern antiseptic standards and nursing care. We can still discern amid what William Fergusson called the 'noise and confusion of a public ward' the changes through which hospitals passed in the first decades of the nineteenth century.[2]

'New hospitals contrive': the hospitals of Edinburgh and London

Hospitals were not simply aggregations of doctors and patients. They formed large, complex and dynamic communities within the wider society of the metropolis. Each institution not only required a large staff to function, but also attracted hangers-on living in a symbiotic relationship with it. Hospitals were run by boards of governors, generally local business people and gentry patronised by nobility. They both sustained the institution by contributions and were nourished by it socially as their benevolence became known. Middle class families supported Samaritan societies raising money for artificial limbs or collecting used linen for dressings. The hospital's day-to-day administration devolved upon bursars, treasurers and secretaries, who became brokers in the economy of institutional power. Hospitals naturally required physicians and surgeons but also apothecaries, druggists, demonstrators in anatomy, librarians and curators of pathological collections, many of whom required or professed to need assistants. The operating room employed a surgeryman and his boys, the apothecary a laboratory-man. Though not entirely responsible for what we would regard as nursing care, each hospital employed a matron and a number of nurses, each ward often under its own sister. Local clergymen might serve as chaplains,

131

variously willing or suborned. A hospital needed domestic servants – cooks and skivvies, butlers, laundry maids, cleaners, bed-bug exterminators, barbers, coal-carriers, lamp trimmers – and a housekeeper to direct them. Access to the buildings required watchmen or beadles. Maintaining their fabric demanded carpenters and boiler men. The movement of beds and their occupants depended upon porters and even the dead needed a man to attend to them. The hospital provided a focus for the hundreds of students who walked its wards, who paid the fees that sustained its professional staff and who in turn supplied much of the clinical care in the wards. The students also offered a market for the small-scale entrepreneurs who lived off them dealing in second-hand text-books and instruments. Beyond the hospital's walls a wider community fed on it: the tradesmen and their families who supplied its food and drink, the cutlers who made its instruments, the proprietors of the students' digs and the chop-houses and taverns in which they drank and dined. Hawkers and traders plied patients and their families with food and drink often passing through the wards on regular rounds. Local undertakers relied on hospitals for a steady income while they and compliant sextons and church-wardens supplied the dissecting rooms with 'things' for the surgeon.

The first half of the century saw many hospitals founded, enlarged or improved, becoming places assisting healing as well as easing death. Thomas Hood, in a satire on Malthus's gloomy theory of population, bemoaned how 'New hospitals contrive/ For keeping life alive' (and concluded that 'we ought to *import* the *Cholera Morbus*').[3] London had a dozen such little worlds; most provincial cities and towns one. Edinburgh possessed only two. One was one of the largest, oldest and most complex hospitals in the kingdom; the other, although among the smallest, was also for a time one of the best.

The Royal Infirmary of Edinburgh had been founded in 1729. Its internal life is perhaps better known than any other thanks to complementary studies by Lisa Rosner and Gunter Risse.[4] As the only surgical hospital in the Scottish capital until the 1820s it naturally occupied a central place in medical education and its managers, the Town Council and Edinburgh's surgeons enjoyed a close but often fraught triangular relationship. The Infirmary managers' periodic attempts to control surgeons' access to the hospital's wards led to bitter controversy particularly in the first half of the nineteenth century. Like other hospitals conditions varied depending upon financial and managerial competence. In 1817

Figure 5.1

James Syme's clinic Minto House, Edinburgh, scene of Syme's operation upon Allie, from Alexander Peddie's Recollections of Dr John Brown. The site of the hospital, in Chambers Street, is now occupied approximately by the Royal Museum of Scotland.

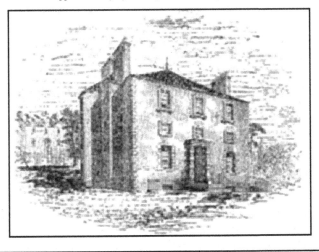

Leonard Horner, the Whig linen manufacturer-cum-gentleman geologist testified to the 'filthiness' of patients' beds, the 'scantiness & bad quality' of their food and the 'neglect' of its nurses. He resolved that the Infirmary 'should keep pace with the latest improvements in every hospital throughout the world'.[5] The aspiration appears to have succeeded. An English visitor later commented on the Infirmary's 'beautiful exterior and well-regulated interior' which in the early 1830s included a large operating theatre able to seat five hundred spectators, 'capitally contrived'.[6]

Edinburgh's other surgical hospital was Minto House in which Allie had lost her breast and her life in 1830. Opened by James Syme (after the managers had banned him from the wards of the Royal Infirmary) it operated as a 24-bed public hospital from 1829 to 1833 and as a 12-bed private hospital from 1837 to 1852. In its first period it treated over 8000 surgical cases. Over the fifteen years of its second incarnation more than 1100 in-patients were treated in its wards and nearly 60,000 out-patients used its public dispensary.[7]

During the first half of the nineteenth century ten major hospitals served London's population of almost two million, all but one located within two miles of St Paul's Cathedral. St

Bartholomew's was the largest with the most students and arguably, in John Abernethy, the most distinguished teacher. Bart's asserted a primacy accepted by the newer hospitals in the west but disputed by St Thomas's and Guy's south of the river. These 'United Hospitals' of the Borough (i.e. of Southwark) separated in the mid-1820s over a combination of the nepotism of Astley Cooper and the ambition of Benjamin Harrison, its imperious but effective Treasurer for fifty years from 1793. The London Hospital in Mile End Road opened its medical school at the instigation of Sir William Blizard in 1785, the first associated with a hospital. At the 'west end of town' were three hospitals founded in the eighteenth century which grew in the nineteenth. St George's Hospital opposite Hyde Park opened a new building begun in 1827. The Westminster Infirmary, opened in 1715 as London's first voluntarily supported hospital, was also enlarged in 1834. The smaller Middlesex Hospital also founded its own medical school in 1834. In the course of the first half of the century several other hospitals were established. King's College Hospital, the medical school of the Anglican foundation of that name, opened in 1840 in the former St Clement Danes Workhouse. University College Hospital (formerly the North London) was established as part of the medical school of the University of London in 1828. The Charing Cross Hospital, founded in 1818, also opened new buildings in 1834 treating 'cases of Accident and dangerous emergency' which were an 'hourly occurrence' in the capital's busy streets.[8] The London General Institution for the Gratuitous Care of Malignant Diseases opened in 1828, known, rather more succinctly, after 1837 as the Royal Free Hospital.

By the mid-1840s some thirty dispensaries treated over 100,000 poor out-patients annually, some (such as the St Giles's or the Worship Street children's dispensary) with two staff, others such as the Western General at Lisson Grove or the Aldersgate Dispensary, with ten or more.[9] Over the first half of the nineteenth century the capital also acquired many smaller, more specialised hospitals. They included the Royal Westminster Ophthalmic Hospital (which the *Lancet* ridiculed as a 'blind manufactory'[10]) and the Lock Hospital for venereal cases. John Cunningham Saunders's London Dispensary for the Relief of the Poor Afflicted with Ear and Eye Diseases, established in 1804, offered a model for specialist clinics. Its lead was followed by Frederick Salmon who founded the Infirmary for the Relief of the Poor afflicted with Fistula and other Diseases of the Rectum in 1835. Other more specialised institutions were founded; Protheroe Smith's Hospital for Women opened in Red Lion Square in 1842 and what became the Hospital for Sick Children in 1851. By the 1860s more than sixty specialist hospitals had been established in London with others in the provinces.[11] A number of private practitioners established 'institutes' or 'infirmaries'. These smaller, private clinics shaded into varying degrees of respectability and profit: James Yearsley's Ear Institution, for example, seems to have been regarded rather doubtfully.

In Scotland hospitals opened between 1794 and 1807 in Glasgow, Dundee, Inverness, Paisley and Elgin. The English provinces mirrored this growth with hospitals and infirmaries established in smaller towns and cities. In the 1820s associations of citizens in seven English provincial towns and cities subscribed to establish new hospitals; in Liverpool, Bath, Chichester, Gloucester, Brighton, Stamford and Shrewsbury. In the 1830s, a decade of growth in London hospitals, no fewer than sixteen more were built outside the capital. Smaller hospitals tended to echo changes in metropolitan institutions albeit more slowly.

None of these institutions remained static. The range of technology they used, for example, reflected the growth of Britain as an industrial power. The London Hospital was proud of its iron bedsteads, in themselves a means of deterring infection. By 1800 St Thomas's pumped water into wards using 'an engine', installed water closets in 1815 and gas lighting in 1817.[12] Other hospitals also introduced water and light. It is true, as Barry Smith shows in *The People's Health,* that drains could be as insanitary as cesspits and that water was not necessarily used for washing.[13] Equally, though, throughout the period existing and the new hospitals gradually changed in response to dissemination of scientific knowledge and theories of medical practice. They were the arenas in which the dramas of treatment and healing occurred.

Before examining how these hospitals treated surgical patients it is useful to be reminded of patients in one hospital at one moment in time. The Library of the Royal Australasian College of Surgeons in Melbourne holds a manuscript 'Journal' of James Syme's three wards of the Edinburgh Royal Infirmary for three months of 1844. The patients were James Syme's; the notes were made by his clerk, or dresser, Joseph Lister, later Syme's son-in-law and Lord Lister, the instigator of antiseptic surgery. Syme's wards treated 86 patients suffering from a wide range of complaints. At any one time about twenty patients occupied the three small wards about a third of whom were girls and women. Sixty six were discharged 'cured' or 'in process of cure'; six merely 'relieved'; three were allowed to go 'with

135

advice' i.e. to return to the care of local doctors. Six remained obstinately 'in statu quo' and four were regarded as 'incurable' and were dismissed. On average patients remained in hospital for just under a month with the shortest stay being a few days and the longest some months. Treating these 86 patients called for 17 operations – Syme countenanced no indiscriminate recourse to the knife. Four patients (less than five per cent of those admitted) died in hospital. What was ward life like for patients like Syme's?

'Nothing particularly dirty': hospital routine

Even though the capital's hospitals could accommodate and treat up to two thousand patients at any one time, the great majority of those coming into contact with a hospital did so as out-patients. They attended in huge numbers although exact counts only became mandatory at the end of the century. At the beginning of the nineteenth century St Thomas's treated almost 3,000 in-patients and around 4,500 out-patients.[14] The Middlesex in the 1830s treated 1,600 in- and 5,000 out-patients.[15] By 1845 King's College Hospital was treating 17,093 patients, all but 1,160 as out-patients.[16] The out-patients rooms were open for only a few days in the week when they must have been bedlam. The dispensary movement, which took rudimentary medical care to the districts where the sick poor lived, probably made inroads into the numbers seeking treatment at hospitals. Even so every 'taking-in day' desperately ill people resignedly waited in their hundreds on hard, backless benches for treatment – perhaps a tot or a pill of a few standard doses of physic and perhaps admission. Figures kept by Guy's in the 1830s suggest that they stood no better than a one-in-four chance of gaining a bed.[17]

Even for the manifestly ill, except for accident cases (and not always then), admission was by no means assured. In almost all hospitals besides the Royal Free, admission was controlled by a system of tickets issued by a hospital's subscribers or governors. Securing a ticket could in itself take days of walking and soliciting, waiting at back doors and calling on the servants or employees of subscribers. Hospital rules often excluded as many sufferers as they admitted. Young children, pregnant women, 'incurables' with cancer or tuberculosis, those with venereal infections or with contagious fevers would often be refused treatment, while the dirty, disorderly or drunk would be seen off by porters at the gates. Even those who met the stipulated criteria and had obtained a governor's ticket were often turned away for want of beds. In 1835 a gentleman complained to

The Times of the bureaucratic rectitude which had fatally affected the treatment of a young woman he had brought to London in the hope of obtaining treatment. 'T.W.H.' arrived with a 'poor sick creature' suffering from fistula, inflammation of the brain and consumption. They arrived at Guy's on a Monday only to learn that 'taking in' day was Friday. Returning on the right day they arrived ten minutes late and were informed that Guy's would not admit patients unless they were punctual to the minute (this in a society in which timekeeping varied locally and few carried watches, especially those likely to seek admission to a hospital). As they remonstrated they saw an aged man refused entry for the third time. Weeping, the young woman and her guardian returned to the country where she died soon after.[18] The case was not unusual: St Thomas's rules stipulated that 'The Time of admitting Patients is at Ten o'Clock Tuesday Morning precisely'.[19]

Having surmounted the obstacles to obtain admission or having been carried in as an emergency or accident victim, a patient would have been housed in a bed in a ward with ten to thirty others. Hospital wards were rarely cheerful and were often hideous and distressing. Dickens, who took his readers into a ward in one of his *Sketches by Boz*, described a casualty ward one night in the late 1830s. Ushered in by dressers smelling strongly of tobacco, he saw in a dim light the 'ghastly appearance' of the patients in long rows of beds. In one a child, half-consumed by fire, lay enveloped in bandages. In another a woman badly injured in an accident lay 'beating her clenched fists on the coverlet, in pain'.[20] In the daytime wards were easy-going often rough-and-ready places. In many ways their function was to collect patients for the convenience of medical practitioners and their students rather than for the ease and treatment of the sick. Patients looked after themselves and each other even being inveigled into helping the porters make adhesive plasters. Friends or relatives brought night-clothes, bedding, and food to supplement the limited and poor fare provided by the hospital kitchen. Patients' diets were always basic and often inadequate comprising combinations of weak beer, gruel, broth and boiled meat with vegetables a rarity. A patient confined for several months without the support of friends or family could risk malnutrition or scurvy. Access to the wards was often open to hawkers and traders including vendors of strong drink and pawnbrokers. At Guy's no tea was provided and hawkers sold patients watercress and periwinkles, to mutual advantage.[21]

John Bell reflected on the common atmosphere of the hospitals he knew at the end of the eighteenth century with their 'noise, confusion and noxious air'. He imagined what 'agonies of mind' a patient must have endured while lying in such a place. He would hear the cries of those being operated upon (in many hospitals minor procedures were performed in the wards often in sight of other patients). He would see other patients carried to the theatre or 'carried back in solemnity and silence' and would hear their 'dying groans'. 'Scenes like these' Bell concluded 'must be a subject of conversation ... among those ... most liable to become patients', the poor.[22] Even so changes to the practice of hospitals and the architecture occurred throughout the period. Thomas Percival urged his colleagues to respect their patients' privacy. A patient, he wrote, 'should not have his mind agitated by the knowledge of the sufferings of another'. He advised surgeons to change aprons and to clean the table and instruments between operations 'when besmeared' to avoid 'every thing that may excite terror'.[23]

The state of hospitals before the almost simultaneous innovations in nursing and hygiene which occurred in the last three decades of the nineteenth century remains debatable. They are often represented as smelly, dark, dirty, squalid and dangerous. Whether this is so demands re-examination. While none approached the standards of cleanliness or order expected and imposed by hospitals in later decades of the century it is important to recognise that they did not always conform to the stereotype too easily assumed. For example, the Sydney Hospital, in New South Wales, opened in 1819 and for its first three years, under the direction of D'Arcy Wentworth, it conformed to the conventional view of the eighteenth century hospital. Patients were housed indiscriminately – men and women, surgical and medical – in wards locked at night and with closed windows, cooking and washing without privies. However, from 1821, under James Bowman, conditions altered immediately and dramatically. Patients were segregated by gender and treatment. Nurses and porters enforced order; food was cooked in kitchens; windows were bolted open, linen was changed and wards were washed out daily. By later standards it was still dirty and unhealthy – scrubbing floors soaked them and encouraged damp; outbreaks of erysipelas occurred; vermin infested the wall cavities and rats invaded the dead house – but it was cleaner and more orderly than is often conceded.[24]

For much of the early decades of the century standards of care and hygiene ranged from the rudimentary to the neglectful. At St Thomas's John Flint South could be expected to examine two hundred patients on one day's rounds as an assistant surgeon.[25] Some

Figure 5.2

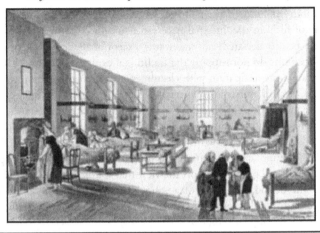

*Though it cannot convey sound or smell,
this 1808 depiction of a ward in the Middlesex Hospital appears to
confound the modern expectation that hospitals were disorderly.*

patients could lie unattended for days. In 1825 in St George's Hospital visitors discovered mushrooms growing and maggots squirming in the damp, soiled sheets of a patient with a compound fracture. The patient had not complained and the men in adjoining beds, expecting nothing better, had regarded the bed as 'nothing particularly dirty'.[26] Against these instances however must be set the procedures in Guy's, St Thomas's and Bart's, recorded in detail by the Charity Commissioners in the 1830s, which suggest at least standards of care against which these abuses were measured.[27]

By the 1840s, though, at Guy's when Samuel Wilkes was a student the wards were still 'mean and comfortless' but through 'continual scrubbing' were markedly cleaner than the 'squalid, dirty barracks' of previous decades.[28] Evidence can be found across a range of provincial and metropolitan hospitals to suggest a greater concern with cleanliness than has been previously allowed. The clearest evidence that a change occurred in expectations of cleanliness earlier than, say, the 1870s, comes from the Royal Infirmary in Edinburgh. A continuous record exists in the managers' Visiting Book.[29] These reports, compiled week-by-week, provide a detailed picture of the state of the wards as the infirmary's lay governors found them. Two seemingly paradoxical conclusions are evident. First, that over several decades reports consistently disclose that the wards were 'exceptionally clean', 'in excellent order', 'clean, orderly and comfortable' or 'in the best Order' with 'all the patients expressing emphatically their Satisfaction'. Second, that many reports also draw attention to dirty sheets, 'a want of ventilation', water closets 'in a bad state' or 'filthy' and broken hot water systems. The reports present a conundrum. Indeed the manager who in 1830 found a 'disgusting state of filth' in the 'internal necessaries' on one visit, had only the week before declared 'all the wards exceptionally clean'. Critical observations do not support the traditional explanation: rather they indicate a preoccupation with cleanliness rather than apathy toward dirt. Certainly nurses and porters needed to be repeatedly reminded of the more exacting standards expected and often left their wards, in a manager's ambiguous phrase, 'unexceptionally clean' but it is impossible to portray the infirmary as dirty in the stereotyped view.

Contemporary illustrations of hospital wards, while perhaps unreliable and partial, support the view that wards became less awful over the period. Drawings of a women's ward in the Middlesex in 1808 and a male ward in Bart's in 1832 qualify the impression of squalor. In both the windows are large, the beds are well-spaced and fitted with curtains and fires heat the ward – a nurse warms a poultice, perhaps, at the stove. Despite the presence of a chamber pot beneath one bed it is possible that sympathetic artists removed the detail of dirt and stains and, of course, it is impossible to convey smell on paper. Nor can the artists have been equal to depicting the feelings of anxiety or pain that surely preoccupied many of the patients in the beds. Still, the drawings support the suggestion that the physical appearance and organisation of wards was more regulated than many later writers asserted.

Joseph Wilde included in his poem *The Hospital* an impression of the routine prevailing in the Devon and Exeter Hospital at the beginning of the century. As a small county hospital its senior medical staff appear to have been more diligent than were their metropolitan colleagues. Wilde described the morning rounds of the medical staff:

Through every ward, t'enquire, the state of each;
To learn their wants; to know if ought amiss
Demands redress ...
To cheer the sad; to chide the querelous;
The careless warn; th' irregular reprove;
And wholesome counsel kindly give to all.[30]

Figure 5.3

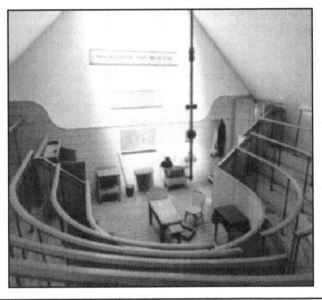

The Women's Operating Theatre of Old St Thomas's Hospital, 1821-62. While partly conjectural, the reconstruction of the operating room, in the roof of the old St Thomas's Church, in Southwark, gives us as authentic idea of an operating theatre of the 1820s as we are ever likely to obtain.

This was clearly an orderly and well-managed institution: other hospitals were less so. Some aspects of hospital life of course remain eternal: Wilde complained that daytime in the ward was one 'continual interruption' while at night the patients were put to bed too early 'even if I had been free of pain' and left in darkness.

'Not so quiet': the operating room

Many patients, especially the well-to-do, underwent operations at home: their experience is virtually invisible. The poor and those with 'interesting' conditions faced surgery in the operating rooms of the great hospitals. As with many other aspects of medical practice no consistent pattern can be found in hospitals' policies toward operating rooms. Some hospitals allowed spectators into the theatre, others forbade entry to all but students and guests, and then only professionals. In Dublin James Cusack was supposed to have charged admittance, erecting a proscenium arch and curtains and issuing tickets.[31] Bart's allowed spectators without restraint or charge. In 1831 the violin virtuoso Signor Paganini had a fancy to see a 'terrible operation' and joined the large crowd which had assembled in anticipation – disappointed on the day – of the removal of Mrs Cave's tumour.[32]

The rise of the medical school created the large, tiered operating theatre: before 1821 operations in Dorcas, one of the women's wards at St Thomas's, were conducted behind a screen in the ward.[33] Even so most operating rooms were crowded: Bransby Cooper's theatre at Guy's was an 'ill-ventilated, inconvenient hole'.[34] John Flint South recalled St Thomas's in the Regency. The scramble for seats reminded him of 'the rush and scuffle to get a place in the pit or gallery of a dramatic theatre'.[35] St Thomas's had two theatres, for men and women respectively. Both were found to be too small and a new women's theatre was opened built in the roof of the adjoining St Thomas's Church. This, now the 'Old Operating Theatre', has been preserved, the only part of the hospital to survive its removal in the 1860s to a site opposite the Houses of Parliament. This room gives a moving impression of the general arrangement of operating theatres. The table stood under a large, translucent skylight illuminating the operating area much more clearly than candles or later gas lamps. For this reason most operations occurred in the daytime, usually in the afternoon. Rows of benches or 'standings' rose in a horseshoe around the table. Here the students stood crushed in 'like herrings in a barrel,' South recalled, 'but not so quiet'.

By mid-century however virtually all operating rooms had become larger and better lit. In most hospitals built during the nineteenth century operating theatres – most included tiers to accommodate students and visitors – were accorded a higher status. The new Westminster Hospital, for example, which opened in 1834 was designed as a shallow U-shape of five floors (including basement and attic). Large, spacious wards ran off the broad central corridor each 'ingeniously arranged' with windows and ventilators. At the centre of the U on the upper floor was the large operating theatre. Surgeons – even before anaesthesia rendered their work less shocking – had attained a symbolic centrality denied their adversaries the physicians. Although larger and more imposing, their theatres were uniformly intimidating: James Crichton-Browne remembered Edinburgh's later in the century as 'rather grim and terrifying': how much more so it must have been before 1850 we can only speculate.[36]

We might imagine that contemporaries casually subjected patients to the gaze of dozens and or possibly hundreds of curious spectators. However surgeons at Guy's told the Charity Commissioners in the 1830s that they respected 'the wishes of a patient ... who expresses a disinclination to be operated upon in public'. Moreover, sensitive to modesty, they arranged women's operations, especially gynaecological, ones in smaller rooms from which idle spectators were excluded.[37] Whether surgeons in other hospitals entertained similar scruples is uncertain.

The operating theatre was the province of the Surgeryman and his assistants. We might presume that the employees of a hospital would be poeple who could find work nowhere else, who accepted the uncongenial, unpleasant and even dangerous work because they could find no other. Samuel Wilkes's and George Bettany's description of Monson Hill, Guy's Hospital's Surgeryman, suggests otherwise. Hill was medically unqualified but was recommended by a physician as a 'cupper' – one who formed the blisters that were a part of the prevailing anti-phlogistic regime. Hill was responsible for the good order and administration of the operating room. Known as the 'Governor' he oversaw much of the routine work of the dressers, becoming a friend and confidante to generations of students. He was often called at night by dressers perplexed by insensible patients and saved them embarrassment and criticism by dropping a hint or a quiet suggestion. A model of modest Victorian achievement, Hill saw one son succeed him and another qualify as a doctor before his death in 1853.[38] Although it was not hinted at in his eulogy he may have been one of the links between Guy's and the resurrection men who, through much of his tenure, supplied its dissecting rooms. Nor was it made clear that Hill's strength would often have been called upon to restrain a struggling patient in the grim and disorderly choreography of the operating room.

A certain etiquette prevailed in most hospital operating rooms. The floor closest to the table was reserved for distinguished visitors to the hospital who sat on specially-placed chairs. Medical staff of the hospital and their dressers sat in the lower tier. The upper tiers held students and visiting medical men in general. Spectators were, as Charles Bell wrote, 'bound to certain rules' not to intervene. Watching a botched operation at the Middlesex Hospital, he wrote that as 'a spectator merely, it was torture to me'.[39] The etiquette that prevented Bell from intervening, however, did not prevail in all operating rooms. Medical periodicals repeatedly carried letters complaining that 'strangers' intruded into the vicinity of the table, that students wearing hats obscured the view of those behind them and that dressers got in everyone's way. At Bart's calls of 'heads' were often heard from pupils on the upper tiers.[40] 'Spectator' complained to the *Lancet* in 1831 that at St Thomas's, students' cries of 'dressers' heads' so irritated Joseph Green that he stopped while excising a tumour from a boy's neck to deliver a brief homily correcting their conduct.[41]

The operating room witnessed terrible scenes of suffering. Indeed its distinguishing characteristic would have been the noise heard within and beyond it. Astley Cooper's new wife, Mary, lived within Guy's and could hear the cries of patients across the courtyard. It is possible that sound carried both ways. When the Edinburgh Royal Infirmary had its surgical block in the old Edinburgh High School, operations proceeded 'amidst the very audible shouts and laughter of happy children' playing in a yard below.[42] Could the children hear patients screaming in the operating room above them?

'Attention and solicitude': post-operative treatment

Closing and bandaging a wound did not, of course, mean the end of treatment or even of surgical intervention and certainly not the end of pain. Arteries not properly closed obliged surgeons to re-enter the wound to suture them. This, Samuel Cooper lamented, was most unfortunate. Removing the dressings to close an inflamed incision was 'a very painful proceeding'. Indeed 'nothing can exceed the suffering' of a patient compelled to endure such a procedure. Even worse, a badly-fashioned stump or a wound tied so as to irritate a nerve could entail a second operation. Cooper warned that this would prove 'exceedingly unpleasant' – for the surgeon, he meant – because patients were 'apt to suspect' that the first had not been properly managed (possibly with some justice).[43]

The time a patient remained in hospital, or at least under the surgeon's care, depended on several considerations. Those being nursed at home generally recovered more swiftly; those in hospital usually suffered from infection. Fundamentally, healing depended upon the quality of post-operative care. Contesting the prevailing ethos of the heroic surgeon, John Erichsen acknowledged that it was not so much surgical skill as post-operative treatment that made the difference between survival and death.[44] Surgeons attempting union could hope for a wound to close in perhaps a month. When subjected to 'heavy' dressings or when wounds were, as Samuel Cooper put it, 'stuffed with lint', healing could take two or more months.[45] Increasingly, the emphasis on lighter dressings and healing by first intention – although often confounded by the physical environment of a ward – resulted in patients' stays in hospital becoming shorter.

Figure 5.4

This engraving of Rahere Ward, St Bartholomew's Hospital, 1832
suggests how critical nursing care was to the operation of a hospital
decades before the transformation wrought by Florence Nightingale.

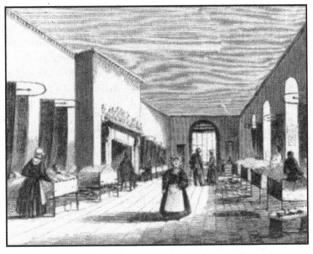

The changes in post-operative care have been attributed to
changes in nursing care. In the decades before Florence Nightingale
effected the dramatic changes from about 1860 nurses have often
been unfairly regarded as slatterns and drunkards. The impression
persists defying abundant evidence to the contrary. The power of the
Nightingale legend still obscures or distorts the character of nurses
before 1860. Nurses have been regarded as essentially hospital
domestics. However, besides removing 'all dust and nastiness' from a
ward and keeping it 'neat and clean', the 1816 regulations in
Edinburgh also made clear that nurses were to 'give or apply the
medicines' and to remain 'attentive to the state and symptoms of the
patients'.[46]

Nightingale's own statistics (from fifteen London hospitals)
disclose that far from being old Gamps or teenage skivvies the great
majority were aged between 25 and 40. If they had not chosen
nursing as a vocation these women at least practised it as an
occupation.[47] Ward sisters maintained positions of standing within
hospital communities. The chief nurse on each ward at Guy's was
called 'The Sister of the Ward': one was Mrs Clarke, the widow of a
disgraced army physician, in reduced but still respectable

circumstances.[48] At Bart's the ward sisters were traditionally known by the name of the ward for which they were responsible; 'Sister Charity' or 'Sister Rahere'. John Chandler, Surgeon at St Thomas's early in the century, was celebrated for treating its nurses 'as if they had been ladies'.[49] The hospital's matron Mrs Sarah Savory explained to the Charity Commissioners that St Thomas's sisters were 'of a much higher class' in the mid-1830s than she had found on her appointment in 1816. 'They are far better educated & much more competent to discharge [an] office of trust & responsibility'.[50]

Examples of the characteristic Nightingalean virtues are apparent before her innovation. St Bartholomew's *Rules and Orders* of 1833 enjoined its nurses to 'watch and attend the sick and weak Patients, and ... give such Night Medicines as are required'.[51] George Guthrie, in describing the post-operative treatment of an aneurism, mentioned – without suggesting it was exceptional – how two nurses at Charing Cross Hospital gently rubbed a patient's leg for three days and nights.[52] It is evident that surgeons valued nurses' experience and skill. Mary Owen, 'Sister Rahere' at Bart's, 'taught an erring house-surgeon how to compress a posterior tibial artery'.[53] At St George's Hospital in 1832 there was 'an old nurse' who 'from long experience understood these matters'(in this case the proper care of aneurism).[54]

Like surgery itself, then, post-operative care underwent a modest transformation before 1850. A.J. Youngson in *The Scientific Revolution in Victorian Medicine* argues that before the Listerian transformation of the 1870s and '80s surgeons were not much interested in the patient's welfare after surgery. This may have been so especially earlier in the period but the evidence suggests a growing commitment to post-operative care, by students as well as surgeons. As often as not in earlier decades the care of patients after operations would have been casual and entrusted to unsupervised students. Increasingly, surgeons complied with Samuel Cooper's injunction that a surgeon ought to 'extend his attention and solicitude' to those in his care as well as merely operating upon them.[55] This growing concern for welfare is part of the 'rise of respectable society' discernible in nineteenth century Britain. It is manifest in such phenomena as opposition to slavery, the factory reform movement, the movement to abolish flogging in the services and the greater paternalism of local charity. The abuses publicised in the early decades of the century became part of the process of their elimination. In hospitals the key development in improving post-operative treatment may have been a result of the hospital's greater teaching role which made available a large workforce of carers –

admittedly indifferently skilled and variably motivated – in the form of students. Despite their efforts, however, patients continued to contract a range of surgical fevers.

'Surgical fevers': erysipelas, pyaemia and gangrene

Surgical fever came in many forms and much of the surgeon's training was directed to detecting and defeating it. They learned to identify it by its appearance and accompanying symptoms, by its smell and even its feel. The most common post-operative infections were erysipelas, pyaemia and gangrene.

Erysipelas turned the patient's skin bright red, clear and shiny: it was known among Scottish students as 'the rose'.[56] Around 1829 Samuel Cooper candidly admitted that 'we absolutely know nothing about the immediate cause' of the infection although he suspected it to be contagious.[57] James Syme writing fifteen years later acknowledged that 'this alarming state ... may be regarded from the first as all but incurable'

Characteristically surgeons adopted divergent and competing treatments for erysipelas. At the North London Hospital in the 1830s four house surgeons advocated and practised four methods of treatment.[58] One applied nitrate of silver; another favoured mercurial ointment; a third lines of lunar caustic; a fourth fomentations and applications of flour. The four surgeons discussed the remedies in their lectures to the hospital's students. Although they mostly maintained either civility or silence in commenting on the others' cases Robert Liston (who favoured the older treatment of fomentations) could not resist saying some 'very uncivil and very bitter things'. He ridiculed the use of nitrate of silver – 'turning a white man into a nigger' – and sarcastically doubted the use of lunar caustic, 'drawing lines horizontally, perpendicularly and slantingularly over a patient's body'. Other surgeons adopted more direct methods. James Syme grew doubtful of the benefits of 'leaching, puncturing or scarifying' but still prescribed the common treatment of cutting incisions along limbs affected by erysipelas. The cuts could be repeated twice daily.[59] Robert Druitt decried small punctures as ineffective and causing 'considerable pain' but endorsed incisions of up to five inches 'as often as necessary'.[60] John Macfarlane of the Glasgow Royal Infirmary went further, making ten-inch incisions and claiming to see the infection 'instantly arrested'.[61]

Suppuration, or pyaemia, had long been considered unavoidable and even necessary and desirable to the process of healing. 'The old surgeons', Samuel Cooper explained to a generation which no longer

147

entirely accepted the laudability of pus, spoke of 'digestion' in the healing of wounds. By this they meant 'bringing [a wound] into a state in which it formed healthy pus'.[62] Joseph Pancoast contested the acceptance of this idea arguing that surgeons 'since the time of Hunter had considered that this opinion is founded merely on prejudice'.[63] From about 1790 surgeons increasingly sought to promote union by first intention. William Hey writing at the end of the eighteenth century declared that surgeons who preferred the doctrine of laudatory pus to be 'defective either in knowledge or humanity' and by the 1840s James Syme was able to claim that healing by first intention was 'always sought for in this country'.[64] The notion became one of the distinguishing features of British surgery. Samuel Cooper described union by first intention as 'the pride of English surgery', one of the greatest 'advances to perfection' ever made in a time of rapid and significant progress.[65] Conversely the Continental practice of packing wounds with lint charpie, often soaked in oil, became associated with unduly prolonged healing. Because suppuration remained so common, however, the idea of 'laudable pus' died hard. Even so surgeons increasingly regarded the inflammation they encountered in the hospital wards as aberrant and undesirable rather than normal and desirable.

Gangrene was then, and remains, the most feared post-operative infection. It has lodged in the imaginations of generations of fiction and screen writers as the representative pre-modern infection: possibly because it is easier to spell than erysipelas. Gangrene was rightly dreaded.* Benjamin Brodie described a 'sloughing stump'. It became inflamed, swollen, painful and tender. The surgeon would loosen the bandages and would see – and smell – a dirty discharge soaking through the dressings. Removing the dressing he would find entire surfaces ulcerated and rotting. The tissue turned to a black slime with the bone either showing through or projecting depending on the wound. The condition progressed seemingly inexorably with cold sweats, palpitations, convulsions.[66] Delirium was rare as Robert

---

* We might suppose that the 'gangrene' these surgeons confronted to be the same as the mortification seen in the Great War. In fact, the later kind – 'gas gangrene' was much more virulent. Earlier surgeons saw 'Phagendaena Gangrenosa', a suppurating ulcer, though one still intractable. See H. Home Blackadder, *Observations in Phagendaena Gangrenosa* (Edinburgh: Balfour & Clarke, 1818) and Anthony Bowlby, *The Hunterian Oration on British Military Surgery in the Time of Hunter and in the Great War* (London: Arnold & Sons, 1919).

Druitt pointed out so the patient retained 'a miserable consciousness of suffering till the end'.[67] Even distinguished surgeons who must have seen gangrene often differed on one of its supposedly classical symptoms: the two Coopers, Astley and Samuel, disagreed over whether hiccoughing constituted a 'characteristic' sign (as Astley claimed) of the condition and whether it inevitably heralded death (which Samuel did not).[68] Samuel Cooper, writing in the 1820s, conceded after describing its symptoms and treatment in detail that ultimately gangrene remained a 'perfect mystery' despite, in insisting on cleanliness so that the wound remained 'perfectly free from contamination', favouring the route to its defeat.[69]

Soon after, however, the consensus of surgical thought identified the spread of gangrene (though not its cause) in crowding patients together, by 'inattention to cleanliness and comfort, and to free ventilation'. This, George Guthrie concluded reflecting on his wartime experience, 'was too firmly established ... to be a matter of doubt'.[70] The hospital regime Robert Druitt recommended indicated the extent of change within wards. He advised ventilating wards and washing patients, with frequent changes of linen and bedclothes and the 'instant removal of all excrements and filth'.[71] He urged 'the most scrupulous care' in washing bandages in boiling water if they were to be re-used but recommended their immediate destruction and the use of disposable tow or lint dressings. Patients with gangrene should be separated from others and 'the utmost care' taken not to convey infection from them by 'sponges or dressings, or even by the fingers or instruments of the surgeon'. Druitt was not unusual: other writers recommended boiling water 'sufficient for the purification of whatever it can be made to touch'.[72]

The regime Druitt advocated became commonplace and the gangrene that Brodie had described became an increasingly unusual sight or smell in the hospitals of Britain ('hardly to be seen now' a student noted in one of Robert Liston's lectures).[73] Already by the late 1820s Samuel Cooper could justifiably claim that in England at least surgeons lost few patients to gangrene. In 1836 an English student in Dublin heard a local surgeon describing gangrene as 'seldom met with in the present day'.[74] James Syme, in his *Principles of Surgery* published in 1842, devoted only a cursory three pages to gangrene (even though, as his ward journals disclose, he continued to lose patients to it). By the 1860s – still 10 years before the acceptance of antiseptic surgery and still, according to the conventional interpretation, in the 'dirty' era – erysipelas and gangrene remained an occasional though diminishing feature of hospital life. The

149

transformation relied above all on the material used for dressings and its usage. Early in the century dressings often comprised discarded linen. The Royal Infirmary repeatedly appealed to Edinburgh's middle class for 'Linen Rags, Old Sheets, Shirts or Table Cloths' while Charles James Fox sent his linen to St George's Hospital.[75] Later tow was adopted which could not be used as often. By the 1840s sponges were rarely seen and seldom used to dress more than one patient and tow dressings were burned after use.[76] Even in the 1840s St Thomas's used 800 pounds of disposable tow a year.[77] John Bristowe and Timothy Holmes, in their comprehensive report on English hospitals in 1864, reported on the widespread use of disposable dressings and the abandonment of sponges. They believed that the most important disposing factors were 'dirt and especially the negligent dressing of wounds', a conclusion they found 'well established'. They learned that at St George's (despite its poor reputation, perhaps founded on Fox's used underwear) erysipelas had been no more than 'sporadic' over fifteen years. Hospital after hospital they found 'free from hospital odour'[78]

The degree to which the surgery of the period was 'dirty' or 'clean' remains a contested question. It is not difficult to find instances to support the view that operators and hospitals were filthy. Even though he idolised his uncle, Bransby Cooper described how Astley Cooper met George IV wearing a blood-stained shirt and with blood-stained hands.[79] Alfred Poland, Aston Key's apprentice from 1839 and assistant surgeon at Guy's from 1849, was so careless of his appearance that he would leave the dissecting room without changing his coat. (Naturally he suffered from, among half-a-dozen other conditions, chronic pus-forming infections.)[80] Lacking a germ theory until the 1870s it would seem likely that 'modern surgeons' did not have a modern understanding of the causes of infection and its transmission. Still the desire for cleanliness – perhaps honoured as often in the breach – gradually grew. Naval surgeons, for example, insisted on cleanliness from the 1790s. It was 'indispensably necessary for the preservation of health' and ships' orders strove to impose it.[81] As early as 1807 naval surgeons such as William Beatty directed that dressing sponges be used once and discarded 'together with the water'.[82] By the 1840s clear signs of change were apparent: in hospitals urging surgeons to clean operating coats and bedding and to ban the performance of post-mortems before surgery.[83] Thomas Pettigrew marvelled that his predecessors had devised treatments that might have been intended to impede rather than assist the processes of nature. 'It almost appears miraculous', he wrote loftily, 'that they ever ... produced union of any wound whatever'.[84]

Even so, the cleanest hospitals still suffered from outbreaks of seemingly intractable infection: it suffused the very fabric of the building. Patient after patient would succumb to erysipelas, pyaemia or gangrene, sometimes one after another in the same bed. Wards would be closed, aired, scrubbed, fumigated and whitewashed in an attempt to be rid of the scourge. Sometimes the infection would be suppressed. More often it would return when patients and, more importantly, surgeons and other staff returned. It lived on them: in the threads of their aprons and operating coats, in the very dirt under their fingernails. As long as they remained unaware of the nature of infection they would unknowingly threaten their patients' lives. Benjamin Brodie told a story about a country girl who one summer entered St George's Hospital for a medical condition. On the journey to London the whalebone in her corset 'slightly chafed' her breast. Within days of arriving at the hospital erysipelas had spread across her chest. The skin became gangrenous and she died in a state of 'complete mortification'.[85] As A.J. Youngson pointed out, the increasing concern over 'hospitalism' – the seemingly ineradicable mortality attributable to hospitals – meant that Lister's antiseptic regime competed with hospitals which were witnessing diminishing mortality rates anyway because they were being kept cleaner.[86]

Lister's understanding of the nature of gangrene had been shaped while a dresser under James Syme in the 1840s. An example taken from Syme's case books illustrates the difficulty in treating gangrene. John Seaman, a 39-year-old carter, had been driving a wagon loaded with cinders up a hill when the wagon struck him on the thigh inflicting a two-inch wound on the inner surface of his left leg and fracturing his tibia. Bandaged and splinted, he was carried to the Infirmary on 17 April 1844. Complaining of 'a good deal' of pain in his swollen foot, he slept with the help of opiates. A week later, 'very restless', his lower leg remained swollen and inflamed with fragments of bone pressing on the skin although a couple of days later Lister optimistically noted that the wound seemed to be cleaner. By 28 April, however, Seaman's foot began to turn blue while the distinctive red line of separation above the ankle told of gangrene. 'His countenance' Lister noted 'has an expression of great anxiety'. By the next day the pain in his mortifying foot had ceased and Syme decided to offer him 'the only chance which remains of saving his life': amputation. Later that day Syme performed a double-flap operation at mid-thigh. Seaman bore the operation well losing little blood. Afterwards, though, his pulse remained feeble despite taking an ounce of wine each hour and later whisky and wine in turns. In the early hours of 30 April he was seized with a convulsion and died.[87] We may suppose that his was a common fate, and so it was, but John Seaman was statistically unlucky.

'Not all dead?': hospital mortality

In August 1792 a satirist published a verse in *The Times* 'on the dissolution of a Partnership, between a Surgeon and Undertaker'. The poet's conceit, occasioned by a dramatic fall in the annual bills of mortality, was that they had 'dwelt in one house, they carved meat for each other': 'whom one potion'd to Death, was tenant for brother'.[88] The surgical mortality before the acceptance of Lister's antiseptic regime appalls us. Mortality rates of up to 50% or higher – often represented as typical of the period – lead us to regard surgery as having been irresponsibly dangerous. Medical writers at the time were also understandably preoccupied with the proportion of deaths. The *Lancet* published a conversation alleged to have occurred at Guy's in which Aston Key asked a dresser about one of his patients. 'Dead, Sir', the dresser replied:

> Mr K. 'How is the man in the next ward?
> Dresser 'Dead, Sir.'
> Mr K 'Oh, very well! [A pause] How is the patient in the other ward?'
> Dresser 'Dead, Sir.' ...
> Mr K. 'Why they're not all dead?
> Dresser 'Yes, Sir, they are'.
> 'That's strange!' Key remarked. 'Not at all' a 'sepulchral' voice replied.[89]

One of the defining characteristics of modern surgery was that patients ought to survive it. By the 1830s the former acceptance of high rates of mortality as inescapable had begun to be supplanted by an awareness that deaths could be avoided. The satirical jibe at Key was conceivable because two conditions had altered. The spirit of reform which the *Lancet* represented prompted a dig at a dictatorial surgeon believed to have secured his position through influence. The ostensible subject of the attack – the surgical mortality at Guy's – was likewise possible only because medical authorities and the profession as a whole had ceased to accept high mortality as inescapable.

The growing body of statistics increasingly maintained requires specialised analysis but they reveal a broadly apparent trend: surgery became less dangerous as the century advanced. Forbes Winslow provided figures for two institutions – the combined hospitals of Guy's and St Thomas's – which make the point impressively. In 1741 the ratio of deaths to 'cures' (by which he meant living discharges) was 1 to 10. In 1780 it had dropped to 1: 14; in 1813 to 1:16 and by 1827 1: 48.[90] In other words, in the previous quarter-century a hospital stay had become five times safer than it had been when the Hunters practised. Comparable figures from naval hospitals – 1 in 8 dead in 1780, 1 in 30 in 1812, 1 in 72 in 1830 – substantiate the impression that 'something like a revolution in hygiene and treatment' occurred around the turn of the eighteenth century.[91]

It is important to distinguish between types of operations and their venues and to recognise that mortality rates changed over time. Rates of mortality varied markedly between hospitals and between surgeons within hospitals. At University College Hospital in the 1840s mortality from amputations prompted by injury averaged 31%, ranging from almost perfect survival rates for operations on the arms to nearly 60% mortality for amputations at the thigh. Similar operations motivated by disease, however, averaged only 19%, with mortality from amputations at the thigh amounting to 20%[92] Earlier in the century of 77 operations Astley Cooper performed for hernia, one in two had died and yet he had written the textbook. By 1842-43 though, in six operations for hernia at St George's Hospital, despite surgeons removing portions of the intestines, regarded as certain death in earlier decades, five survived.[93] The statistics are, therefore, bewilderingly diverse and merit specialist analysis rather than spot inspection. E.M. Sigsworth's revisionist view of hospitals based on the York County Hospital suggests a considerable variance with the conventional view. He found that in the 1820s and '30s the percentage of patients dying in hospital did not exceed 6.3% and that mortality for a range of operations in several hospitals varied between 8 and 17%: hardly the 40% supposedly widespread.[94]

In general, then, mortality rates declined but boldness in innovation resulted in high rates of mortality for novel operations such as hernia, some aneurism operations, hip amputations and ovariotomies. Even so, the figures were bad enough and they remained unacceptable long after the introduction of anaesthesia. Although sceptical of Lister's antiseptic theories James Simpson conceded in 1869 that 'the man laid on an operating table in one of our surgical hospitals' was 'exposed to more chances of death than the English soldier on the field of Waterloo'.[95] Setting aside the difficulties of comparing different figures at different times at different hospitals the mortality rates make gloomy reading. The variations suggest the difficulty of drawing universal conclusions across the period and between hospitals. But generally, because of more effective post-operative care and greater attention to cleanliness, mortality decreased albeit gradually and all too slowly.

Notes.

1. E.M. Sigsworth, 'Gateways to death?: Medicine, Hospitals and Mortality, 1700–1850', in Peter Mathias (ed.) *Science and Society 1600–1900* (Cambridge: CUP, 1972), 97–110.
2. 'Statement to the Managers of the Royal Infirmary', 2 July 1834, Add Ms 84, RCSEng.
3. Thomas Hood, *Hood's Own: or, Laughter from Year to Year* (London: A.H. Baily & Co., 1839), 267–69.
4. Guenter Risse, *Hospital Life in Enlightenment Scotland: Care and Teaching at the Royal Infirmary of Edinburgh* (Cambridge: CUP, 1986); Lisa Rosner, *Medical Education in the Age of Improvement: Edinburgh Students and Apprentices 1760–1826* (Edinburgh: Edinburgh University Press, 1991).
5. Leonard Horner to Dr Marcet, 13 December 1817, Ms 9818, f. 75, NLS.
6. 'Notes of a Northern Tour by a Southern Lecturer', *Lancet*, 1833–34, Vol. I, 899.
7. Robert Paterson, *Memorials of the Life of James Syme* (Edinburgh: Edmonston & Douglas, 1874), 48.
8. Benjamin Golding, *The Origin, Plan and Operations of the Charing Cross Hospital* (London: W.H. Allen, 1867), 77.
9. *Lancet*, 1843–44, Vol. I, 326–27.
10. J.F. Clarke, *Autobiographical Recollections* (London: J. & A. Churchill, 1874), 259.
11. Lindsay Granshaw, '"Fame and fortune by means of bricks and mortar": the medical profession and specialist hospitals in Britain, 1800–1948', in Lindsay Granshaw & Roy Porter, *The Hospital in History* (London: Routledge, 1989), 199–220, 199–220.
12. F.G. Parsons, *The History of St Thomas's Hospital*, 3 vols (London: Methuen, 1936), *Vol. III*,, 5; 42; 44.
13. F.B. Smith, *The People's Health 1830–1910* (London: Croom Helm, 1979), 267.
14. John Ford (ed.), *A Medical Student at St Thomas's Hospital, 1801–1802 The Weekes Family Letters* (London: Wellcome Institute for the History of Medicine, 1987), 24.
15. Smith, *op. cit.* (note 13), 251.
16. *The Times*, 26 February 1846, 5e.

17. PP 1840, Vol. XIX, 32nd Report of the Charity Commissioners [into Guy's Hospital], Table II, 746.

18. *The Times*, 11 July 1835, 3f.

19. St Thomas's admission ticket, CHAR/2, 387, PRO.

20. 'The Hospital Patient', in Charles Dickens, *Sketches by Boz: Illustrative of Every-Day Life & Every-Day People*, 'The Hospital Patient' (London: John Macrone, 1836).

21. 'In Memoriam Samuel Wilks', *Guy's Hospital Reports*, Vol. LXVII (3rd Series), 1913, 3.

22. John Bell, *The Principles of Surgery*, 2 vols (Edinburgh: T. Cadell & W. Davies, 1801), Vol. III, 292–93.

23. Thomas Percival, *Medical Ethics, or A Code of Institutes and Precepts* ... (Oxford: J.H. Parker, 1849), 39.

24. J. Frederick Watson, *The History of Sydney Hospital from 1811 to 1911* (Sydney: W.A. Gullick, 1911), 42–44; 59–61; 108.

25. St Thomas's Hospital, CHAR/2, 387, PRO.

26. Smith, *op. cit.* (note 13), 262.

27. PP 1840, Vol. XIX, 32nd Report of the Charity Commissioners.

28. 'In Memoriam Samuel Wilks', *Guy's Hospital Reports*, Vol. LXVII (3rd Series), 1913, 3.

29. Managers Visiting Books, 1818–71, LHB/1/6/1, LHSA.

30. J. Wilde, *The Hospital, a Poem in Three Books, Written in the Devon and Exeter Hospital*, (Norwich: Stevenson, Matchett & Stevenson, 1809), 37.

31. *Lancet*, 1825–26, Vol. II, 178.

32. *The Times*, 6 December 1831, 1e.

33. Ford, *op. cit.* (note 14), 17.

34. Clarke, *op. cit.* (note 10), 523.

35. John Flint South, *Memorials of John Flint South* (Fontwell: Centaur Press, 1970), 27.

36. James Crichton-Browne, *Victorian Jottings from an Old Commonplace Book* (London: Etchells & Macdonald, 1926), 121.

37. PP 1840, Vol XIX, 32nd Report of the Charity Commissioners [into Guy's Hospital], 740.

38. Samuel Wilks & G.T. Bettany, *A Biographical History of Guy's Hospital* (London: Ward & Lock, London, 1892), 422–25.

39. Charles Bell to George Bell, 23 March 1805 George Joseph Bell, (ed.), *Letters of Sir George Bell* (London: John Murray, 1870), 40.

40. *Lancet*, 1831–32, Vol. I, 379.

41. *Ibid*, 229.

42. Crichton-Browne, *op. cit.* (note 36), 121.

43. Samuel Cooper, *A Dictionary of Practical Surgery* (London: Longman, Hurst, Rees, Orme & Brown, 1829), 80–81.

44. John Erichsen, *On the Study of Surgery* (London: Taylor, Walton & Maberly, 1850), 29–30 .

45. Cooper, *op. cit.* (note 43), 302–03.

46. Royal Infirmary of Edinburgh, *Regulations respecting Nurses* (Edinburgh: 1816), 1–4.

47. Note A 'On the Mortality of Hospital Nurses', in Florence Nightingale, *Notes on Hospitals* (London: John Parker & Sons, 1863), 20 .

48. Bransby Cooper, *The Life of Sir Astley Cooper, Bart.*, 2 vols (London: John Parker, 1843), Vol. I, 148.

49. Parsons, *op. cit.* (note 12), Vol. III, 37.

50. Evidence of Mrs Savory, St Thomas's Hospital, CHAR/2, 387, PRO.

51. *Rules and Orders for the Government of St Bartholomew's Hospital*, 1833, 89, CHAR/2, 386, PRO.

52. George Guthrie, *Commentaries on the Surgery of the War in Portugal, Spain, France, and the Netherlands* (London: Renshaw, 1853), 256.

53. Geoffrey Yeo, *Nursing at Bart's: A History of Nursing Service and Nurse Education at St Bartholomew's Hospital, London* (London: St Bartholomew's and Princess Alexandra and Newham College of Nursing, 1995), 20.

54. *Lancet*, 1831–32, Vol. II, 265.

55. Cooper, *op. cit.* (note 43), 216.

56. James Gregory, *Additional Memorial to the Managers of the Royal Infirmary* (Edinburgh: Murray & Cochrane, 1803), 340.

57. Cooper, *op. cit.* (note 43), 453–54.

58. Clarke, *op. cit.* (note 10), 312–13.

59. James Syme, *Principles of Surgery* (Edinburgh: Sutherland & Knox, 1842), 441–42.

60. Robert Druitt, *The Principles and Practice of Modern Surgery* (Philadelphia: Lea & Blanchard, 1842), 85–86.

61. John Macfarlane, *Clinical Reports of the Surgical Practice of the Royal Infirmary* (Glasgow: D. Roberston, 1832), 257–58.

62. Cooper, *op. cit.* (note 43), 374.

63. Joseph Pancoast, *A Treatise on Operative Surgery* (Philadelphia: Carey & Hart, 1852), 137.

64. William Hey, *Practical Observations in Surgery* (London: T. Cadell Jnr & W. Davies, [1803; 1814]), p. 526; Syme, op. cit. (note 59), 148.

65. Cooper, *op. cit.* (note 43), 78; 152.

66. Benjamin Brodie, *Clinical Lectures on Surgery* (Philadelphia: Lea & Blanchard, 1846), 42; Cooper, *op. cit.* (note 43),, 868–73.

67. Druitt, *op. cit.* (note 60), 98.

68. Astley Cooper & Frederick Tyrrell, *The Lectures of Sir Astley Cooper, Bart.* ... (London: Thomas Tegg, 1824), 215; Cooper, *op. cit.* (note 43), 873.

69. Cooper, *op. cit.* (note 43), 145; 700–03.

70. Guthrie, *op. cit.* (note 52), 156.

71. Druitt, *op. cit.* (note 60), 100–102.

72. James Fergusson, (ed.), *Notes and Recollections of a Professional Life* (London: Longman, Brown, Green & Longmans, 1846), 97.

73. H. McBean's 'Notes from the Surgical Lectures of Mr Robert Liston', Edinburgh, 1831–32, DK.4.23, UEA.

74. Notebook of R. Jones, December 1836, MS 6061, WIMH.

75. J. Blomfield, *St George's 1733–1933* (London: Medici Society, 1933), 35.

76. James Miller, *A Probationary Essay on the Dressing of Wounds* (Edinburgh: 1840), 18–19 .

77. PP 1840, Vol. XIX, 32nd Report of the Charity Commissioners [into St Thomas's Hospital], p. 708.

78. Bristowe and Holmes, PP XXVIII 1864, 475, 477, 577 .

79. Cooper, *op. cit.* (note 48), Vol. II, 234.

80. Wilks & Bettany, *op. cit.* (note 38), 353.

81. Alexander Stewart, *Medical Discipline, or Rules and Regulations for the More Effectual Preservation of Health* ... (London: Murray & Highley, 1798), np; Orders and Regulations, HMS Egmont, 1794–97, Mss 118, RNM.

82. 'Measures recommended for the eradication and prevention of Disease on board the Elizabeth', November 1807, Orders and Letters of Sir William Beattie [sic], Ms 417/88(2), RNM.

83. Guenter Risse, *Mending Bodies, Saving Souls: A History of Hospitals* (New York: OUP, 1999), 366.

84. Thomas Pettigrew, *On Superstitions Connected With the History and Practice of Medicine and Surgery* (London: J. Churchill, 1844), 163.

85. Brodie, *op. cit.* (note 66), 44.

86. A.J. Youngson, *The Scientific Revolution in Victorian Medicine* (New York: Croom Helm, 1979), 220–21.

87. Case no. 42, 'Journal of Surgical Wards, 1844...', RACS.

88. *The Times*, 15 August 1792, 3c.

89. *Lancet*, 1833–34, Vol. II, 176.

90. Forbes Winslow, *Physic and Physicians: A Medical Sketch Book*, 2 vols

(London: Longman, Orme, Brown, 1839), Vol. I, 40.

91. Christopher Lloyd, *The British Seaman 1200–1860: A Social Survey* (London: Paladin, 1970), 239 .

92. John Erichsen, *The Science and Art of Surgery* (London: Walton & Maberly, 1853), 60.

93. J.Y. Simpson, *Ovariotomy Is It – or Is It Not – an Operation Justifiable upon the Common Principles of Surgery?* (Edinburgh: Sutherland & Knox, 1846), 6.

94. Sigsworth, *op. cit.* (note 1), 110.

95. Simpson, 'Our existing system of hospitalism and its effects', *Edinburgh Medical Journal,* Mar 1869, 818.

6

'Gennelmen!':
Medical Students

A student who saw it often, described John Abernethy's customary 'irresistibly droll' entrance into the lecture theatre at Bart's.[1] He would slouch in, hands in pockets, often whistling. Throwing himself into a chair, he would swing a leg over its arm and begin lecturing. His calculated idiosyncrasy captured the attention of Bart's students for over twenty years. Once he stood in silence before the new students crowding the lecture hall, regarded them for a time and said 'God help you all'.[2] His apprehensions (a contemporary claims that he added 'What is to become of you?') were surely justified.[3]

The first half of the nineteenth century saw a decisive change in the nature of medical education. Formerly doctors had acquired the book learning and practical skills of what had been regarded as a trade by being apprenticed to a master. By mid-century the hospital and medical school had supplanted the independent practitioner and his apprentice. Medical studies increasingly came to comprise formal courses of lectures, classes in dissection, periods spent walking hospital wards, attendance at surgical operations and, for some, terms as 'dressers'. These studies culminated in examinations by the colleges governing admission to the profession.

'His secrets keep': apprenticeship

Some apprentices started very young. Edwin Lankester was not unusual in being indentured at twelve, while a surgery boy of fourteen could be mistaken for a student.[4] Andrew Combe recalled that on his first day of his apprenticeship at fifteen, he had to be dragged to the master's surgery.[5] The articles of indenture of a medical apprenticeship closely resembled those of a tradesman. William Getty in the 1820s promised 'his said Master' – his father or uncle – to 'faithfully ... serve, his secrets keep, his lawful commands ... gladly do'.[6] George Moreton's indentures which bound him in 1833 could have served him as well as a blacksmith or a cooper.[7] Not all ventured upon the business of medicine with any firm belief in the mission of healing. John Brown's description of an apprentice he met in Chatham could apply to many of his fellows: 'a good-natured

159

young man, with no great depth either of thought or feeling'.[8] It would perhaps be unreasonable to expect otherwise from students in any generation.

William Chamberlaine, in his *Dissertation on the Duties of Youth Apprenticed to the Medical Profession*, offered advice to doctors contemplating taking on apprentices and counselled young men pondering a medical career. He described the stench of dressing a neglected ulcer or carious bone and advised young men that 'if you cannot bear these things, put Surgery out of your head, and go be apprentice to a man-milliner or perfumer'.[9] Apprenticeship entailed much drudgery but also confronted young men with the realities of surgery. James Paget who became an eminent pioneer of pathology recalled the first operation he saw as an apprentice in 1830. He was called to attend while his master treated a young boatman with an injured arm and leg. Paget reflected that the boatman bore the amputations 'very bravely'. The apprentice retained his composure through the amputation of the thigh but found that 'when the first intense curiosity was over' he felt more opportunity for sympathy. As his master began operating on the man's arm Paget felt 'very faint, and had to stand aside, useless'.[10]

Apprentices notoriously displayed little desire to study and enjoyed many opportunities for distraction. Chamberlaine felt little regard for them or the system of medical education which produced them. He offered a compelling picture of idleness, describing the apprentice, who 'sits at his desk with his Pharmacopoeia before him ... over which he places ... the Newgate Kalendar ... or some book much worse than a silly Novel'. This, he complained, 'he makes <u>his</u> Study, and which, with a sleight-of-hand ... he ... whips under his seat when he hears his master's approach'.[11] Chamberlaine's poor opinion of apprentices perhaps reflected his misgivings about a system in which responsibility for teaching medicine fell on men often struggling to earn a living and often lacking either facilities or aptitude for instruction. At the same time his complaints of apprentices' shortcomings ring true and were certainly based on observation and hard-earned experience: 'Is he destructive of glassware?' he asked. 'Is he an early riser?' Above all 'IS HE APT TO GIVE SAUCY ANSWERS?'[12]

Apprenticeship sufficed as long as medicine resembled a trade in which doctors acquired and employed a relatively narrow range of clinical skills based on an equally circumscribed body of knowledge. As medical knowledge increased – indeed, as doctors recognised that the rate of increase was itself accelerating – it became desirable for specialised teachers to impart that knowledge. Young men seeking to become doctors needed to gain a wider clinical education that would have been possible within the limits of an apothecary's practice. The trend away from apprenticeship and toward institutional training became clearly marked. Early in the century more doctors qualified through apprenticeships than from the schools and even in 1850 many students had served several years as apprentices before finishing their training in a hospital. Increasingly, however, the medical school became established as the central institution by which young men became doctors and from which a few graduated to become surgeons.

'The art of cobbling': medical schools and courses

From the 1790s hospitals became finishing schools for medical apprentices. Aspiring doctors acquired both knowledge and skills by studying in one of the medical schools of the capitals in London, Edinburgh or Dublin, at Glasgow or the ten English provincial schools established between 1824 and 1834.[13] The numbers studying at any time were large. In 1786 130 students were studying in Edinburgh. By 1806 the number had risen to 366 and in 1826 to 574.[14] London hosted 800 students in the 1820s and by the 1840s perhaps 1,500 enrolled in the capital's hospitals and private schools at any time.[15] They came from all over the kingdom, the empire and the world. A list of graduands of Edinburgh in 1835 makes the point. Quaintly rendering their native places in Latin, of the 114 young men only 38 were identified as 'Scotus'. Thirty and 31 hailed from 'Hibernus' and 'Anglus' with five 'Ex India Orientalis' and four from 'Canadensis' or 'Neobrunsvicensis'[16] Lists from Glasgow in the early 1840s show that men of 'Hibernus' outnumbered those of 'Scotus' by about three to one and that like Edinburgh it attracted students from places as distant as 'Polonus', 'Jamaicensus', 'Americanis' and 'Mexicanus'.[17]

The preliminary qualifications required by the English and Scottish colleges were complex and often unclear. They differed between institutions, changed over time and were subject of public contention and private negotiation. By the 1840s there existed twenty ways of obtaining accreditation to practise medicine.[18] In essence, however, candidates intending to become general practitioners could have trained for four years. It struck some as curious that while a tailor or a shoemaker could not be regarded as fully trained in fewer than five or even seven years, 'four years ... are supposed to perfect a young gentleman in the art of cobbling the stomachs, skins and bones of his fellow creatures'.[19] The purely surgical component of this training was in any case much shorter.

The duration of the London syllabus set by the college, which included only anatomy, surgery and hospital attendance, was only sixteen months. The syllabus set by the Edinburgh college appeared longer and more varied but the Edinburgh year was even shorter than London's and comparing the two remains as difficult in retrospect as it was at the time. Against Edinburgh's range of subjects which gave students the broad training that would lead to the acceptance of the 'general practitioner', stood the advantage of range of cases available in London's wards.[20] Edinburgh also held the advantage of variety available through the 'extra-mural' schools affiliated with the university whose lecturers and demonstrators maintained high standards, enforced by open competition.

In either case medical education remained relatively superficial: Henry Spry, preparing to qualify as an Assistant Surgeon with the East India Company, told his patron that with nine months of study he could 'perfect myself in Surgery & Anatomy etc. etc..'[21] At the time, however, a full course of study in a good metropolitan hospital provided as thorough a grounding in medicine as a young man could obtain. By 1846 those students who attended King's College for the full three year course could expect to cover anatomy, physiology, 'materia medica', chemistry and botany in their first year. In the second more anatomy and physiology followed as well as dissection and pharmacy. In the third came surgery, midwifery and forensic medicine together with a growing emphasis on 'the practical pursuits of the hospital' through terms spent in the wards.[22]

Students arrived in London or Edinburgh ready for the commencement of the 'anatomical season' on 1 October. They had selected the hospital in which they would study on the recommendation of friends or family, by proximity to lodgings, increasingly by the reputation of its best-known surgeons or – how often – at random. The *Lancet* counselled prospective students to take care, publishing reports intended to correct abuses. In 1833 Guy's Hospital, with its handsome exterior, 'airy and inviting' entrance and 'lofty and well-ventilated' wards, might have appeared superficially attractive but Thomas Wakley warned against it. 'Alas!', he lamented, its surgeons attended irregularly and pupils had become the objects of insult even from hospital servants. St Thomas's, though less pleasing externally, offered better opportunities for surgical instruction. Its students were treated with 'liberality' and its wards were open to them up to seven hours a day. A Bart's student objected to its Dead House or mortuary, likening it to a pig-sty especially when half-a-dozen dressers were 'feeding' there. 'To describe it,' he claimed, 'would disgust your readers'. St George's seems to have represented the nadir. A pupil at the hospital, 'The Student's Friend', wrote exposing abuses there. He described surgeons and physicians as 'grossly irregular' in attending and claimed that the surgeons in particular were so seriously at loggerheads as to imperil the functioning of the hospital. From the perspective of St George's Board, though, the students' disorderly conduct led them to appoint 'spies' among the pupils.[23] As we have seen, medical politics intruded even into teaching.

Though assiduous students were known to attend lectures at other hospitals, most tended to remain within their own institution for the several years they spent in London. Students of one hospital were sometimes entitled to attend lectures and operations at others, drawn by the reputations of their surgeons or the advertisement of notable cases. Until the schism of the mid-1820s, St Thomas's and Guy's were effectively one institution while, as Sir Anthony Carlisle explained, there was 'a courtesy at the west end of town'.[24] In the 1830s the Westminster, St George's and the Middlesex hospitals, and in the 1840s students of University College and the Middlesex enjoyed reciprocal access to each others' wards.[25] They manifested an acute awareness of their interests, both economic and pedagogic. In 1836, for example, a large group of students met at the Crown and Anchor tavern in the Strand to deplore injustices in the examinations at Apothecaries Hall and, addressed by their hero Wakley, to urge the cause of medical reform generally.[26]

With medical education an important function of the metropolitan hospitals most maintained facilities and teachers to instruct students. Many of the honorary surgeons on their staffs were also professors, expected to devote part of their time to clinical instruction. St George's and the Westminster hospitals had no formal schools of their own and depended upon ancillary private schools in Great Windmill Street, effectively the Middlesex's school, from about 1812 until its decline in the 1830s. Although a consortium of the staff at the Westminster bought the Dean Street School in 1834 the hospital's board declined to support it and it remained only informally associated with the hospital for nearly two decades.[27] These private anatomical schools – the 'mushroom schools' as the *Lancet* called them – offered a fertile field for imaginative and competitive advertising, retailing what it described as the 'puffing and chicanery of self-created professors'.[28] They included Joseph Carpue's Dean Street School in Soho, Edward and Richard Grainger's in Webb Street, Frederick Tyrrell and William Lawrence's

Aldersgate School in the City, Joshua Brookes's at Blenheim Street and Lane's School in Pimlico. All but Brookes's school closed for the summer. Brookes's – notoriously filthy – remained open, keeping cadavers bearable by injecting them with nitre, consequently always smelling like a pork butcher's.

New students, Benjamin Brodie observed, seemed 'bewildered' by the world they encountered.[29] Like all new students, intimidated, entranced or distracted by the novelty of independent life in the metropolis. They entered studies guided imperfectly by family, friends and relations and were confronted by a diversity of choice possibly for the first time. Few besides those with medical fathers or uncles arrived with much idea of what to expect. Nor were they advised in advance of what they would face. The senior surgeons who delivered commencement addresses to the students of their institutions often had their remarks printed. They rarely, and then only obliquely, referred to the trauma into which their training would bring them.

'A great mixture of persons': medical students

The educational background of many students was, as James Wardrop lamented, 'very deficient'.[30] As the products of grammar schools, most possessed some classical learning. Not all teachers required such a facility. Sir Anthony Carlisle deprecated its value. He loftily observed that 'neither Hippocrates, Galen or Celcus, would be admitted to our diploma': if examined on the circulation of the blood, he explained, they would be failed.[31]

Investment in a medical education could have imposed a considerable burden on many students' families. At the most basic level many would attend hospitals for only a year ('all that our College requires' said Benjamin Brodie).[32] The cost of this would be perhaps twenty guineas tuition plus the cost of lodgings, food and additional courses at private schools. As a student in 1815 Thomas Wakley had an allowance of £80 a year, regarded as the minimum which a student needed.[33]. Richard Grainger, a private teacher of anatomy (and therefore more familiar with students' circumstances than their eminent hospital teachers), estimated that students were likely to have to find close to five hundred pounds for a reasonable course of study. At the same time he had known 'some gentlemen' pay a thousand pounds to 'distinguished surgeons in the Borough' for a five-year course, one that promised to give them both excellent medical training and useful patronage.[34]

Students remained characteristically hard up. Many made the

Figure 6.1

A London medical student in 1840, depicting the raffish
demeanour many medical students affected. Though dating from a
decade after the passing of the Anatomy Act the artist has added the
epigram 'We murder to dissect', reflecting the enduring popular
suspicion of medical students.

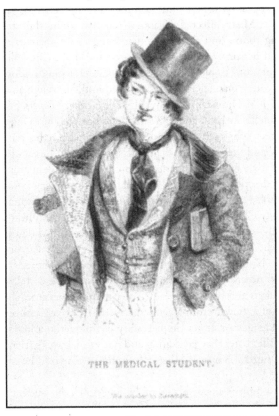

THE MEDICAL STUDENT.

acquaintance of 'uncle' within a month of term beginning, with
dissecting cases and tooth-drawing instruments appearing in pawnbrokers' windows in November followed shortly by watches.[35] The
typical student's plaint was that sent by Mungo Park (son of the
African explorer and a student at Edinburgh) to his uncle, a Scottish
provincial surgeon. 'If you could conveniently send me some money
… it would be very acceptable'.[36]

London's medical students constituted a distinct community

within the metropolis. 'In a medical school,' Benjamin Brodie reflected, 'there is a great mixture of persons'.[37] Recognisable by their top hats and raffish dress, by their impecunious habits – and perhaps by the odour of the dissecting room – they congregated in the cheap lodging and chop-houses surrounding the great teaching hospitals. In the 1840s they were described as 'a rough-looking lot', dressed flashily and fashionably though with notably grimy shirts, their faces adorned by moustaches and exuding 'an all-pervading smell of tobacco'.[38] Many affected cigars, to combat both the stench in dissecting rooms and the smells that hung about their irregularly-laundered persons.[39] Astley Cooper lamented that many fell prey to the 'temptations to pleasure and vice so numerous in London'.[40]

As a young man Charles Dickens lived in the Borough among the students of St Thomas's and Guy's. In *The Pickwick Papers*, published in instalments in 1836 and 1837, he described the cheap lodgings of Lant Street inhabited by transient tenants, where the rents were 'dubious' and the water was frequently cut off. Lant Street's residents included two medical students, Bob Sawyer and Benjamin Allen. Dickens describes them with heavy-handed irony. They lounge, feet on the table, smoking cigars, drinking neat brandy and eating oysters on a frosty Christmas morning. They discuss dissection heartily and too loudly to impress Mr Pickwick. 'Have you finished that leg yet?' asks Allen. 'Nearly,' replies Sawyer, 'it's a very muscular one for a child's ... Nothing like dissecting to give one an appetite.' The two students describe an operation with braggadocio telling the Pickwickians and two young ladies 'an agreeable anecdote' about the removal of a growth from a gentleman's head. Sawyer, 'enlivened' by the brandy, demonstrates the necessary technique on a loaf with an oyster knife. Later they go skating and one of Pickwick's friends falls. 'Are you hurt?,' Benjamin Allen asks him. 'I wish you'd let me bleed you ....'[41]

Albert Smith's characters, notably 'Joe Muff', the student hero of a series in *Punch's* first volume, offers another fictional prototype. [42] Corroboration is not hard to find, not least in their pranks. Bransby Cooper recorded how Astley Cooper's apprentices once placed a monkey's entrails in a box of hair powder laughing with 'immoderate effect' when Cooper's hairdresser plunged his hand into it.[43] William Gibney terrified his landlady's maid by writing 'REPENT' on her bedroom wall in phosphorus only visible in the dark.[44] Many students participated in body-snatching expeditions out of unthinking bravado. Much of the misconduct attributed to medical students stemmed from their youth and immaturity, many little

more than boys, facing an appalling reality. John Flint South recalled
that he and his fellows behaved like 'a parcel of schoolboys'.[45] Astley
Cooper recalled a telling exchange with a fellow student. 'Lord!
Cooper, what do you think I have done?' he asked. He had in fact
punctured a patient's radial artery while bleeding him but 'bound
him up and sent him away.'[46]

The physical realities of medical education were believed to
corrupt young men, many barely out of their teens and at liberty in
the metropolis: William Guy warned commencing students in 1846
that their predecessors had made the medical student 'a by-word for
vulgar riot and dissipation'.[47] Obstetrical lectures provoked what a
contemporary called 'shocking indecency' from youths aping the
worldly sophistication of their older colleagues.[48] A fragment of
dialogue in the *Lancet*, surely contrived, reflects both the students'
culture and the banter of the lecture room. Joseph Green was
summoned to examine a student suffering from gonorrhoea. His
lodgings were supposedly in Sutton Street near Guy's new anatomical
theatre. After gazing admiringly at the new building, Green exclaims
'A splendid erection, Sir' to which the student replies 'I can assure
you it is a d____d painful one'.[49] Many coped with the
unaccustomed sights and smells of the dissecting room by cultivating
a hearty indifference. A contemporary regarded 'drinking, smoking
and brawling' as 'the very rational occupations' encouraged by the
dissecting rooms. 'It was no uncommon thing', he claimed, 'to see a
regular battle among the students [with] parts of the human body
forming their weapons'.[50] This 'unseemly jesting', as William Fuller
called it, was a widespread tradition among medical students and has
only been restrained in recent decades.[51]

On the evidence of the introductory addresses delivered in many
hospitals at the beginning of October each year, students deserved
their reputation. Judging from the injunctions to sobriety and
industry and the warnings against idleness and bad company, they
clearly merited the advice. John Abernethy could speak in a
published lecture quite matter-of-factly about a student with a
venereal gleet, while the body of one of Burke and Hare's victims, the
beautiful prostitute Mary Paterson, was recognised by many of
Robert Knox's students.[52] Benjamin Brodie enjoined students at St
George's to 'feel and act as gentlemen': that the reminder was
considered necessary is sufficient evidence that many did not.[53]

Medical students were so much expected to behave badly that in
commending the Edinburgh Medical Society, a writer expressed
surprised pleasure at its student-members' respectability who debated

167

freely 'without deviating into licentiousness'.[54] It is important to acknowledge that the conventional image of the raffish medical student – to which many surely played up – obscured others who dressed drably, lived frugally, worked diligently and behaved quietly. Less obvious than their noisy colleagues, they are represented by H.V. Carter who admonished himself in 1849 with 'twelve directions for forming habits' including 'be simple and neat in your personal habits' and 'let there be no conversations in the hours of study'.[55] Like Benjamin Brodie, in the lecture room and the dissecting room he may have felt 'like a solitary person ... Between myself and the great majority of students there was nothing in common'.[56] There is, of course, no telling whether Carter too sniggered at the obstetrical lectures or played pranks in the dissecting room but he reminds us of the complexity and variety within the medical community.

'Ink-stains and industry': lectures

The best teachers – Abernethy, Liston and Astley Cooper – captured the imagination of their young students. George Macilwain who felt so repulsed by the challenge he faced as a young student at Bart's in 1816, saw in Abernethy's expression something consoling. 'I almost fancied,' he recalled forty years later, 'that he could have sympathised with the melancholy with which I felt oppressed'.[57] Despite Abernethy's reputation as sharp and cantankerous, for years after his death fond and possibly apocryphal anecdotes were still being recounted by his former students.[58] Indeed, alone of the surgical teachers of the period, reverberations of Abernethy were transmitted from generation to generation among Bart's men until by the end of the twentieth century they remained like a faint echo from deep space. In training aspiring practitioners the personality of the teacher was paramount in attracting, retaining and educating students. In Edinburgh Robert Knox rehearsed his witty anatomical lectures choosing his dress and adornments as carefully as an actor. Their generally long careers and the large numbers crowding their lecture halls gave them widespread and long-lasting influence: it was calculated that Astley Cooper had lectured to 8,000 pupils.[59] His students thronged the steps of Guy's awaiting his arrival and as he commenced each lecture with 'Gennelmen!', sat silently, the only sound heard being, as John Flint South recalled, the 'subdued pen-scratching of the note-takers.[60]

Each taught to an individual, often idiosyncratic syllabus but they generally expected students to record lectures verbatim as the numerous surviving students' notes attest. Contemporaries tended to regard the very lack of uniformity as a virtue, a sturdy testament to a healthy diversity of opinion as well as a reflection of the contingent nature of much contemporary medical knowledge. Students, however loyal to their teachers' doctrines, suffered from their dogmatism. Charles Aston Key boasted that it was his custom to assert and not retract: pupils, he insisted, 'did not understand doubts' and those entertaining them, he said, went away uninstructed.[61] Joseph Carpue, the 'chalk lecturer' of the Dean Street School, made pupils recite his own descriptions of bones and structures back to him learning by rote from a blackboard.[62] Patrick Watson, who had perhaps suffered for his teachers' unjustified certainty as a student at Edinburgh in the early 1850s, bemoaned that lecturers often differed markedly. Students would hear from one 'that blood-letting is a panacea, from another that it is nothing short of manslaughter'.[63] William Fergusson introduced a note of common sense in his *System of Practical Surgery* deploring the futility of dogmatic assertion prevalent in lecture theatres. 'The student may go from hospital to hospital' he counselled 'and see excellent stumps' formed by adherents of either of the predominant schools.[64]

Not all medical lecturers possessed the popular appeal of Abernethy. Dr Charles Balham who held the Chair in the Theory and Practice of Medicine at Glasgow notoriously indulged his taste for literary studies spending weeks criticising poetry and describing his continental travels.[65] Not that lecturing would ever have been easy. A correspondent to *The Times* in 1819 condemned 'Medical Dandyism' alleging that even those who attended lectures spent more time handing about snuff-boxes, adjusting their cravats and arranging the evening's amusements.[66] A letter to the *Lancet* a few years later described students as throwing paper balls and apple cores at each other and irritating those sitting on the tiered benches below them.[67] In the 1840s Joe Muff chose a seat out of the lecturer's eye-line so he could play cribbage with a neighbour.

Young men at large in London could not all be expected to work diligently. Study did not necessarily entail long hours over books. The marks of 'ink-stains and industry' visible on the fingers of Joe Muff's colleagues in the first weeks of the term often faded to be replaced by nicotine stains. Forbes Winslow complained that many worked just enough to pass their examinations.[68] Only when the examinations approached for the Society of Apothecaries or the College of Surgeons (the 'Hall' and the 'College') did many bend to fourteen-hour days sustained by snuff and coffee.

•

Figure 6.2

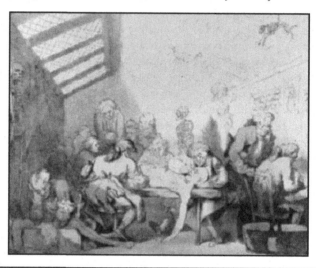

Thomas Rowlandson's 'The Dissecting Room', showing the chaotic
and cramped conditions in which anatomists and students worked in
private anatomical schools, and their intimacy with corpses.

'Such a stinck': dissection

In old age Benjamin Brodie mused that many acquaintances had
presumed that he had discovered as a student 'a particular taste or
liking for my profession'. He contradicted them confessing that he at
first found his medical studies 'disagreeable' and even 'repulsive'. [69]
Nor was he alone. Along with many of his contemporaries Brodie
found anatomical dissection repellent, perhaps even more so than
watching operations. The discoveries of the Hunters and their
disciples had, however, confirmed the centrality of anatomical
dissection as the foundation of medical and surgical education and it
was an experience all students underwent.

Students typically enrolled in a course of lectures and
demonstrations in anatomy given by teachers in one of the many
private schools serving the needs of hospital pupils. The courses were
always held over the winter term to ensure that students got full value
out a cadaver before decomposition reduced its pedagogic worth.
The growth of formal medical education from the last decade of the
eighteenth century placed cadavers at a premium. 'In London,'

William Dent of Guy's wrote to his mother in 1809, 'we could not get a dead body [for] under three guineas'.[70] Twenty years later – just before the Anatomy Act that legalised and regulated the supply of corpses – the demand had driven prices higher to 9 or even 16 guineas.[71] Bob Sawyer and his friends formed a syndicate to go shares in a corpse. The shortage generated tension within the profession especially among students less able to pay the going rates. In 1832 students met at a tavern in Covent Garden to protest against the partiality of parish authorities in apparently favouring students at Bart's and King's College (presumably because they were willing to pay higher prices). 'Riotous scenes' ensued with aggrieved students employing 'language of the most violent character'. To report the details of the melée, *The Times* decided, would 'ill serve the interests of science'.[72]

Hampton Weekes, in his first weeks as a student at St Thomas's in the autumn of 1801, self-consciously showed a friend from Sussex around 'his' hospital. After cautiously peeking into the dissecting room his friend expostulated that he had 'never smell't such a stinck in my life'.[73] Weekes's apothecary father admonished him not to show 'every country fellow' the dissecting room, because it 'makes such a noise ... ab[ou]t cutting up human subjects'.[74]. John Flint South described the same room as he recalled it in 1813. It was a square chamber illuminated by two external windows and a skylight. One end held high glass-fronted cases containing preparations used by the demonstrators in anatomy. On one wall stood a fireplace and a copper used to prepare specimens and a sink 'indiscriminately used for washing hands and discharging all the filth' of the room. The room contained about a dozen tables on which cadavers would be laid out. Around each table stood six or eight students clad in what South described as 'filthy linen or stuff dissecting gowns'.[75] Eighty or more men and up to a dozen corpses filled the room. The stench of bodies, even during the autumn and winter months, must have been overpowering.

William Bowman began his studies in 1832 at the age of sixteen. Being of an unusually reflective turn he delivered a paper to fellow members of the King's College Medical and Scientific Society in his second year as a student. Bowman recalled his recent experience of entering a dissecting room for the first time. Even if prepared, he wrote, a person would very likely feel an 'impression of disgust ... so powerful as to produce transitory faintness and perhaps vomiting'. Bowman spoke of the 'revolting scene' which excited his 'deepest disgust'. He found that he could not eradicate the 'peculiar odour' of

Figure 6.3

*This caricature of James Syme reducing a fracture in the
Royal Infirmary of Edinburgh suggests how students populated the
wards of a major hospital, observing or – in this case –
ignoring operations and procedures.*

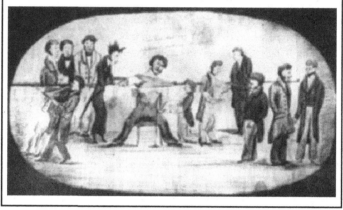

the cadaver from his hands despite frequent washing.[76] (A notice in
the *Lancet* passed on a hint from French colleagues at La Pitié:
rubbing the hands well with charcoal before washing would 'dispel
the usual stench of dissection'.[77])

Dissecting rooms represented a major source of danger. Many
students and sometimes their demonstrators were infected from
accidental cuts while working on cadavers. Among Astley Cooper's
proteges alone, Thomas Callaway, Frederick Tyrrell and John Scott
were all wounded in conducting one post-mortem examination and
Scott was disabled by blood-poisoning for months, while the
promising David Babington fell 'a victim to his professional zeal'.[78]
Some evaded dissection as best they could. Thomas Goldie Scott of
Edinburgh lamented the death of a classmate who had 'always
expressed a great dread of it' and expressed his relief at avoiding 'a risk
that has proved fatal to many'.[79] Others survived more by luck than
judgement: William Gibney, about 1810, washed down sandwiches
and porter at the dissecting tables in Edinburgh while a friend
recalled how John Epps, a student in the Borough in the 1790s, cut
his lunch with his dissecting knife.[80] No wonder John Abernethy
referred to the 'disgusting and health-destroying avocations of the
dissecting room'.[81]

•

'Walking the wards': hospital practice

Most courses obliged students to spend time 'walking the wards'. This experience left students, alone or in groups, at liberty in the often chaotic wards of large hospitals. Benjamin Brodie recalled how his impression was 'at first all is confusion ... quite inexplicable'. In the beginning he saw everything 'through a mist'.[82] At length, Brodie found a way of making sense of these random encounters with the sick and injured. To do so depended largely upon the student's individual resource. William Guy, Physician to King's College Hospital, enjoined his students to cultivate habits of 'fixed, thoughtful, and earnest attention', not the 'listless attention of the mere spectator'.[83] William Bowman recalled students in the wards as resembling 'travellers in a strange country'.[84]

Students in the wards became 'wondering spectators' at operations, gazers upon 'each strange or fearful accident or disease'.[85] In doing so they also acquired and exercised important clinical skills. Students practised bleeding and bandaging. Skill in bleeding became obsolete in that the practice declined throughout the period until by mid-century depletion became the stigma of the old-fashioned practitioner. Bandaging, however, has been much under-rated as a skill; perhaps because with the introduction of professionally trained nurses it became regarded as women's work. Cooper's *Dictionary* discloses how important bandaging was particularly through its role in promoting union and encouraging healing.[86] Given the difficulty of suturing a struggling patient it is not surprising that some surgeons decided to stitch as little as possible in favour of careful bandaging. The 'art' of bandaging, wrote Robert Druitt, was not to be learned from books but acquired in hospital practice. John Abernethy demonstrated on his long-suffering surgerymen, binding them like mummies, to his students' amusement.[87]

Time that should have been spent walking the wards allowed indifferent students to stand 'idling in the passages'.[88] The students' propensity to harass patients especially young women was well established by 1803 when Thomas Percival urged that to 'sport with their feelings' was cruel. He advised his colleagues, with some justice, to remind students of their responsibilities 'forcibly and repeatedly'.[89] Hampton Weekes made light of attending obstetric cases at St Thomas's as 'going to Groanings': the women he observed 'stared at me & seemed a little difident'.[90] Conscientious young men, however, used their time on the wards not only to further their clinical knowledge and skills but to learn the realities of hospital care. The evidence is sketchy but it would appear that the more serious students spent time dressing wounds and watching over patients in their crises: 'caretaking' as South put it.[91] Edinburgh's students were explicitly enjoined to be mindful of the 'sacred and important trust' for the 'comfort and welfare of the Patients'.[92] Indeed, the medical staff at the Middlesex Hospital (in a memorial seeking to establish a medical school) argued that a hospital could not properly function without students to 'administer much comfort and assistance to the patients'.[93] The Charity Commissioners' report of 1837 noted the 'constant presence' of students in the wards of Guy's.[94] The testimonials which students routinely obtained from their seniors suggest that they learned attitudes of care as well as techniques of treatment. Robert Quain and Robert Liston at University College Hospital signed a certificate to testify that George Moreton had 'discharged the duties of dresser with much care and ability'. At the same time Quain signed an individual reference commending Moreton's 'unvarying kindness towards the Patients'.[95] Even if these were conventional phrases they suggest solicitude as well as technical proficiency.

'A very hard trial': surgery

Surgery could not be easily taught by theory. As a reviewer of George Ballingall's *Surgical Cases* pointed out, it was scarcely possible to conceive 'how great a distance separated surgery as it was taught in books and lectures and surgery as it appeared in practice'.[96] An anonymous contributor to the *Edinburgh Medical and Surgical Journal* emphasised how different was an actual operation to the descriptions of demonstrators and lecturers. The pupil, he claimed, need only attend an operation for a few moments to be 'instantly struck with the difference'. In the classroom 'all is smooth, all natural, and most easily dissected' but in the theatre 'all is agitation'. The operator and his assistants would obscure the patient's body; the patient's cries would 'melt the heart of the most obdurate'.[97]

Despite embarking on a career in which witnessing and then inflicting pain would be unavoidable, few were mentally prepared for their first operation. The opening weeks of the term exposed students who had not served an apprenticeship to a severe trial of endurance. Few forgot the sight of their first operation. William Wilde who became an ophthalmologist, recalled the first time he observed the excision of the eyeball; 'so horrible and distressing a scene that the impression it made still lingers in my recollection'.[98] In a detailed memoir written in old age John Flint South recalled with clarity and

honesty his first months at St Thomas's. Its operating room was small
and poorly ventilated and, with the wartime increase in medical
students, usually crowded. Although writing six decades later South
still vividly recollected it. 'This was for me,' he recalled, 'a very hard
trial'. As for others it was not so much the bloodshed which
disturbed him but the sight, and especially the sound, of patients in
pain. 'So long as the patient did not make much noise I got on very
well'. If the patient's cries were great and especially if it were a child
South became 'quickly upset, and had to leave the theatre'. Like
many others he often left the room or fainted. If, on recovering, the
operation continued (further evidence if it were needed that
operations were not over in seconds) he would return to see it out.[99]
One who also returned was James Simpson, who had been so
distressed by watching the amputation of a woman's breast in his first
weeks at Edinburgh (as a fourteen-year-old) that he walked out,
intending to seek a legal career, before resolving to return.[100]
Hampton Weekes described his first operation in a letter to his father.
Watching from the tiers above the table, he felt 'something
indescribable' and fainted. 'I shall soon get callous to it all' he rightly
predicted. A fortnight later he reported having witnessed several
more operations and now 'mind nothing about it ... the more the
poor devils cry ye more I laugh with the rest of them'.[101]

Students were not obliged to attend operations throughout their
training except during the terms devoted to surgery. Indeed not all
medical educators considered that students could gain much from
attending the theatre at all. Thomas Alcock cautioned students
against 'running after extraordinary cases and operations'. General
practitioners, he warned, were more likely to be called upon to
bandage and bleed than to perform lithotomies, to make new noses
or to tie the aorta.[102] Abernethy's biographer, his student George
Macilwain, condemned 'exhibitions' as 'more calculated to give
publicity to the surgeon than ... to ... chasten the feelings of men
about to enter a profession'. It is significant that Abernethy himself
disliked operating, placing his faith in 'regimen'. Perhaps he inspired
Macilwain's view that students regarding operations as a spectacle
could hardly be then expected to see them as a serious duty. For all
its power – or perhaps because of it – relatively few described or
analysed their reactions to surgery, in print at least, and we are left to
infer from hints and asides and others' observations how they reacted
to the trial of the operating room. Operations acquired a centrality in
student culture: 'pupils will flock the thickest,' George Macilwain
observed bluntly, 'where they expect to see most operations'.[103]

Despite the shock of seeing and hearing operations those who persisted did overcome their horror and disgust. So completely did some adjust to the scene that William Gibson – himself an experienced operator – confessed that he had often been bemused by his students 'delight' in surgery.[104] Young men such as these had failed to develop the 'surgical tact' which Henry Bigelow hoped to see mature in his students: the ability to see beyond the blood and the cries to discern what surgeons needed to do, and how.[105] And yet their seniors did not seriously expect them to acquire useful knowledge or practical skills: it was to accustom them to the pain and discomfort inevitably accompanying medical or surgical procedures. George Wilson, who knew surgery as both student and patient, acknowledged in an address to Edinburgh's students in 1855 that the distress of witnessing surgery could be 'deadened by repetition'.[106] A student witnessing operations would eventually become used to the scene which would, George Macilwain brusquely remarked, 'blind him to any association with pain and suffering'. By the time he became a dresser or qualified himself he would have acquired 'an indifference to everything save adroitness of manipulation and mechanical display'.[107] James Paget who had felt faint and useless at his first operation advised younger colleagues that they should 'strive for such control of will ... to be able to divert the attention, as much and as often, from the watching of pain'.[108] Students, increasingly entranced by the lure of 'modern surgery', could not be dissuaded from crowding the operating room.

'To follow the box': dressers

Each term a few senior students with surgical aspirations were accepted as 'dressers'. As with therapeutic techniques and operative procedures the selection and duties of dressers varied between hospitals. In some, securing a position as a dresser was, as John Warren put it, 'merely a matter of money down'.[109] 'They are not chosen for talent or proficiency', the Charity Commissioners learned of Guy's in the 1830s, 'but in consideration of the payment of an additional fee'.[110] A dresser's appointment placed those who sought surgical experience in the most advantageous situation to obtain it. Those who could not afford to pay for the experience sought it informally, by assisting a private practitioner or by 'moonlighting' in treating the poor. *Punch* advised medical students to walk the railways instead of the wards suggesting that the number of accidents would enable them to complete their education unusually rapidly.[111]

Dressers were eponymously required to dress wounds. Their

'principal duty' wrote James Miller in 1840, was 'attention to
cleanliness', a revealing reminder of their importance in ensuring
healing without suppuration.[112] They were said to carry or follow 'the
box'. In many hospitals their responsibility was embodied by the
'plaister box' holding the bandages, pledgets, plasters, linseed meal,
sponges and all the requisites of their office. In the Edinburgh Royal
Infirmary dressers wore aprons with pockets for instruments and
carried a box for fresh dressings and a pail for old.[113] They would
officiate at the scramble of 'taking in' day, attend to accident cases
brought to the hospital's gates and perform simple procedures such
as poulticing, lancing abscesses and bleeding. Most would assist at
operations, although exactly what they were expected or permitted to
do depended upon the surgeon. At the Westminster they merely
watched surgeons dressing.[114] In some hospitals they would hold
patients, instruments or limbs; in others they would suture incisions
or tie arteries.

Dressers attempted little more than assisting before qualifying
and the only operations most performed were upon the 'dead
subject'. Indeed the one part of surgery which neither dressers nor
any other student would be allowed to attempt was the cutting part
itself. Many – perhaps most – would not trouble on that account and
would not, unless compelled, take up the scalpel or saw in general
practice. A few, however, particularly, those seeking to become
hospital surgeons wished to attempt surgery themselves. This – 'the
ingeneous student' as Charles Bell described him – was inspired by
the novel and daring surgery open to him weekly in the operating
rooms of the great hospitals. Such a man, Bell wrote, 'makes up his
mind to practise that which is the most curiously complex and
fanciful'.[115] Surgical aspirations were common enough for William
Gibson to denounce the presumption of young surgeons in his often-
reprinted text *Institutes and Practice of Surgery*. Because amputations
were regarded as among the easiest of operations, Gibson wrote they
were 'too often' the first attempt of the 'young and inexperienced'
thinking that they effect a 'brilliant exhibition of dexterity' by ' a few
flourishes of the knife'. Few older surgeons, he averred, would deny
that they too had committed such mistakes.[116]

A story told by Astley Cooper in one of his celebrated
Introductory Lectures offered the students of Guy's Hospital a complex
cautionary tale.[117] 'A few years' earlier (the lecture was published in
the first issue of Wakley's *Lancet* in 1823) one of Guy's dressers very
much wished to perform an operation. He sought out a surgery boy
who happened to have an infected leg saying bluntly 'Abraham, I

should like to cut off your leg'. 'Indeed!' Abraham replied – he comes across as mentally retarded – 'I should not like it'. 'Oh,' said the dresser winningly, 'it will never be of any use to you ... you had better be without it'. The student offered to pay and lodge the boy and at length wore him down. Recruiting a friend, on the appointed day the dresser set about amputating the boy's leg. As he cut, the wound bled freely. 'Screw the tourniquet tighter' the dresser called but the screw broke. The dresser lost his composure, vainly trying to compress the limb by hand, panicking as his sleeve filled with blood. Had not another student called by and pressed the door-key to the femoral artery Abraham would have bled to death. Cooper failed to say what happened to either the dresser or the unfortunate surgery boy. He ostensibly told the story hoping to persuade his listeners of the need to take anatomical study seriously but it seems also to have been a caution to those who imprudently hoped to operate before they were qualified or ready. That Guy's employed a surgery boy with a chronically infected sore passed without comment.

'Speak up, Sir!': examinations

Success in examinations for both the apothecaries' licentiate or the college's diploma depended for many on 'grinding' or cramming. Qualified men familiar with the curriculum and, more importantly, the personalities and preoccupations of the examiners would, for a fee, coach weaker students not so much in the art of healing, as in the art of passing examinations. Wakley's *Lancet* denounced these 'grinders' as the bastard offspring of the medical corporations. *Punch's* Joe Muff resorted to one before sitting his examination before the college. He described its atmosphere as 'fragrant with the amalgamated odours of stale tobacco-smoke, varnished bones, leaky preparations, and gin-and-water'. Asked by the grinder what he would do if confronted by a man with a 'bad incised wound' the student replied 'send for the nearest doctor'.[118]

The examination in London was held before the college's Court of Examiners: ten members of the Council who acted as the gatekeepers of the profession. A candidate expressed his intention to sit for the diploma, sent in his testimonials and waited on the college. On the evening of the examination he was summoned to appear and was shown to a room in which stood a large horseshoe-shaped table. One of the Court adopted the role of principal examiner; another recorded and assisted ensuring that both question and answer were clear.

Figure 6.4

'The Examination of a Young Surgeon' at the
Royal College of Surgeons' horse-shoe table satirised by George
Cruikshank in 1811. Though requiring the candidate to
describe the organs of hearing, several of the examiners are
depicted as hard of hearing.

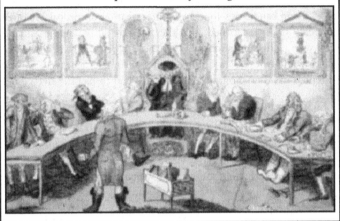

Although 'a more respectable ordeal' than what *Punch* called the
'jalap and rhubarb botheration' held at Apothecaries' Hall, the
surgeons' examination remained a poor test of the knowledge and
skill aspiring doctors were supposed to have acquired over several
years of study. John Scott, later Surgeon to the London Hospital,
recalled his own examination in the 1820s as dealing only with
surgery and anatomy and lasting only half an hour.[119] Others passed
on even less rigorous testing. It became notorious that patronage
remained instrumental in determining the outcome of examinations.
Wakley alleged that an exchange had been heard at the college
between an examiner and a candidate:

'Whose pupil had he been?'
'Mr _____'s'
'Oh! very well ... I taught him; so there is no occasion to ask you
any questions.'[120]

Failed candidates were known to allege that examiners hard of
hearing had ruined their chances: 'Speak up, Sir!' was heard more
than once. Some examiners were believed to be notoriously hard,
others easy. Sir William Blizard 'delighted in terrorising the

179

candidate' while George Chandler of St Thomas's had been known to have failed only one candidate and had then not slept for a fortnight: an odd tenderness for a man whose living involved cutting conscious patients.[121] As ever, connections helped: Hampton Weekes judiciously mentioned his father's name twice and overheard the examiner commend him to the Master of the College with 'this gentleman has pass[ed] a very good examn. indeed, very well, sir ....'[122] Some candidates found the interrogation an ordeal. 'It often happens,' Guthrie testified, 'that they faint, or sit like statues, unable to answer a single question'. Those unable to proceed were allowed to wait a while before continuing and if still tongue-tied, were advised to return in a few months. But they still had to pay the five guinea fee.[123]

Predicated as it was on seniority, the college's Council and Court of Examiners included 'ancient members' who had qualified and grown old before the Hunterian revolution had inaugurated the period of 'modern surgery'. Many failed to keep pace with the discoveries, theories and innovations which their younger colleagues taught in clinical lectures. Candidates could be reprimanded or even failed for espousing novel rather than conventional responses. Richard Grainger claimed that a young man, 'one of the most industrious students' he had ever taught, had been failed because he had not recommended an obsolescent treatment for traumatic gangrene. The student, familiar with Larrey's work on gangrene, contradicted what had been the conventional wisdom (that until a 'line of separation' marked the extent of a gangrenous infection amputation should not be attempted) and was accordingly failed. Not realising that he could have appealed on the spot (and presumably overawed by the assembled court) he gave way, learning too late that John Abernethy had corrected the court's ignorance.[124]

Success was likely if not guaranteed. In the decade 1823-1832 4,164 students sought a diploma and only 262 – just over six per cent – were rejected. In the 1840s the college's examiners became more rigorous with just over 11% of the 1,776 aspirants failing.[125] Those 'plucked' or failed were free to return after further grinding. Some took their failure hard. In 1818 a student assaulted a member of the Edinburgh college who had failed him while in 1826 another sent anonymous threatening letters to a strict examiner. Hard examiners could be hissed in the lecture room.[126] The great majority might have pondered John Bell's verdict on the examination system at the beginning of the century. Bell had seen ignorant men answer fluently and men of ability appear as fools. 'Examinations', he declared, 'are no more a test of medical skill, than … torture is a test of truth'.[127]

'What is to become of you?': Paget's students

James Paget the nauseous apprentice who had graduated from Bart's in 1836 at last answered John Abernethy's question 'What is to become of you?' In 1869 he published in the *Hospital Reports* of Abernethy's old institution, Bart's, an account of over a thousand students who had enrolled in his classes between 1843 and 1859.[128] Paget had traced the fate of almost all of his students and classified them according to whether, in his view, they had succeeded or failed. Forty one young men died before qualifying, four of fevers after dissecting, two from suicide. Fifty six had 'failed entirely' to qualify through 'idleness or listlessness, … ill-health or misadventure or 'habits of intemperance and dissipation'. About one in ten had attained 'distinguished' or 'considerable' success. Most – just over 500 – had achieved 'fair' success. A further ten per cent, 'erratic men', were barely making a living. The residue interested him most. Ninety six – nearly as many as had achieved notable success – had left the profession: some (16) had been expelled or removed; others after inheriting money. Regrettably, in Paget's eyes, three became actors (one 'well esteemed in genteel comedy'); seven entered the army and seven took holy orders., To Paget's disgust three became homoeopaths. Almost as many (87) had died within twelve years of graduation. In his papers he added pungent comments on many: 'idle, dissolute, extravagant, vulgar & stupid'; 'right-minded, good-hearted & of fair abilities'; 'he married a prostitute'; 'active, persevering, pushing little Welchman'; 'commonplace but steady'. His terse comments are a eulogy on the diversity of students Paget and his fellow teachers helped to become doctors.[129]

Students learned more in lecture theatres and wards besides how to recognise and treat the injuries and ailments to which the human body is prone. They learned ways of being doctors. They learned that healing required technical skill and anatomical knowledge but also humanity. It demanded toughness but also compassion and, above all perhaps, resilience; the capacity to see and hear what was required but also the ability not to notice or heed that which interfered with the task. They learned these attitudes from their teachers and from each other.

Notes

1. John Flint South, *Memorials of John Flint South* (Fontwell: Centaur Press, 1970), 85.
2. Thomas Pettigrew, *Biographical Memoirs of the Most Celebrated Physicians, Surgeons, etc., etc.*, 3 vols (London: Fisher, Son & Co., 1839–40), Vol. II, 4–5.
3. Forbes Winslow, *Physic and Physicians: A Medical Sketch Book*, 2 vols (London: Longman, Orme, Brown, 1839), Vol. I, 119 .
4. Mary English, *Victorian Values: The Life and Times of Dr Edwin Lankester* (Bristol: Biopress, 1990), xv; W.T. Gairdner, *Medical Education, Character, and Conduct* (Glasgow: Maclehose & Sons, 1883), 10.
5. George Combe (ed.), *The Life and Correspondence of Andrew Combe, MD* (Edinburgh: Machlachlan & Stewart, 1850), 18.
6. 'Indenture of Wm Getty', A3970, ML,S.
7. 'Testimonials of Dr G.F. Moreton', V1008, MLSA .
8. John Brown to William Broome, 26 October 1831, John Brown, *Letters of John Brown* (London: A.& C. Black, 1907), 13 .
9. William Chamberlain, *Tirocinium Medicum, or a Dissertation on the Duties of Youth Apprenticed to the Medical Profession* (London: William Chamberlain, 1812), 52.
10. Stephen Paget (ed.), *Memoirs and Letters of Sir James Paget* (London: Longmans & Co., 1902), 23.
11. Chamberlaine, *op. cit.* (note 9), 13.
12. *Ibid.*, 222 .
13. William Porter, *The Medical School in Sheffield, 1828–1928* (Sheffield: Northend, 1928), 2. Schools also opened at Manchester, Birmingham, Leeds, Hull, Newcastle, Bristol, Liverpool and York.
14. 'Medical Education', *Edinburgh Medical & Surgical Journal*, 1826, Vol. 26, 308.
15. PP 1828, Vol. VII, Part 1, Report of the Select Committee on Anatomy, 4.
16. List of Graduands, Edinburgh, 1835, Mss Eur F133/5 OIOC, BL.
17. PP 1846, Vol. XXXIII, 479–80.
18. Amédée Pichot, *The Life and Labours of Sir Charles Bell* (London: R. Bentley, 1860), 172n.
19. Patrick Herron Watson, *Introductory Address Delivered at Surgeons' Hall, Edinburgh* (Edinburgh: Edinburgh Medical Journal, 1867), 22.
20. Evidence of George Guthrie to the Select Committee of Medical Education, PP 1834, Vol. XIII, 17.
21. Henry Spry to H. Pennington, [nd: 1824?'], Photo. Eur 308, BL,

OIOC .

22. William Augustus Guy, *On Medical Education* (London: Henry Renshaw, 1846), 14.

23. *Lancet*, 1833–34, Vol. I, 22, Vol. I, 757, Vol. II, 94–95.

24. PP, 1834, Vol. XIII, 148.

25. H. Campbell Thomson, *The Story of the Middlesex Hospital Medical School* (London: John Murray, 1935), 45.

26. *The Times*, 19 January 1836, 6a; 22 January 1836, 1e.

27. W.C. Spencer, *Westminster Hospital - An Outline of its History* (London: H.J. Glaisher, 1924), 107-09.

28. *Lancet*, 1833–34, Vol. II, p. 59; *Lancet*, 1832–33, Vol. I, 12.

29. Benjamin Brodie, *An Introductory Discourse on the Duties and Conduct of Medical Students and Practitioners* (London: Longman & Co., 1843), 13.

30. Evidence of James Wardrop, PP 1834, Vol. XIII, 169.

31. Evidence of Anthony Carlisle, PP 1834, Vol. XIII, 149.

32. Evidence of Benjamin Brodie, PP, 1834, Vol. XIII, 118.

33. S. Squire Sprigge, *The Life and Times of Thomas Wakley* (London: Longmans, 1899), 22. Even so, this was perhaps twice the annual wage of an artisan.

34. Evidence of Richard Grainger, PP 1834, Vol. XIII, 198.

35. 'The Physiology of the London Medical Student', *Punch*, 23 October 1841, 177.

36. Mungo Park to Thomas Anderson, 23 February 1819, NLS, Ms 20311.

37. Benjamin Brodie, (C. Hawking, ed.), *Autobiography*, (London: Longmans & Co., 1865), 25.

38. *Cornhill Magazine*, Vol. III, February 1861, 246.

39. *Lancet*, 1830–31, Vol. I, 313.

40. Evidence of Astley Cooper, PP 1834, Vol. VIII, 87.

41. Charles Dickens, *The Pickwick Papers* (London: Chapman & Hall, 1857), Chapter XXX.

42. 'The Physiology of the London Medical Student', *Punch*, 2 October - 18 December 1841.

43. Bransby Cooper, *The Life of Sir Astley Cooper, Bart.*, 2 vols (London: John Parker, 1843), Vol. I, 325.

44. R.D. Gibney, (ed.), *Eighty Years Ago, or the Recollections of an Old Army Doctor* (London: Bellairs & Co., 1896), 18.

45. South, *op. cit.* (note 1), 39.

46. *Lancet*, 1823–24, Vol. I, 385.

47. Guy, *op. cit.* (note 22), 23.

48. William Dale, quoted in Charles Newman, *The Evolution of Medical Education in the Nineteenth Century* (London: OUP, 1957), 42.

49. *Lancet*, 1825–26, Vol. I, 500.

50. Newman, *op. cit.* (note 48), 42.

51. Henry Willam Fuller, *Advice to Medical Students* (London: John Churchill, 1857), 22.

52. John Abernethy, *The Surgical Works*, 3 vols (London: Longman, 1811), Vol. I, 190.

53. Brodie, *op. cit.* (note 29), 30–31.

54. W.P. Alison, *History of Medicine* (London: Blackwood, 1833), lxxi.

55. Journal of H.V. Carter, MS 5817, WIHM.

56. Brodie, *op. cit.* (note 37), 24–25.

57. George Macilwain, *Memoirs of John Abernethy*, 2 vols (London: Hurst & Blackett, 1854), Vol. I, xi.

58. Frederic Skey, *Operative Surgery* (London: John Churchill, 1850), 11.

59. *Blackwood's Magazine*, April 1849, Vol. 65, Part I, 49.

60. South, *op. cit.* (note 1), 32; 84.

61. J.F. Clarke, *Autobiographical Recollections* (London: J. & A. Churchill, 1874), 525.

62. Victor Plarr, *Lives of the Fellows of the Royal College of Surgeons*, 2 vols (London: Simpkin, Marshall Ltd, 1930), Vol. I, 198–99.

63. Watson, *op. cit.* (note 19), 22.

64. William Fergusson, *A System of Practical Surgery* (London: John Churchill, 1846), 170.

65. *Lancet*, 1832–33, Vol. I, 63.

66. *The Times*, 11 March 1819, 3e.

67. *Lancet*, 1823–24, Vol. I, 290.

68. Winslow, *op. cit.* (note 3), Vol. II, 348.

69. Brodie, *op. cit.* (note 37), 20-21.

70. William Dent to his mother, 5 March 1809, Letters of William Dent, 7008-11, NAM.

71. Evidence of Astley Cooper and J.H. Green before the Select Committee on Anatomy, PP 1840, vol. VII, Part 1, 6, 37.

72. *The Times*, 4 December 1832, 2f.

73. Hampton Weekes to Richard Weekes, 10 October 1801, John Ford (ed.), *A Medical Student at St Thomas's Hospital, 1801–1802 The Weekes Family Letters* (London: Wellcome Institute for the History of Medicine, 1987), 51.

74. Richard Weekes to Hampton Weekes, 9 November 1801, *ibid.*, 68.

75. South, *op. cit.* (note 1), 28–29.

76. J. Burton-Sanderson & J.W. Hulke, *The Collected papers of Sir W. Bowman,* 2 vols (London: Harrison & Sons, 1892) , Vol. II, 39; 48.

77. *Lancet,* 1833–34, Vol. II, 277.

78. Astley Cooper & Frederick Tyrrell, *The Lectures of Sir Astley Cooper, Bart.* ... (London: Thomas Tegg, 1824) , Vol. I, p. 21; Vol. II, 261.

79. Thomas Goldie Scott to his father, William, 18 January 1843, NLS, Acc. 9266/1.

80. Gibney, *op. cit.* (note 44), 52; Ellen Epps (ed.), *Diary of the Late John Epps, MD* (London: Kent & Co., [1875]), 204.

81. John Abernethy, *Introductory Lectures Exhibiting Some of Mr Hunter's Opinions Respecting Life Diseases* (London: Longman, Hurst, Rees, Orme & Brown, 1819), 4.

82. Brodie, *op. cit.* (note 37), 44–45.

83. Guy, *op. cit.* (note 22), 39.

84. Bowman, 'Thoughts for the Medical Student', in Burdon-Sanderson & Hulke, *op. cit.* (note 76), Vol. II, 64.

85. Charles West, *The Profession of Medicine* (London: Longman, 1850), 17.

86. Samuel Cooper, *A Dictionary of Practical Surgery* (London: Longman, Hurst, Rees, Orme & Brown, 1829), 222–23.

87. Robert Druitt, *The Principles and Practice of Modern Surgery* (Philadelphia: Lea & Blanchard, 1842), 487.

88. Watson, *op. cit.* (note 19), 23.

89. Thomas Percival, *Medical Ethics, or A Code of Institutes and Precepts* ... (Oxford: J.H. Parker, 1849), 29.

90. Hampton Weekes to Richard Weekes, 1 November 1801, Ford, *op. cit.* (note 73), 59.

91. South, *op. cit.* (note 1), 27.

92. Royal Infirmary of Edinburgh, *Regulations respecting Clerks* (Edinburgh: 1816), 1.

93. Thomson, *op. cit.* (note 25), 26–27.

94. Guy's Hospital, CHAR/2, 385, PRO.

95. 'Testimonials of Dr G.F. Moreton', V1008, MLSA.

96. 'Review of Dr Ballingall's Surgical Cases, *Edinburgh Medical & Surgical Journal,* Vol. 27, 1827, 433.

97. 'Dr Buchanan's History of the Glasgow Royal Infirmary', *Edinburgh Medical & Surgical Journal,* Vol. 39, 433.

98. T.G. Wilson, *Victorian Doctor, Being the Life of Sir William Wilde* (London: Methuen, 1942), 90.

99. South, *op. cit.* (note 1), 36.

100. J. Duns, *Memoir of Sir James Y. Simpson, Bart.* (Edinburgh:

Edmonston & Douglas, 1873), 27.

101. Hampton Weekes to Richard Weekes, 24 Sep 1801; 8 October 1801, in Ford, *op. cit.* (note 73), 44; 49.

102. Thomas Alcock, 'An Essay on the Education and Duties of the General Practitioner in Medicine and Surgery' in *Transactions of the Associated Apothecaries and Surgeon Apothecaries of England and Wales* (London: the Society, 1823), 61.

103. Macilwain, *op. cit.* (note 57), Vol. II, 224;222.

104. William Gibson, *Institutes and Practice of Surgery* (Philadelphia: J. Kay, Jnr & Brother, 1841), vii.

105. Henry Jacob Bigelow, *An Introductory Lecture delivered at Massachusetts Medical College* (Boston: David Clapp, 1850), 9.

106. Jessie Aitken Wilson, *Memoir of George Wilson*, (Edinburgh: Edmonston & Douglas, 1860), 35.

107. Macilwain, *op. cit.* (note 57), Vol. II, 224.

108. James Paget, *Studies of Old Case Books* (London: Longmans & Co., 1891), 160.

109. James Mumford, *Surgical Memoirs, and other essays* (New York: Moffat, Yard & Co., 1908), 202.

110. Guy's Hospital, CHAR/2, 385, PRO.

111. *The Times*, 6 September 1845, 8a.

112. James Miller, *A Probationary Essay on the Dressing of Wounds* (Edinburgh: 1840), 18.

113. Royal Infirmary of Edinburgh, *Regulations respecting Dressers* (Edinburgh: 1816; 1831), 3.

114. Evidence of Anthony Carlisle, PP 1834, Vol. XIII, 148.

115. Charles Bell, *Illustrations of the Great Operations of Surgery* (London: Longman, 1821), 47.

116. Gibson, *op. cit.* (note 104), Vol. I, 503.

117. *Lancet*, 1823-34, Vol. I, 4.

118. 'The Physiology of the London Medical Student', *Punch*, 18 December 1841, 265.

119. Evidence of John Scott, PP 1834, Vol. VIII, 182.

120. *Lancet*, 1833–34, Vol. I, 407.

121. South, *op. cit.* (note 1), 46.

122. Hampton Weekes to Richard Weekes, 4 June 1802, Ford, *op. cit.* (note 73), 172–73.

123. Evidence of George Guthrie, PP 1834, Vol. XIII, 42.

124. Evidence of Richard Grainger, PP 1834, Vol. VIII, 199.

125. 'An Account of the Number of Persons who have obtained Diplomas from the Royal College of Surgeons', PP 1833, Vol. XXXIV, 117;

'Returns from the Colleges of Physicians and Surgeons'; PP 1846, Vol. XXXIII, 474.

126. Clarendon Creswell, *The Royal College of Surgeons of Edinburgh Historical Notes from 1505 to 1905* (Edinburgh: Oliver & Boyd, 1926), 187–89.

127. James Bell, *Memorial Concerning the Present State of Military and Naval Surgery* (Edinburgh: Mundell & Son, 1800), 18.

128. 'What becomes of Medical Students', *St Bartholomew's Hospital Reports*, Vol. 5, 1869, 238–42.

129. 'Medical students at St Bartholomew's Hospital', 330(16), RCSEng.

7

'The living subject':
Surgeons and Patients

It is almost impossible to understand the experience of painful surgery at second hand. Operations were devised and practised upon cadavers but they were performed upon what medical texts described as 'the living subject'. We must also recognise that clinical accounts rarely describe or explicitly reflect surgeons' reactions to or feelings about their work. Though painful surgery appears as shocking and while it was so to novices, contemporary observers knew no alternative and largely accepted pain as unavoidable. It appears that students became accustomed to the sight and sound of surgery relatively rapidly. How then can we enter into an experience which most participants took for granted?

'Testing himself': a surgeon's first operations

Obtaining a college's diploma, of course, did not necessarily imply a determination to become an operator. Indeed a student's training up to that point largely tested only whether he understood surgical techniques in theory – or at best on 'the dead subject'- and whether he could bear the sight and sound of the operating room. Even dressers were required to hold and hand and help rather than cut. The most a dresser should have attempted was the amputation of a finger, and then under supervision.[1] Whether a young man had a talent for operative surgery was difficult for anyone – student or teacher – to establish. James Wardrop found himself a qualified and seemingly well-educated surgeon at 22 without having performed an operation. He had studied at Edinburgh under John Barclay, in London at Guy's and St Thomas's, under Henry Cline, Astley Cooper and John Abernethy, and in France at the Ecole de Medicine. Back in Edinburgh and aware of a 'predilection to surgery' he 'made the experiment', performing an operation to discover whether he possessed 'the temperament which would enable him to undertake the practice of surgery with comfort to himself'. He evidently found in favour for very soon after Wardrop attempted an amputation of the thigh, 'testing himself', as an early biographer put it.[2]

Young men 'of little caution and no experience,' as Samuel

189

Cooper described them, felt pressure to perform operations that might establish their reputation leading to referrals and the beginning of a career.[3] Anthony Carlisle denounced them as 'young anatomists, flushed with dissecting room assurance' who ventured operations at which more experienced surgeons balked.[4] It was incontrovertible that an aspiring surgeon became an experienced operator only by making errors: George Guthrie drew the ire of the *Lancet* for admitting that before a man could operate successfully for cataract he must 'spoil a hatful of eyes'.[5] Experienced operators stressed, probably without exaggeration, the contrast between operating on the dead and the living subject. Carlisle spoke of the differences between cutting into 'natural' and 'diseased' tissues and between 'moving, bleeding flesh and a passive carcass'. He could not 'transmit these important details to posterity' he said.

William Fergusson grasped the essential difference between the procedures attempted as a student and the awesome responsibility of operating as a supposedly qualified surgeon: 'measurements by inches may do very well in the dead subject'.[6] While surgeons used dead subjects to rehearse operations (John Simon practised unfamiliar operations on cadavers a dozen times), the living subject presented them with many greater challenges.[7] John Bell evoked the anxiety of a young man in this predicament in memorable descriptions. He described the desperate uncertainty of the inexperienced operator who found himself committed to operating, hoping that 'the blood and the cries will hide everything that is wrong'. He remembered how he trembled, thinking of what he had to do. 'Faltering and disconcerted ... hesitating at every step', 'like a blind man ... bewildered and lost'. Bell had seen other young surgeons in the same confused and distressed plight, 'turning round to their friends ... holding consultations amidst the cries of the patient' who lay 'bleeding in great pain and awful expectation'.[8]

'Do unto others': the decision to operate

Operations were such perilous undertakings that in civil practice it was rare for them to proceed on the approval of only one surgeon, however senior. Early in the century surgeons often required the concurrence of a physician before operating. As surgeons gained confidence, however, they resisted that subordination. Despite the lonely eminence of the heroic surgeon it remained customary for a colleague to second the decision to operate and confer validation in the event of failure or criticism. 'Humanitas' denounced an operation at the Middlesex Hospital in 1836 when George Mayo amputated a girl's leg at the thigh, ostensibly to cure 'neuralgia' in the stump for which the unfortunate patient had already endured three operations. Three established surgeons – Charles Bell, James Arnott and Edward Tuson – had already declined to remove the leg to ease the pain but a relatively junior surgeon had decided to attempt a bold and uncertain procedure. He was said to have justified his willingness because 'the poor patient desired it' but 'Humanitas' alleged that 'for months and months the most specious arguments and solicitations have been employed to obtain the poor girl's consent'.[9] As today, obtaining a patient's consent was considered important as much for the protection of the surgeon as for the safety of the patient.

Experienced surgeons sometimes took the decision out of the hands of patients, at least for minor procedures. Astley Cooper would sometimes use the knife 'under pretence of mere examination'. His nephew Bransby recounted a patient's reaction:

> Sir, you had no right to do that without consulting me; God bless
> my soul! Sir, the pain is intolerable; if you had asked me I don't think
> I should have submitted.

Cooper tartly replied that the patient would be well in the time it would have taken him to decide whether to submit or not.[10]

Whether a surgeon proposed a capital operation depended on the answers to many questions. Samuel Cooper suggested half a dozen, the burden of which impressed on surgeons a prudence in contrast to their reputation for 'lopping off' limbs at will. He asked; is the affliction curable?; can diseased parts be removed safely?; is there any chance of cure by other means?; what is the best chance of life? Having decided on surgery Cooper enjoined consideration: he advised keeping the interval between informing the patent and performing the operation short, keeping instruments out of sight and reminded that an operation needed to be performed well rather than quickly.[11] Astley Cooper urged his students to ponder whether 'we should choose to submit to the pain and danger we are about to inflict'.[12] Abernethy likewise told his students that there was 'but one rule in surgery ... Do unto others ....'.[13] Surgeons themselves, however, appear to have submitted rarely to their colleagues' knives. The only account of an operation written by a surgeon – Canadian John Stephenson – of the cleft palate that Philibert Roux repaired in

---

*The operation lasted an hour, and took 'all his skill and all my endurance', Stephenson wrote (originally in Latin). He 'suffered less from the pain than from the irritation and tickling caused by the introduction of the needles'.

1819 is brief and evasive.'[14]

'To submit or not': the patient's decision to consent

Patients facing the prospect of surgery confronted a terrible choice in which, as Henry Bigelow put it, 'fear of pain co-operated with a fear of death'.[15] To some surgeons the decision could appear simple. Benjamin Brodie put the forceful view. A man has a stone in the bladder: he suffers torture and without surgery can only anticipate a painful and slow death. As the lesser of two evils he can submit to three minutes on the table and within forty eight hours could be declared perfectly safe and cured.[16] Of course the choice was rarely so simple and Brodie knew it. An accomplished operator, he advised caution, reckoning that in only one in sixty cases did he recommend surgery for schirrous breast. Brodie's caution may have been due as much to patients' reactions as to clinical indicators of likely success. He believed in making the patient acquainted with all that the surgeon knew on the subject.

Just as patients pondered whether to submit, so surgeons wondered whether to urge or accept the necessity for operating. Surgeons certain of their diagnosis and skills could bring considerable persuasion to bear, arguments difficult for a patient to resist. The surgeon's reputation for independence, if not arrogance, might be supposed to be rooted in the traditions of the heroic age when the operator assumed his lonely and oppressive responsibility. It comes as something of a surprise, then, to find that surgeons placed before their patients candid impressions of the likely outcome of the procedures in question. Frederic Skey urged his colleagues not to 'conceal or withhold' details which would help patients decide nor 'contend by argument or entreaty' to influence them.[17] 'The patient', said even Brodie, 'must decide for himself'.[18]

The case book of Maurice Collis provides an example of a patient who did just that. In 1830 a young woman named Alicia Syme consulted Collis, Surgeon of the Meath Hospital in Dublin. Miss Syme had lost her nose at the age of nine ten years before to 'a species of herpetic ulceration'. She had no hopes of having it relieved but rather sought treatment for an eye infection. Collis, however, had read in the *Edinburgh Medical and Surgical Journal* of Robert Liston's attempts to restore lost noses and he broached the subject with her. Miss Syme ('of a low stature, ... rather robust') was no lady but Collis, by his account, gave her every opportunity to give what we would describe as informed consent. He described to her the reasons why an operation could be attempted as well as 'all the objections against it'

Figure 7.1

John Abernethy (1764-1831) about 1825,
one of at least a dozen prints of him sold at the height of his career.
The portrait suggests something of Abernethy's ability to command the
attention of his students and the confidence of his patients.

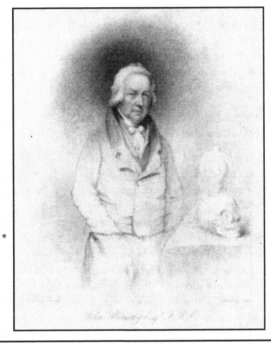

and gave her Liston's description of his case. 'I left her to her own decision to submit or not' he said. Miss Syme decided to consent. Collis cut a graft from her forehead in a painful operation in which she was 'excessively irritable and unsteady,' doubtless rueing her decision. Although cured of an 'unpleasant and disgusting deformity' Miss Syme remained an object of pity, at least in winter, when her cheeks became pink but her nose remained white: Collis could not look at her without laughing.[19] Though his work might be used to help a patient to decide, Liston himself was loath to induce. 'I won't try to persuade the patient', he told James Miller, 'it is too serious ... to promise a successful result'. This private communication between friends is a long way from the overbearing figure of legend.[20]

Psychological insights, however intuitive, informed many surgeons' attitude toward patients awaiting surgery. John Green

Crosse advised students to 'manage the minds of your patients'.[21] John Abernethy detailed the means of that management: he told his students that surgeons had 'but two holds' over patients' minds– fear and hope. 'I use both of them' he said.[22] Abernethy's brusquerie became legendary – so much celebrated that, imitated by his numerous pupils, he may have unwittingly encouraged the arrogance still apparent in some surgeons today, generations removed from the medical world of Georgian London. Abernethy's direct manner is captured by dialogue he reproduced in his lectures of his response to a patient suffering from a stricture of the urethra. He produces a bougie and proposes to employ it to enlarge the diameter of the patient's urethra:

> 'Oh Lord, Sir, you frighten me; you could not, I am sure'
> 'We will try, if you please'.[23]

Aston Key was less subtle. Told by a lady to whose house he had come to cut out a tumour in the neck that 'I don't think I can have it done' Key, after remonstrating repeatedly, used 'a very decided though unparliamentary expression' and left in disgust.[24] Just as we need to appreciate the variety of surgical operations and the range of techniques, we also need to free ourselves of the assumption that all patients approached surgery in the same frame of mind.

Some patients chose to decline surgery even when given a reasonable chance of surviving. In 1836 the Edinburgh Eye Infirmary recorded in its annual reports the number of 'operations recommended but not consented to': they equalled the number of operations performed.[25] The choice was no easy one. A country gentleman consulted Astley Cooper over a stone in the bladder. Cooper recommended lithotomy, at his hands a quick and relatively safe, though excruciatingly painful, operation. The man considered whether he possessed the resources to undergo the trial. 'I never can submit to an operation' he told Cooper simply, and returned to the country where he died shortly after.[26] This was a legitimate and very real choice and the patient's desire to confront it with dignity was respected in a society which admired 'bottom', the capacity to endure travail.

'The friends at last consented': families and surgery[27]

Deciding to submit to surgery was for many a collective rather than an individual decision. At the very least a family would be involved in weighing up the risks and benefits and often the term 'friends' had a literal meaning. Surgeons often preferred to communicate with the patient through intermediaries because it resulted in 'calmer' and more 'disinterested' resolution.[28] In 1830 John Macdonald entered James Syme's Edinburgh Surgical Hospital with a swollen thigh exuding a foul discharge, the result of an injury five years before when he had suffered a compound fracture, now incurable. Macdonald's friends asked after the possibility of amputation. They were told that it offered the smallest chance of success and would be 'extremely unpleasant'; there was 'no small probability' that he would die on the table. Everyone who saw him considered his death as certain and close. Syme felt that 'it seemed proper to state the matter fully to the friends' who, against the odds, 'decided on making the trial'. In removing the leg, in a double flap operation high up at the trochanter, Syme discovered the cause of the discharge – diseased bone. Though Macdonald took soup and cordials after the operation he survived just seven hours. In this case 'the friends' accepted responsibility for the operation: as Syme was careful to make clear in his clinical report.[29] And yet, involving the friends also entailed risk. 'The friends should never have the opportunity', said Brodie from experience, 'of turning round ... afterwards, and saying, "you said there was no danger, and here my wife, my husband, or my friend is dead"'.[30]

Indeed the burden of grief in the event of failure was evenly distributed between those electing surgery, those performing it and the chance inherent in the event. John Scott at the London Hospital operated to remove a painful tumour from the clavicle of a fourteen-year-old girl whose mother had decided that surgery was preferable to the continuing pain of the tumour. Scott cut around the tumour and attempted to remove it with his fingers. It burst exuding 'a large quantity of cheesy scrofulous matter'. The tumour had enveloped a blood vessel which then burst and she died within three-quarters of an hour. It is impossible to say who should have been held accountable.[31]

Despite John Brown's memorable description of James restraining the growling Rab in Minto House, it was rare for members of the family to remain during the operation especially in hospitals. In rural emergencies the household members and servants could be asked to assist however. Robert Liston, summoned to treat a farmer whose arm had been 'crushed to jelly' in a machine, found the household 'terrified to death' (quite possibly of Liston) and 'worse than useless'. They refused to remain in the house, much less in the room, and Liston was obliged to amputate with the help of a pupil and his post-

195

Figure 7.2

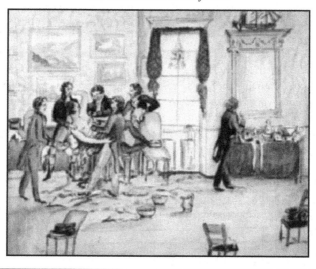

*This rare watercolour depicts surgeons performing an
operation on an 'R. Power' in 1817. Many operations were performed
in private homes, especially of the middle and upper classes, though it
is unlikely that any of these men is related to the patient.
The man died thirteen days later.*

chaise driver.[32] Apart from the distress they would feel the
practicalities of the operating room prevented loved ones offering
comfort during the process. However, patients' relatives sometimes
attended 'private' operations. In August 1846 Charlotte Brontë
accompanied her father, the Rev. Patrick Brontë, to a surgeon in
Manchester to support him during an operation for cataract.
Charlotte remained in the room at her father's wish. She wrote home
to Haworth that during the fifteen-minute operation in which her
father displayed 'extraordinary patience and firmness', she 'neither
spoke nor moved', feeling that 'the less I said, either to papa or the
surgeons, the better'. During her father's month-long convalescence
in Manchester Charlotte began to write *Jane Eyre*.[33]

The consequences of allowing loved ones even near the operating
room is illustrated by the story told by the Australian writer Mary
Gilmore. Growing up in rural New South Wales in the 1860s she
heard a visiting Englishman and former clergyman tell a story in
which 'the agony in his voice' remained with her still. Years before,

the man's young wife developed breast cancer and submitted to an operation. She had asked her husband to remain with her 'for she thought that with him there she could endure'. Her cries so unnerved the young man that he put his hands to his ears and ran. His wife died on the table. Suffering from 'brain-fever' he abandoned his vocation and emigrated to Australia where he lived a wandering life. A macabre souvenir marked the depth of his distress. He carried in his pocket her tanned breast, soft as velvet and ivory-coloured from his sweat.[34] Gilmore's story may be apocryphal but it loses none of its power as a symbol of the trauma an operation might cause to loved ones obliged to impotently observe it.

'Dread': anticipating surgery

Patients came to the operating table by several routes. The victims of industrial, domestic or road accidents came involuntarily, carried to infirmaries by cabs or in barrows or brought on doors hastily unhung for the purpose. Soldiers and sailors, as we have seen, reached the surgeons of a ship or a regiment hardly willingly but with equal urgency. Only in civil surgery did patients confront not only a choice over whether they would consent to surgery – the contemporary expression being to 'submit' – but also a delay between diagnosis and treatment which added apprehension to the burden of physical suffering. Thomas Graham, Baron of Lynedoch, having heard his surgeon's arguments took up his pen and wrote in an assured hand to his apothecary, 'My dear Sir I have settled with Mr Alexander to have the operation performed on my eyes at 12 o'clock on Wednesday next'.[35] He had several days to contemplate the ordeal to come.

Understandably, fear of pain deterred many sufferers from seeking relief by surgical treatment. Too often their reluctance aggravated conditions which eventually compelled recourse to surgery anyway. Tumours grew until their bulk or pain obliged consultation. Stones lay painfully in bladders growing larger and more difficult to remove. Aneurisms grew weaker, left untreated until on the verge of bursting. Diseased joints brought pain and debility. Lesions suppurated, diminishing the prospect of cure while increasing the likelihood of operation. Patients would go from one practitioner to another and often quacks of various colours, seeking assurance that treatment other than surgery would alleviate or cure their condition. Samuel Cooper described the pathetic plight of women suffering from uterine polyps who would take tonics and astringents, seeing one practitioner after another 'till, at length, the uterus is examined, and a polypus is discovered'.[36] 'All this fatal procrastination', James Miller mused, 'because the sufferer could not brook the thought of pain *under the knife*.[37] The tough-minded William Fergusson wondered that 'some patients will suffer any pain to avoid a cutting instrument', describing the case of 'a timid old lady' who consented to the application of strong caustic potassa fusa to remove a 'fungoid-looking tumour' that Fergusson could have excised swiftly.[38] Other surgeons, such as John Erichsen, expressed similar contempt for 'persons of an irritable and anxious mind'. His response to a patient exhibiting 'ignorance or timidity' was simply 'to compel him'.[39]

A surgeon's disdain for the timid could rest as much on clinical theory as moral judgement. 'Fear', William Falconer asserted in his prize-winning essay of 1791, was 'a debilitating passion'.[40] It diminished the force of the heart, weakened the pulse, induced 'paleness, shivering, and faintness': all understandable responses to the prospect of surgery. Fear, however, also provoked diarrhoea, jaundice, schirrous and gangrene and made patients more liable to 'contagious distempers'. The case of a Mrs Appleyard seemed to substantiate Falconer's theory. William Hey recalled how awareness of an imminent operation to extirpate a tumour in her breast intensified her suffering. The operation had to be deferred on account of Mrs Appleyard's 'sickness and frequent retching' which began immediately after she had consented to surgery. Hey noticed that her 'uneasiness of mind ... seemed to be the sole cause' of her complaints. He relieved the symptoms with 'aromatic and volatile medicines' and proceeded to remove a large tumour weighing over four pounds. Unfortunately the growth recurred and she died after a second such operation.[41] Such anxiety could even become fatal. In 1831 Glasgow surgeons reported John Macbride's 'sudden death from dread of operation'. Having crushed his arm between two cart-wheels the week before, Macbride was unanimously advised to consent to amputation. He seemed 'extremely depressed, began to shake, and earnestly declared he could never submit'. The following day he died, of no discernible cause except fear.[42]

Our horror of painful surgery is such that we tend to imagine that all patients came to the operating room unwillingly. Frederic Skey, however, in describing his *New Operation for the Cure of Lateral Curvature of the Spine* insisted that in these cases young patients in particular often implored surgeons to attempt the operation. These patients, he maintained, clung to hope of relief however slight offering 'ready consent and even solicitation' to sway the 'wavering decision of the operator'. They counted the pain of 'disappointed expectation' greater than the pain of the operation.[43] Likewise one surgeon reported that a woman suffering from a scirrhous breast not only 'demanded an operation with great earnestness' but having lost the breast 'demanded a new trial'.[44]

Having accepted the inevitable the patient lay composing his or her self as best they could for the ordeal to come. Wilde, having watched the practice of the Devon and Exeter Hospital, observed how the hospital's surgeons 'out of the hearing of the timid patient' reached the decision for surgery: 'th' unhappy man (His own consent first gain'd)' was then

... removed
To a remote apartment, far from noise,
Which might distract him in his sad affliction ... [45]

Despite his reputation for self-possession and arrogance it was Liston who wrote in the opening pages of his authoritative *Elements of Surgery* that surgeons should 'attend to the state of the patient's mind and feelings'.[46] In this Liston echoed Thomas Percival's injunction in *Medical Ethics* to consider patients' 'feelings and emotions' as much as the symptoms they exhibited.[47] It was a commonplace of operative procedure, as Everard Home stressed in his lecture notes, that operations should be deferred ''til both the body & mind of the patient are prepared'.[48]

As the appointed day neared patients became aware of the necessity for preparation which can only have aggravated their dread. Some operations required dressings to be made to fit a particular wound and patients would be measured to enable the manufacture of pads, trusses or special dressings. Worse still, some surgeons planning particularly difficult operations felt justified in marking their patients' skin to guide the incisions. Major amputations requiring the shaping of flaps involved problems in three-dimensional geometry. Skey wrote that it had been his practice 'for many years' 'to sketch out a map of the parts implicated' with pen and ink upon the skin.[49] Samuel Cooper likewise recommended marking guides on patients' bodies.[50] Nathan Smith's method of measuring incisions and flaps must have placed unusual strain on his patients. He would encircle the limb in paper at what the text-books called the 'place of election' measuring its circumference. He would then fold the paper and shape it to make the semi-circular arcs which described the flaps and then transfer its profile to the limb in crayon.[51] The patients' thoughts while contemplating those crayon and ink marks on the day before the operation can only be imagined.

Despite the diversity of attitude and practice there must still have been a moment of decision at which the patient accepted that the operation would proceed. Detailed examples from British sources are scanty. A surgeon who had watched John Collins Warren at the Massachusetts General Hospital described his practice. Warren would stand at the patient's head so he could be heard but not seen and ask "Will you have your leg off?" (as it might have been) "or will you not ...?". If the patient declined to proceed Warren would without further argument or recrimination have the patient returned to the ward. If the patient consented several assistants would secure him and Warren would proceed with the operation, continuing despite protest, struggle or entreaty.[52] The practice in Paris was not to compel patients to submit but those declining surgery would be obliged to leave hospital.[53] It was said that Robert Liston, having obtained a patient's consent, once pursued him into the privies and broke down the door to carry him back to the operating room after he had reneged.[54]

Other surgeons allowed a choice up to the point of incision – or acknowledged the impossibility of compulsion. William Squires, Liston's assistant at the first operation using ether in England, recalled that as Frederick Churchill came to he looked about and, not realising the operation was over, uttered 'the patient's old cry ... "I can't have it done, I must die as I am"'.[55] James Miller remembered operations curtailed 'from want of courage and self control' by the patient. He described one of Liston's patients in Edinburgh, a 'lady of rank' suffering from a tumour deep in her neck, who had set and broken many appointments to have it excised at her house. At last, one morning Liston arrived to find the lady sitting, apparently composed and attired in suitable loose clothing for the operation. With everyone anxious and an assistant kneeling before her (ready to restrain her) Liston prepared to make the first incision. The lady shrieked and overturned the table with its instruments and hot water. The assistant, kicked in the stomach, lay heaving on the carpet while the patient fled the room.[56] A surgeon's response might be irritation, philosophic resignation, or even relief. William Cooper, Astley's uncle, remarked as a would-be patient, alarmed by the sight of the instruments, fled the theatre 'By God I am glad he is gone'.[57]

James Miller, who over twenty years saw hundreds of patients in the operating room, displayed an unusual gift in imagining the ordeal from the patient's perspective. In advocating the adoption of chloroform he described the experience of painful surgery. Miller imagined the patient entering the theatre perhaps walking, perhaps carried, his nerves 'screwed to a pitch of unnatural tension ... preternaturally acute'. He would have heard the hum of voices of the waiting students, seen the glare of light from the great skylight which illuminated many operating rooms, the glitter of instruments, and 'the ominous table, vacant ....' He may have taken in the steam rising from pitchers of hot water, the dressers in their aprons, the piles of clean linen and towels and even the 'crowd of eager faces' on the surrounding benches. There were some, Miller recalled, who displayed no alarm or unease and who met the prospect with bravado. Most, though, of either sex 'quail under it'. At this point some lost heart and fled. Others submitted to the preparations suffering alarm and 'an amount of shock equal to that which the operation itself might produce'. Miller had seen youths brought unwillingly to the theatre, their progress able to be traced by frightful yells, or 'sobs of deep distress'. Occasionally 'a plurality of stout assistants' could scarcely drag the unwilling patient into the operating room. All this, Miller considered, was 'bad; painful, injurious and unseemly': and this before the cutting began.[58]

'My life in your hands': confidence

In his *Medical Ethics* (first published in 1803 and re-printed several times before 1850) Thomas Percival made clear the connection between a surgeon's demeanour and his patient's ability to bear an operation and even make a recovery. He urged his colleagues to 'unite tenderness with steadiness, and condescension with authority'. This, he believed, would excite in his patients 'gratitude, respect, and confidence'.[59] Of the three, confidence made the most difference. James Gregory believed that a practitioner 'unfeeling and rough in his manners' – the epitome of the conventional image of the surgeon – could 'make ... his heart sink within him, as ... one who comes to pronounce his doom'.[60] Samuel Cooper was unusually aware of the moral dimension of operating. He approved of anything that tended to 'calm, assuage and relax' believing that it could even retard mortification.[61] Frederic Skey believed that 'the larger the ... confidence entertained by the patient in the skill and resources of the surgeon, the more fully he will divest his mind of apprehension'.[62] Allowing for the adulation Cooper attracted from contemporaries and especially his nephew Bransby, they did recognise his capacity to reassure patients as among his most distinctive gifts. A man about to undergo an operation for aneurism is reported to have said 'I place my life in your hands ... anything you wish I will submit to'. The man survived only forty hours.[63]

We are permitted very few glimpses of what passed between surgeon and patient. We can only hear their words mediated by the few snippets recorded. We cannot see the looks they exchanged or the way glances were avoided. We cannot hear the breathing of either party, see the sweat beading their brows or soaking their armpits or smell the fear hanging over both. But we can sense from the little we have that, in the heightened emotion attending the event, surgeons and patients could build a bond of trust which might carry both through the ordeal before them. Charles Bell suggested something of the reciprocal relationship; even obligation. 'If a patient says '"In your hands I believe myself safe"', he wrote, 'I think the obligation binding'.[64]

The very words a surgeon spoke and his manner could carry a profound message of reassurance or – conversely – of indifference. Those suffering acutely from the conditions demanding surgical alleviation may have responded profoundly to such an invocation. George Macilwain, student of John Abernethy, recalled him 'as usual' in speaking a few words of encouragement to a woman patient. After a few seconds she said 'very earnestly but firmly', 'I hope, Sir, it will not be too long'. Abernethy replied with equal gravity 'No indeed, ... that would be too horrible'.[65] Thomas Percival thought it 'humane and salutary' for assistants in the course of an operation to 'speak occasionally' to the patient to comfort him and assure him, 'if consistent with truth', that the operation went well and would soon end.[66] Astley Cooper was more comfortable with dissembling to ease a patient's mind: 'It is your duty ... to support hope' he told his students 'even when you are still doubtful of the issue'.[67]

The effect of this attitude in practice is suggested by a detailed report of George Guthrie's operation to remove a large malignant tumour from the face of a Hertfordshire woman named Mary Brown. Mrs Brown, forty five years old and with fourteen children, had entered the Westminster Hospital in 1835. In October Guthrie cut out the tumour in a long and difficult operation involving a large incision and complex and 'tedious' dissection. During the operation the maxillary artery ruptured and haemorrhaged 'which occasioned a good deal of distress to the patient'. Mrs Brown, however, bore the 45-minute operation in silence and with 'noble courage'. The *Lancet's* correspondent recorded both Guthrie's 'highly censurable' calls to his assistants ('a knife!', 'I want something that will cut here!', 'a hook!', 'a sponge!') but also his words of encouragement. While directing his dressers peremptorily, Guthrie also spoke to the patient evidently in a different tone. 'You bear it very well, my dear lady!' he said. 'It is almost done!' and 'By the blessing of God, my dear soul, it is nearly over'. The reporter felt that Guthrie's good intentions were marred somewhat by the clanking of instruments in a pewter bowl at the patient's ear but the report indicates how strong the nexus could be between a surgeon speaking encouragingly and a patient demonstrating ideal courage.[68]

'Shakes, swears or sweats': the strain of operating

Nor was it only the patient who needed courage. It is in considering how surgeons felt about their work that we encounter dissension in the available evidence. Testimony supporting that traditional view tends to be couched in the general: surgeons were 'rough, strong and quick, and very indifferent to pain': that, though, from Sir Frederick Treves, a nineteenth century witness, but one who never saw an operation performed without anaesthetic.[69] The evidence suggesting that surgeons were powerfully affected by their responsibility – which they generally nevertheless continued – usually relates to particular men. Here the 'great man' paradigm so pervasive in medical history can be productively subverted. Biographies, memoirs and writings of the great surgeons of the period provide ample testimony that even the boldest operators harboured misgivings and anxieties. James Crichton-Browne who, like Treves, never saw an operation performed without anaesthesia, passed on a saying from his teachers who claimed 'every great surgeon, it used to be said, shakes, swears or sweats'.[70]

James Miller, one of the most candid surgeons, listed the sources of a surgeon's anxiety as he stood before a patient on the table. First he dreaded the pain he was about to inflict. Next came the difficulty of the operation, the ensuing unforeseen complications and the risk of failure. These could equally affect the patient's life and the surgeon's reputation.[71] The desire to finish an operation quickly (whether from concern for the patient or for reputation) imposed a peculiar strain on operators. Some expressed this tension by shouting at the patient, colleagues or dressers. The tension showed in the haste with which, as Samuel Cooper said, surgeons sawed through bone with 'short, very rapid, and almost convulsive strokes'.[72]

Many surgeons, like John Scott of the London Hospital, reacted to the strain of operating with an 'irritable and uncertain temper'.[73] Everard Home when exasperated was 'violent in his language'.[74] John Flint South was 'easily roused to wrath and did not then measure his language'.[75] Charles Mayo, 'blunt, outspoken, and testy', often

203

exploded with 'half-humorous vituperative epithets of the quaintest and most original description'.[76] It is apparent – and perhaps understandable – that in the crisis of an operation many surgeons swore aggressively, the more so because the culture of the wards accepted anger and crudity as a part of everyday occurrence. Those who recalled Charles Aston Key's 'dictatorial' manner excused it by pointing out that the 'brusqueness and roughness' was the habit and that the use of 'strong words and oaths' towards patients and subordinates was 'not all uncommon'. Once, finding that a steward had not signed for wine, Key turned white with rage, abused the steward, nurses and pupils and, after writing 'C.A.K.' in gigantic letters on the relevant form crushed the pen to splinters.[77]

Some surgeons undoubtedly conformed to the popular stereotype exhibiting (as Charles Bell put it after observation) 'coarseness, want of feeling, and stupidity' perhaps even insobriety.[78] Although as a physician and a malicious insinuator his evidence is suspect, it is no wonder that James Gregory reported that surgeons at the Edinburgh Infirmary worked 'primed with a good dram of brandy'.[79] However, the best surgeons offered (as John Simon wrote) 'brotherhood to the sufferers'.[80] Samuel Cooper acknowledged the desirability of surgeons wishing to 'participate in the pain'.[81] The words and the actions of many contradict the shallow stereotype of the brutal or indifferent surgeon. They were men of great humanity on whom fell the burden of their skill. They exercised that skill to alleviate suffering albeit at the cost of inflicting pain on their patients and conflicting with their humanity.

John Abernethy was one of the period's most noted surgical teachers. He appears often in memoirs and in compilations partly because over thirty years he lectured to thousands of students but also because he was an eccentric, celebrated for his hearty good sense and brusque manner. We have a clearer impression of his reactions to surgery than that of any other operator. A colleague once greeted him casually as he walked to the operating room with a conventional 'How are you?'. 'Sir,' Abernethy replied, 'I feel as if I was going to a hanging'. As he aged Abernethy's dislike of operating deepened. He became 'figetty' and it became 'unpleasant' to assist him although he is said never to have been 'unkind to the patient'.[82] One of Abernethy's students recalled, though, how he had seen him in the retiring room after a severe operation, with tears in his eyes, lamenting 'what he had just been compelled to do by dire necessity and surgical rule'.[83] More bluntly another observer remembered him vomiting after operating.[84]

204

James Arnott who knew Charles Bell as Surgeon to the Middlesex Hospital recalled how Bell went to operations 'with the reluctance of one who has to face an unavoidable evil ... [whose] cheek has been seen to blanch on proceeding to operations performed with the utmost self-possession and skill'.[85] Bell felt the loneliness of the responsibility most and referred to it both in private letters to his wife and brother and in his published works. Even the most skilful, Bell wrote, 'have gone to work with anxious feelings'.[86] A serious operation was 'always severe on me' he told his wife Marion. To his brother George he often confided that, for example, he had 'an anxious operation on my spirits tonight'. The operation failed and three weeks later he told his brother how he had had 'a most miserable time ... I shall regret it as long as I live'. Nor did the burden become easier with time. 'I suffer indescribable anxiety' he told his brother, 'the more I do, the worse'.[87]

Likewise Robert Liston, one of the most 'heroic' of the British surgeons (and the first to use ether anaesthesia), has been described as 'crude, loud, abrasive, insensitive, and brutally rough on his patients'.[88] Liston presented a brash exterior and his reputation for self-possession became legendary. One admirer, Forbes Winslow, described the 'perfect *non chalance*' with which he commenced the most formidable operation preparing the instruments and table 'with as much *sang froid* as a waiter at the London Tavern ... preparing for a dinner party'. Externally Liston conformed to this impression. 'His voice,' Winslow conceded, 'is somewhat harsh and discordant'. In the operating room, however, it became 'music to the sick man's ear'. His hand 'hard as iron' in the operating room became 'soft as down when applied to the throbbing pulse and aching brow'.[89] His friend James Miller revealed after Liston's death that he had 'I well know', lost many an hour's sleep 'and many a meal' from the 'mental anxiety in the prospect of operation'.[90]

Observers detected the tension. George Crabbe, who as a clergyman may have encountered surgeons uneasy with their calling, described in his narrative poem *The Borough* the effects on 'Men who suppress their Feelings but who feel/ The painful Symptoms they delight to heal'.[91] In their portraits can be seen the 'surgeon's mouth', embodied by Joseph Green, 'with its close-shut lips and air of restraint and firmness'.[92] James Miller felt the conflict between 'my brain urging my hands to work freely [and] my heart upbraiding me for causing the poor patient such agony'.[93] A surgeon even admitted in a contribution to the *Lancet* how, when a hernia operation was able to be avoided, that 'I believe I was guilty of entertaining some

Figure 7.3

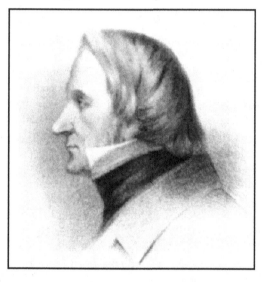

*Joseph Henry Green (1791-1863),
nephew and pupil of Henry Cline, whose portrait
suggests the close-set 'surgeon's mouth'.*

slight sensations of involuntary disappointment'.[94] William Hey junior admitted that he and his colleagues were 'so continually brought into contact' with suffering that 'our sensibilities become blunted'.[95] It was a concern that many surgeons must have shared even if few expressed it in print.

Silas Weir Mitchell knew the extremes: a surgeon who 'fears to hurt ... does too little'. Mitchell urged his colleagues to take 'a larger view of the uses of pain and distress'.[96] Henry Smith who wrote about painful surgery in 1854 argued that the 'firmness of purpose' surgeons were obliged to adopt was yet compatible with 'the most generous and most gentle sympathy'. He believed that feelings of humanity would animate 'the really good surgeon' even though he must occasionally display an 'apparent insensibility' to his patients' suffering.[97] In an address to medical students Bigelow sketched out the qualities of the ideal surgeon: young – at most middle-aged – with a strong, steady hand, ambidextrous, bold, above all devoid of pity. He had to act, Bigelow affirmed, 'as if he was not moved by the shrieks of his patient'. And yet Bigelow decried insensibility and brutality claiming that it was possible to be a 'humane surgeon'.[98] Reflective surgeons struggled with the tension between the desire to heal and the need to hurt. Unreflective surgeons suffered the consequences of unresolved ambiguity, like Gideon Mantell who, after amputating a boy's arm in 1831, 'muddled through the day' oppressed by what he had had to do.[99]

Operative surgeons could not turn aside from the horror of their calling but had to confront it and look beyond it. John Abernethy, though a reluctant operator, was candid. In describing a procedure he began 'I made a wound ...'.[100] Those who cut with assurance and skill were convinced that they caused less suffering than those who wielded the knife half-heartedly. William Fergusson expressed his contempt for the 'amiable sensitiveness' of surgeons who eschewed cutting abscesses in favour of the repeated application of caustics which did their work – and inflicted greater pain for longer – but after the surgeon had left the ward.[101] But contemporaries saw no paradox, much less an oxymoron, in the term used by Pettigrew 'the humane surgeon'.[102] Many sought the least painful way to do what they had to do and deplored unnecessary or unjustifiable procedures. William Fergusson himself questioned the practice of closing incisions four or more hours after operations having 'always remarked the additional distress'.[103] Reactions such as his challenge the picture of the surgeon indifferent to suffering. Charles Bell expressed the realistic attitude which in many surgeons became a gratuitous hardness. They could not, he pronounced, act 'like the foolish maid who holds her apron betwixt her pretty eyes and the object of her horror'.[104] Surgeons looked directly into the face of the living subject.

Notes

1. 32nd Report of the Charity Commissioners [into St Thomas's Hospital], PP 1840, Vol. XIX, 684.

2. Thomas Pettigrew, *Biographical Memoirs of the Most Celebrated Physicians, Surgeons, etc., etc.*, 3 vols (London: Fisher, Son & Co., 1839–40), Vol. II, 2.

3. Samuel Cooper, *A Dictionary of Practical Surgery* (London: Longman, Hurst, Rees, Orme & Brown, 1829), 344.

4. Evidence of Anthony Carlisle to the Select Committee on Medical Education, PP 1834, Vol. XXXIV, 144.

5. George Guthrie, *On the ... Operation for the Extraction of a Cataract* (London: W. Sams, 1834), 1.

6. William Fergusson, *A System of Practical Surgery* (London: John

Churchill, 1846), 170.

7. Royston Lambert, *Sir John Simon 1816–1904 and English Social Administration* (London: Macgibbon & Kee, 1963), 39.

8. John Bell, *The Principles of Surgery*, 2 vols (Edinburgh: T. Cadell & W. Davies, 1801), 6–7.

9. *Lancet*, 1835–36, Vol. II, 187.

10. Bransby Cooper, *The Life of Sir Astley Cooper, Bart.*, 2 vols (London: John Parker, 1843), Vol. II, 320–21.

11. Samuel Cooper, *The First Lines of the Practice of Surgery* (London: Longman, Hurst, Rees, Orme & Brown, 1840), 720–21.

12. 'Case of Ligature of the Aorta', in Astley Cooper & Benjamin Travers, *Surgical Essays* (London: Cox & Son, 1818), 112.

13. John Abernethy, *Lectures on Anatomy, Surgery and Pathology* (London: James Bullock, 1828), 164.

14. Francis, 'Repair of Cleft Palate by Philibert Roux in 1819', *Journal of the History of Medicine and Allied Sciences*, 1963, 213–14.

15. Henry Jacob Bigelow, *An Introductory Lecture delivered at Massachusetts Medical College* (Boston: David Clapp, 1850), 13.

16. Benjamin Brodie, *Clinical Lectures on Surgery* (Philadelphia: Lea & Blanchard, 1846), 31.

17. Frederic Skey, *Operative Surgery* (London: John Churchill, 1850), 13.

18. Brodie, *op. cit.* (note 16), 33.

19. 'Mr Collis's Case in which a nose was supplied', *Edinburgh Medical & Surgical Journal*, 1831, Vol. 36, 62–66.

20. Liston to Miller, 7 May 1835, Ms 6084–95, WIHM .

21. John Green Crosse, *An Inaugural Address, Delivered at the Opening of the Norfolk and Norwich Hospital Museum* (Norwich: Bacon & Co., 1845), 26.

22. Abernethy, *op. cit.* (note 13), 309.

23. *Ibid*, 207.

24. Samuel Wilks & G.T. Bettany, *A Biographical History of Guy's Hospital* (London: Ward & Lock, London, 1892), 334.

25. *Annual Report of the Edinburgh Eye Infirmary* [1836], 5.

26. Pettigrew, *op. cit.* (note 2), 98.

27. Cooper, *op. cit.* (note 3), 158.

28. Skey, *op. cit.* (note 17), 13.

29. 'Seventh Report of the Edinburgh Surgical Hospital', *Edinburgh Medical & Surgical Journal*, 1831, Vol. 36, 238.

30. Brodie, *op. cit.* (note 16), 33.

31. *Lancet*, 1833–34, Vol. I, 224.

32. Robert Liston, *Lectures on the Operations of Surgery* (Philadelphia:

Lea & Blanchard, 1846), 410.

33. Elizabeth Gaskell, *The Life of Charlotte Brontë* (London: J.M. Dent, 1946), 278–281.

34. Mary Gilmore, *Old Days: Old Ways A Book of Recollections* (Sydney: Angus & Robertson, 1934), 162-63.

35. Letter, 11 June 1832, Ms 16428, vii, f.55, NLS.

36. Cooper, *op. cit.* (note 3), ix.

37. James Miller, *Surgical Experience of Chloroform* (Edinburgh: Sutherland & Knox, 1848), 34.

38. Fergusson, *op. cit.* (note 6), 59.

39. John Erichsen, *The Science and Art of Surgery* (London: Walton & Maberly, 1853), 46, 48.

40. William Falconer, *A Dissertation on the Influence of the Passions on the Disorders of the Body* (London: C. Dilly, 1791), 38–39.

41. William Hey, *Practical Observations in Surgery* (London: T. Cadell Jnr & W. Davies, [1803; 1814]), 266.

42. *Glasgow Medical Journal*, Vol. IV, No. XIII, 96–97.

43. Frederic Skey, *On a New Operation for the Cure of Lateral Curvature of the Spine* (London: Longman, Orme, Brown, Green & Longmans, 1841), 49–50.

44. *Lancet*, 1834–35, Vol. I, 154.

45. J. Wilde, *The Hospital, a Poem in Three Books, Written in the Devon and Exeter Hospital*, (Norwich: Stevenson, Matchett & Stevenson, 1809), 40.

46. Robert Liston, *Elements of Surgery* (London: Longman, Orme, Brown, Green & Longmans, 1840), vii.

47. Thomas Percival, *Medical Ethics, or A Code of Institutes and Precepts* … (Oxford: J.H. Parker, 1849), 28.

48. 'On Amputation', 'Sir Everard Home's lectures', 1811, 1f3No. 334, RCSEng.

49. Skey, *op. cit.* (note 17), 32.

50. Cooper, *op. cit.* (note 3), 86.

51. Nathan Smith, *Medical and Surgical Memoirs* (Baltimore: William A. Francis, 1831), 217.

52. James Mumford, *Surgical Memoirs, and other essays* (New York: Moffat, Yard & Co., 1908), 157.

53. F. Campbell Stewart, *The Hospitals and Surgeons of Paris* (Philadelphia: Langley, 1843), 98.

54. Cock, 'Anecdota Listoniensa', *University College Hospital Magazine*, Vol. II, Nov 1911, No. 2, 58.

55. Squires, 'The First Operation under ether in Great Britain', *Lancet*, 1896, 1142–43.

56. Miller, *op. cit.* (note 37), 27–28.
57. Cooper, *op. cit.* (note 10), Vol. I, 301.
58. Miller, *op. cit.* (note 37), 24.
59. Percival, *op. cit.* (note 47), 27.
60. James Gregory, *On the Duties and Qualifications of a Physician* (London: W. Creech, 1805), 19.
61. Cooper, *op. cit.* (note 3), 877.
62. Skey, *op. cit.* (note 17), 3.
63. Cooper, *op. cit.* (note 10), Vol. II, 204.
64. Charles Bell, *Illustrations of the Great Operations of Surgery* (London: Longman, 1821), 116.
65. George Macilwain, *Memoirs of John Abernethy*, 2 vols (London: Hurst & Blackett, 1854), Vol. II, 203.
66. Percival, *op. cit.* (note 47), 38.
67. Astley Cooper & Frederick Tyrrell, *The Lectures of Sir Astley Cooper, Bart.* ... (London: Thomas Tegg, 1824), 30.
68. *Lancet*, 1835–36, Vol. I, 189–91. A letter from an assistant in a subsequent issue contested the accuracy of the report..
69. Frederick James, *The Elephant Man and Other Reminiscences* (London: 1923), 54.
70. James Crichton-Browne, *Victorian Jottings from an Old Commonplace Book* (London: Etchells & Macdonald, 1926), 185.
71. Miller, *op. cit.* (note 37), 29–30.
72. Cooper, *op. cit.* (note 3), 74.
73. Victor Plarr, *Lives of the Fellows of the Royal College of Surgeons*, 2 vols (London: Simpkin, Marshall Ltd, 1930), Vol. II, 274.
74. Cooper, *op. cit.* (note 10), Vol. II, 474.
75 Plarr, *op. cit.* (note 72), Vol. II, 332.
76. *Ibid*, 48.
77. Wilks & Bettany, *op. cit.* (note 24), 334.
78. Charles Bell to George Bell, 28 November 1835, George Jospeh Bell, (ed.), *Letters of Sir George Bell* (London: John Murray, 1870), 346.
79. James Gregory, *Additional Memorial to the Managers of the Royal Infirmary* (Edinburgh: Murray & Cochrane, 1803), 154.
80. Joseph Green, *Spiritual Philosophy: Founded on the Teaching of the Late Samuel Taylor Coleridge*, 2 vols (London: Macmillan, 1865), Vol. I, lii .
81. Cooper, *op. cit.* (note 3), 1061.
82. Macilwain, *op. cit.* (note 65), Vol. II, 204.
83. Victor Medvei & John Thornton, *The Royal Hospital of St Bartholemew (1123–1973* (London: St Bartholemew's Hospital

Medical College, 1974), 207.

84. Agatha Young, *Scalpel: Men who made Surgery* (London: Robert Hale, 1957), 132.

85. J.M. Arnott, quoted in Gordon Gordon-Taylor & E.W. Walls, *Sir Charles Bell: His Life and Times* (Edinburgh: E. & S. Livingstone, 1958), 82.

86. Charles Bell, *A System of Operative Surgery* (London: Longman, Hurst, Rees, Orme & Brown, 1814), 193.

87. Charles Bell to George Bell, 16 February 1826, Bell, *op. cit.* (note 77), 294.

88. Roderick McGrew & Margaret McGrew (eds), *Encyclopaedia of Medical History* (New York: McGraw-Hill, 1985), 325.

89. Forbes Winslow, *Physic and Physicians: A Medical Sketch Book*, 2 vols (London: Longman, Orme, Brown, 1839), Vol. II, 362; 358.

90. Miller, *op. cit.* (note 37), 29.

91. George Crabbe, *The Borough* (London: J. Hatchard, 1810), 93.

92. Plarr, *op. cit.* (note 73), Vol. I, 467.

93. Miller, *op. cit.* (note 37), 51.

94. 'Mr Gower's Professional Reminiscences', *Lancet*, 1830–31, Vol. I, 39.

95. William Hey (jun), *The Retrospective Address in Surgery* (Worcester: Deighton, 1843), 89–90.

96. Silas Wear Mitchell, *Doctor and Patient* (Philadelphia: J.B. Lippincott, 1888), 45.

97. Henry Smith, *The Improvements in Modern Surgery* (London: John Churchill, 1854), 22.

98. Bigelow, *op. cit.* (note 15), 11.

99. C.. Cecil Curwen, (ed.), *The Journal of Gideon Mantell: Surgeon and Geologist* (Oxford: Etchells & Macdonald, OUP, 1940), 99.

100. John Abernethy, *The Surgical Works*, 3 vols (London: Longman, 1811), Vol. II, 259.

101. Fergusson, *op. cit.* (note 6), 55.

102. Pettigrew, *op. cit.* (note 2), 164–65.

103. Fergusson, *op. cit.* (note 6), 171.

104. Bell, *op. cit.* (note 64), vii.

8

'The cutting part':
In the Operating Room

As the patient and the friends composed themselves for the ordeal to come, the surgery boys and junior dressers would prepare the operating room. Central to the operation was the table, as a rule a narrow form and surprisingly low to those encountering it anew. The table needed to be robust. It had to bear not only the patient but also the weight of several assistants restraining his or her struggles. Frederic Skey recalled having seen a table literally come to pieces in the middle of an operation bringing operators and patient to the floor.[1] A contributor to the *Lancet* ascribed the 'scenes of confusion and want of system' prevailing in the operating rooms of even the great London hospitals to the inadequacies of makeshift tables. He expressed grateful interest to James Veitch (who had devised thin ligatures twenty-five years before) for inducing the Admiralty to fund the construction of a new table. Not only strong enough to withstand the stresses of operators and patients upon it, the table also included drawers for instruments. In Veitch's table the instrument drawers were out of sight, obviating the 'most ostentatious and ill-timed display of instruments' which eroded the resolve of those awaiting surgery.[2]

'Secured him well': preparations for surgery

On the appointed 'operating day' the hospital's surgeryman would direct his boys to set out linen, towels, sponges and rags and, if the room lacked piped water or a copper, fetch jugs of hot water. 'Cordials' and water would be placed on a table within arms reach. The surgeon's dressers would prepare the instruments; some the property of the hospital kept in cupboards or drawers in the operating room; others the surgeon's own. Some advised covering them with lint 'to preserve the edges' of the knives.[3] Many concealed them with cloths to avoid alarming the patient while others warmed them to lessen the shock of the incision.[4]

In an adjoining room the surgeon and his assistants would prepare themselves. As they donned aprons or sleeves the senior surgeon would deliver last-minute instructions, allotting places and

213

duties and offering guidance and advice on the 'composure and quietness' he expected would obtain.[5] There is no clear evidence as to what they would have worn. Stories of blood-flecked frock coats and even evening dress appear to belong to the middle decades of the century. Photographs and engravings of surgeons and dressers show a mixture of clothes – shirt sleeves and aprons as well as hand-me-down formal clothes.

Contemporary texts make little reference to aspects of the preparation for operations which would have been inescapable. Few texts discuss the need to shave parts of the body for example. Others, such as James Wardrop, recommended bleeding the patient to faintness before commencing surgery to reduce the sensation of pain although the practice would seem to induce other risks. (John Flint South disagreed: 'unless the operator's object were to finish his patient'.[6]) Again practice differed between hospitals and surgeons: at Bart's in 1835 a sixteen-year-old girl about to undergo a half-hour operation for the excision of a tumour from her jaw was led into the theatre blindfolded, one of the very few descriptions referring to the practice.[7]

Accounts of operations make few references to whether and how patients were restrained. In describing amputation at the thigh Samuel Cooper advised assistants, rather obviously, to hold the patient's hands and to 'keep him from moving too much'.[8] Benjamin Bell referred to patients having to be 'supported' or 'secured' to 'prevent interruptions' in the course of the operation.[9] 'Supported' might appear to be a euphemism: Philip Crampton described an 'ungovernable' woman patient thrashing about in 'terror' unable to be restrained by four strong men.[10] If, however, surgeons were as the evidence suggests, less heartless than they have been portrayed then the term suggests a more humane regime than we may have imagined. Still, the struggles of a patient needed to be restrained lest an operation have to be abandoned and many surgeons routinely adopted a restraint of some kind including straps to tie a patient down. Country surgeons, operating with only the help of an apprentice, a coachman or a farm labourer might note how, as one amputating a 16-year-old boy's arm in a 'wretched cabin' in Ireland 'secured him well' but formal descriptions of cases in hospitals usually omit the details of restraint.[11] Experienced assistants were necessary, as the experience of a Dr Dunn, a county surgeon apothecary, suggests. Dunn confessed how in 1821 when he attempted to excise the bones of a boy's foot he encountered 'a deluge' of blood. The patient fainted. Dunn's two fourteen-year-old apprentices, a local woman and two labouring men called in to hold the patient became 'so sick and alarmed as to desert the room'[12]

The almost entire failure of texts to discuss these aspects demands consideration. As befitted a calling only a generation or two removed from a system of apprentices and masters, much of the detail of surgical procedure was conveyed not formally in manuals but informally. It is likely that surgeons advised their students which restraints worked and which did not and that senior dressers handed on advice to junior dressers.

As the porters placed the patient upon the table they may have been asked whether they wished to be restrained. Some expressed a desire to bear the ordeal without straps or belts. Sometimes, we may be sure, surgeons may have decided to overrule their patients' wishes perhaps signalling to their assistants to seize limbs or hold down a body at the moment they took up the knife. It is important to recall that in many cases patients were offered but declined restraint. While prone to make assumptions about the qualities of 'nervous' or 'timid' subjects, surgeons probably also developed a feel for whether patients would accept or require restraint. Patients' reactions would also change as the moment approached. A patient's resolve might waver when entering the operating room, on seeing the table, or catching a glimpse of the instruments which, Nathan Smith acknowledged, would often 'strike a dread into the mind' of the most composed man or woman.[13] Surgical texts occasionally referred to the need for patients to co-operate with the operator: 'a surgeon must be well assisted by the patient', wrote Robert Liston, 'or he cannot succeed'.[14] In operations for haemorrhoids or cleft palate or even some amputations it was important for patients to strain, hold themselves in particular attitudes or otherwise act in concert to enable the surgeon to complete the operation. Restraint alone could not always ensure that a patient remained still and in the right position. Accounts of operations which commend the patient for displaying fortitude refer not only to the sound that patients did (or rather did not) make but to the fact that they sat or lay still, helping the surgeon to work as rapidly as all desired. We are accustomed to thinking of patients, passive or struggling, as victims of the surgeon's knife. We need to accept that not only could patients volunteer for surgery but could co-operate during the operation.

Unless he practised in a hospital eschewing the device, a dresser would position and tighten the tourniquet. Whether he used a tourniquet or not depended as much on custom as on clinical necessity. William Gibson commented darkly in the early 1840s how

Figure 8.1

A surgeon (dressed in a long apron and sleeves)
with four assistants about to amputate an arm at the shoulder.
Charles Bell advised surgeons to 'appoint them to their places and their
duties'. One will compress the arteries in the neck; another will hold
the arm to be removed. The man on the right is tying a sheet about the
patient to restrain him to the chair; from Bell's,
Illustrations of the Great Operations of Surgery.

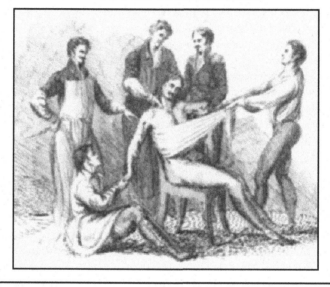

it had become 'fashionable' to trust to 'fingers and assistants':
Benjamin Brodie regarded it as a 'great mistake': Fergusson ascribed
it to 'foolish vanity'.[15]

The surgeon would take up the position most convenient for
his work; standing, occasionally sitting or even kneeling. His
dressers would arrange themselves around depending upon their
allotted duties. Junior dressers or porters might be told to hold the
patient steady, to grasp a limb in readiness for its removal or
sponge away blood from stumps or incisions. More senior
assistants would stand by to retract skin and muscles away from
the site of an incision or to help in tying arteries. Coster
advocated the importance of hospital surgeons employing skilled
assistants lest he 'appear awkward in the eyes of the spectators'.[16]
An inexperienced student dresser, as Everard Home noticed,

might 'actually be afraid of his own hands'.[17]

The operator bore the responsibility – and received the recognition of his colleagues – as the key member of a group. Frederic Skey stressed the importance of his dressers and assistants understanding the purpose and the detail of the operation. They were intended to 'multiply the hands of the operator', ideally to form 'one mind acting by four hands'. Skey advised operating in silence (in a text published in 1850 but clearly articulating ideas developed over years of operating without chloroform).[18] William Fergusson operated so completely without speaking that onlookers imagined him to have fallen out with his colleagues.[19] If directions had to be conveyed Skey advised the surgeon to speak 'plainly, briefly but intelligibly' and to avoid using operations for the purpose of demonstrating to pupils and juniors. John Erichsen, 'educated in the doctrines of Mr Liston', believed that the senior surgeon should indicate his instructions silently by a look or a gesture.[20] The prudent surgeon carefully rehearsed his assistants, for his reputation partly depended upon them: Anthony Carlisle called for 'the dramatic management of all the parties at a violent operation'.[21]

Despite drills and instructions the necessity of working together rapidly but carefully inevitably led to chaos. Liston, himself known to sacrifice care to speed, recalled 'indescribable' and 'under the circumstances, laughable' confusion. He describes a scenario which must surely have been a nightmare to all involved, with a tourniquet strap wrongly threaded, two assistant surgeons climbing onto the table pressing 'with all their might' on the patient's groin to arrest the arterial blood.[22] The disorder usual in some operating rooms rendered confusion even more likely. While 'recognised' assistants held back, their places were taken by 'persons ... unconnected with the ... hospital'.[23] At other times dressers would 'crane over and see what the surgeon is about,' obscuring the spectators' view.[24]

Operations did go wrong. Liston's nightmare represented perhaps the worst case – a haemorrhaging patient and unnerved assistants unable to prevent death. But less dramatic interruptions could disrupt the progress of an operation. 'Who has not seen', Wlliam Gibson asked, 'muscular fibres torn to shreds and tatters by the saw in the midst of a rapid and bungling operation?' by a surgeon trusting to his hands rather than a cloth retractor.[25] It often happened that the operator discovered an unexpected condition in the course of cutting or felt the need to consult senior colleagues to resolve a problem. Skey advised retiring to another room – yet another indication that operations were not over in a few minutes.[26]

217

'One sweep of his knife'?: the incision

Henry Bigelow described the moment of incision. Speaking to an audience whose members had witnessed surgery as operators or spectators he asked them to 'mark the hushed breath, the fearful intensity of silence, when the blade pierces the tissues ...'[27] The best operators cut decisively. 'If a man sets about it hesitatingly he makes some blunder or other' Abernethy admonished.[28] Frederic Skey declared 'Timidity marks the ignorant man at every step'. He described the consequences of his uncertainty and indecision in 'dissecting a little here, and dividing a little there. Heeding the advice of one assistant and then another, he protracts the operation by three or four times.'[29] Flustered by the pressure of the moment others made mistakes, cutting blindly, missing details, confused or surprised by the unexpected. Insights into the tension of the operating room suggest a different complexion to the old surgeons' joke – how 'with one sweep of his knife he cut off the limb of his patient, three fingers of his assistant and the coattail of a spectator'.[30]

With an untrammelled medical press and a profession in ferment it is not surprising to find that the journals freely printed allegations of incompetence and accounts of botched operations. Contemporaries accepted that not all operators could be equally proficient: Samuel Cooper wrote of the mortality attending a 'want of ordinary dexterity'.[31] Some of the errors described by observers (not always rivals or adversaries in the cause of medical reform) appear striking to modern eyes. Charles Bell, William Fergusson and Anthony Carlisle all told of surgeons embarrassed at forgetting saws. Carlisle alleged that a surgeon amputating in a patient's country house had cut to the bone before finding that he had left his saw in town: Bell claimed that William Lynn had to send for the hospital's joiner to obtain one.[32]

'Billy' Lucas, son of a distinguished surgeon of St Thomas's, little resembled his father. Although agreeable and popular, like him, he appears to have been 'not overburdened with brains of any kind' and operated 'generally very badly'.[33] Bransby Cooper (himself an incautious operator) branded him 'rash in the extreme'.[34] John Flint South recalled how these shortcomings 'now and then led him into ugly scrapes'. South regaled a horrifying story he had heard from other students which he believed. Just as Lucas was about to amputate a leg he found himself on the 'wrong' side of the patient (usually the left side). He shifted his position but performed the circular amputation as if her leg were still on the other side. This left the patient with bone projecting from the stump but no covering, and the amputated limb having superfluous flesh.[35] South does not record what Lucas did next but he probably had to perform another incision higher up to obtain enough flesh to fashion a stump. It was perhaps as well that Lucas was hard of hearing.[36]

'The most dreadful part': surgeons and pain

James Miller, among the most reflective of the surgeons of the era, wrote frankly and movingly of his feelings about the infliction of pain. Why was it, he asked, that his colleagues 'grew pale, and sickened, and even fell' while witnessing operations. Not from the mere sight of blood, he replied, nor of the sight of the wounds, but from 'the manifestation of pain and agony emitted by the patient'.[37] For them, as well as for us, it was the pain of surgery which remained the most horrific part of surgery. It was pain that made operations a torment for all concerned: patient, surgeon or student.

Surgeons discussed the reactions of patients to surgical pain in generalities and saw in their capacity to endure pain a relationship to their likelihood of recovering. Chelius, the German authority whose works were translated into English by John Flint South, believed that those who bore pain well were less prone to infection and more likely to survive than those 'excited by the least pain'.[38] Anthony Carlisle, despite his genial exterior and preoccupation with shellfish, acquired a profound depth of humanity through observing his patients' reactions. Their capacity to withstand painful operations, he confessed in a lecture to the London college in 1818, was 'extremely variable'. It did not 'depend upon age, sex, or strength'.[39] Others believed that there existed a hierarchy of sensitivity to pain. Chelius reported that operations were likely to be unfavourable on the very stout, on 'persons of a sanguineous temperament' and, surprisingly perhaps, those very tall and very strong. Paradoxically, 'nervous subjects', those 'very sensitive and excitable' though 'much affected' by the pain of an operation could be sustained by encouragement and comfort and were known to 'quickly perk up' afterwards. James Paget concluded that just as some people have an ear for music so others possessed 'a very fine sensibility to pain'. He was 'sure that the more cultivated races are far more sensitive to pain'. This hierarchy placed blacks at the bottom and 'among ourselves', Irish below English.[40] The only rule Carlisle would venture was that the inhabitants of colder, northerly climes and those who laboured for a living were 'more favourable subjects for severe operations'.

This hierarchy implied that women, particularly gentlewomen, were more sensitive to pain but surgeons differed in their views of women. Benjamin Brodie remained wary. He urged his colleagues not to operate on 'women of the higher classes of society, persons of either sex of a nervous or hysterical predilection or members of families in which 'mania' prevailed. Ladies, he claimed, died in 'a strange and unaccountable manner' after even the most 'trifling operations'.[41] Other surgeons found women more resilient: George Guthrie describing a tumour 'as big as your head' extracted from a woman's abdomen through a fourteen-inch incision jocularly remarked that 'ladies often did take a great deal of killing'.[42] Samuel Warren praised their 'great firmness', their capacity to endure pain which would 'utterly break down the stubborn strength of a man'.[43] Thomas Wakley stated at an inquest that men would 'quiver at the slightest touch' while women would submit to the most painful operations 'without a shudder'. Oddly, he then went on to describe a case of a man bearing an amputation without a word.[44] The evidence suggests that no one group possessed a monopoly on fortitude.

Surgeons often encountered shock and knew its manifestations. They knew too its causes: 'alarm and fear' said James Miller simply.[45] Benjamin Brodie could also describe 'the effect produced on the nervous system by a long, painful, and anxious operation' even 'upon a healthy subject'.[46] Surgical shock was also 'corporeal' as Miller acknowledged. As the operation proceeded patients would often faint. While this might appear to be a blessing syncope, or fainting, carried with it the chance of a dangerous and often fatal lowering of the pulse. Dressers would therefore strive to rouse the swooning patient by sprinkling cold water on the face, administering smelling salts (liquor of caustic ammonia or naptha, Hoffman's spirit of aether) or, most commonly, getting them to take a mouthful of 'cordials'. That surgeons would take the time to revive swooning patients offers yet another argument against the view that operations were ordinarily over within seconds. Operations would often halt while surgeons felt for a pulse and assessed whether a patient required a stimulant; either wine, brandy, whisky or a preparation of ammonia. Fergusson wryly observed that the quantity able to be consumed was often 'remarkable' although administering too much wine would induce vomiting. Operations were unavoidably messy.[47] Nor were patients the only ones to feel faint. Among the gossip circulating in the autumn of 1834 was a rumour of 'a most awful affair in the Borough'. An unnamed surgeon attempting to ligate the femoral artery for a popliteal aneurism 'cut a little awry'. Seeing blood spurting, the operator fell in a swoon. Benjamin Travers took up the instruments and continued as the other was carried out of the theatre.[48]

Accustomed as we are to assuming that surgeons worked insensibly to the pain they caused little attention has been paid to the fact that many surgical writers discussed the need to diminish pain and passed on suggestions about how they could reduce it. 'Pain is the most dreadful part of every operation' Benjamin Bell wrote flatly.[49] The authors of surgical texts repeatedly stressed the desirability of minimising either the intensity of pain or its duration. Authors scrutinised even relatively minor procedures to find improvements. The removal of a toenail, for example, was regarded as one of the most painful procedures, which could be ameliorated by several methods all directed to avoid the tearing which caused the most pain. Even giants such as Syme and Liston, supposedly impervious to their patients' suffering, discussed and advised on improvements to this procedure.

Surgeons taught that not all cuts were equally painful, and that a careful use of the knife could greatly affect a patient's experience of pain. Liston told his students their object should be to make incisions 'with as little pain to the patient as possible'. There was, he said, 'a way in many cases of preventing pain, or rendering it less severe'.[50] Charles Bell passed on one such hint. In opening the abdomen in a hernia operation he instructed students to grip the skin firmly. 'Pinch pretty hard', he advised, 'the pain is nothing'.[51] Robert Druitt reminded his colleagues that to pause mid-operation to enlarge an incision was 'awkward ... and most cruel'.[52] In this lay the operator's central dilemma. Even while condemning undue rapidity James Miller argued that to abridge suffering 'for even moments' would be 'of huge import'.[53] Liston recommended transfixion in amputation specifically because it was less painful. He asked his students to recall the times they had had a bubo – significantly, a venereal symptom – opened by a lancet and to acknowledge that puncturing it and drawing the blade upwards was 'vastly' less painful that drawing the blade across its face.[54] Astley Cooper went further, concerned to keep scarring to a minimum, a consideration that testifies as much to his command of anatomy as to his skill in cutting and stitching.[55]

Surgeons had to strive to inflict less pain because they lacked other means to alleviate it. At the opening of the period James Latta's *A Practical System of Surgery* (1795) and Benjamin Bell's *System of Surgery* (1804) each devoted two pages to chemical and mechanical methods of relieving pain – more than any other texts in the period.

221

The surgeon's resources remained limited and no notable innovation in the relief of pain was available before the possibilities offered by mesmerism in the early 1840s. Opiates, though addictive, were useful in relieving post-operative and chronic pain but they were useless for preparing patients for the acute pain of an operation. In the quantities required they caused severe and inconvenient vomiting ('If the patient vomit', Valentine Mott warned, 'he is apt to die') and did not allay the pain of cutting.[56] Surgeons experimenting with compression of the nerves reported some relief but James Moore's device for compressing nerves also compressed veins and other tissues and few used it.[57] Patients complained that Moore's instrument caused more pain than amputation itself. Samuel Cooper remained lukewarm, thinking that the method of 'stupefying the nerves of a limb' was 'perhaps, not undeserving of further consideration'.[58] James Arnott advocated the use of ice to numb tissues, without success.[59] In 1823 the *Lancet* carried a report on 'acupuncture' but the practice, which required an understanding of the anatomical basis of pain management and careful training, never became generally adopted in the period.[60]

A fundamental difference existed between surgeons as to whether patients ought to be encouraged to cry out or not. On the one hand those who exhibited 'fortitude' were commended. On the other many authorities held that to suppress emotion was to impede healing. William Griffin, in a rare *Essay on the Nature of Pain*, argued that 'moans and tears' were 'a favourable sign' able to bring emotional relief and to 'soften' the parts – that is, to relieve the muscular tension which made cutting living tissue so difficult.[61]

'A few jets of blood': haemorrhage

Unstoppable bleeding remains the surgeon's greatest fear. Samuel Cooper evoked the shock of a surgeon confronted with a serious haemorrhage: 'pale as a corpse, and trembling, he beholds the jet of blood'.[62] It has long been a staple of the conventional view that operations before anaesthesia must have been accompanied by extensive bleeding. Insofar as the popular imagination contemplates surgery, it is likely to include images of surgeons in barns or the cockpits of warships besmeared in gore to the elbows. As we have seen, though, military and naval surgery represents a very different therapeutic dynamic. Civil surgery does not offer the same dramatic images though it is easy to construct a picture of bloody surgery.

Contemporary surgeons feared haemorrhage with good reason. John Bell described in his influential text *The Principles of Surgery*, a patient's death on the table from loss of blood. It was drawn from life and emphasises how, having witnessed such a scene, a surgeon would do all he could to avoid repeating the ordeal. Haemorrhage offered 'the least painful of deaths', wrote Bell, but also 'the most awful'. As the bleeding continued uncontrollably the patient's face – paradoxically – became livid then 'deadly pale'. The lips turned dark and the hands and feet grew cold. As surgeon and dressers desperately tried to stem the flow of bright arterial blood, the patient might faint and revive several times while the pulse fluttered and faded. He would feel sick, gasping and speaking in a low, hoarse voice all the while tossing his arms, 'the most fatal sign of all,' Bell felt. Restlessly the dying patient would raise his head, desperately gulping for air and all the while thrashing his limbs until, drawing long, convulsive sighs, he died. The face, once livid, now appears not transparently pale but of a 'clayey and leaden colour'. 'This fear of haemorrhagy was always uppermost in the mind of the young surgeon' wrote Bell.[63]

So wary were surgeons of what Charles Bell called 'a few jets of blood' that surveying clinical reports in periodicals such as the *Lancet* and the *Edinburgh Medical and Surgical Journal* over the succeeding fifty years suggests that control of haemorrhage became a preoccupation among operators. Some used the danger of haemorrhage to heighten the surgical drama: 'the cry is now! Now! Gentlemen, take care of yourselves! Is all ready? I am about to cut the artery!' Spectators might believe that they had witnessed 'a great and bloody operation'.[64] Again the evidence admits of many qualifications and exceptions. The rapidity of operations generally and the patient's struggles often resulted in surgeons failing to ligate arteries or accidentally cutting them. James Miller conceded 'oozing' to have been 'very frequent' in the operations of even his late friend Liston. The cause in Liston's operations, though, was 'imprudent haste' in closing the stump or the wound when his dressers, vying for their chief's attention and approval, had failed to ligate arteries as carefully as they might. The contest to 'do up' rapidly, Miller believed, derived from the desire to save the patient pain.[65]

It is also true that fashions in operating practice led directly to excessive bleeding. By the late eighteenth century surgeons had adopted an effective screw tourniquet designed to be tightened to compress the major arteries – on the upper thigh, for example, for a leg operation. The ability to control bleeding made a significant difference to their confidence in attempting the more complex operations in the extremities. But tourniquets, being mechanical devices, went wrong. Screws and straps broke, the band could be positioned inexpertly, they could be tightened too late or loosened too early with disastrous consequences. Practices differed markedly between hospitals and between surgeons making generalisation suspect. It is clear, however, that tourniquets were abandoned in the Edinburgh Infirmary from the 1820s while operators revelling in their physical strength, such as Robert Liston and George Guthrie, eschewed them in favour of gripping the arteries with their left hands while cutting with their right. This tour de force enabled them to locate the point of compression more precisely but when judgement erred or strength failed – or the patient moved – the results could be horrific.

Some operations, notably mastectomies and major amputations, were unavoidably vascular. William Fergusson recalled that a spectator had told him, in a striking metaphor, that the sound of bleeding in an amputation 'seemed like the noise of rain falling on a cupola'.[66] The power of Fergusson's image derives partly from its novelty. In practice he also believed that bleeding was 'greatly, perhaps entirely under the control of the surgeon'.[67] The consequence of this dread of haemorrhage and the precautions enjoined in every text and every school was that, barring accidents, relatively few patients died of loss of blood on the table. In 1841 Charles Bell who, in old age, had little patience with bravado, observed that fear of haemorrhage had 'almost disappeared'.[68] Operators considered excessive bleeding to be avoidable, a sign of clumsy and unskilful surgery and reports in the medical press recorded the loss of 'less than an ounce' of blood with approval. Operations in the final decades of painful surgery though often hurried and prone to haemorrhage as a result, were not unduly bloody, certainly not gratuitously so. Surgeons were aware of the danger of haemorrhage and became skilled in preventing or dealing with it.

'The poetry of surgery': operative styles

Perhaps the most bizarre and incongruous aspect of surgery for modern readers is the fact that contemporaries discerned in their work a variety of what can only be called styles. 'Hardly a man will perform a dozen operations in the same manner' wrote George Macilwain.[69] Skilled observers not only recognised in the actions of their fellows technical points but also what can only be regarded as aesthetic attributes. The technicalities can be imagined and need not detain us for long. Frederic Skey identified an 'evil incidental to bad operators' who were wont to 'picking in pieces' structures which ought to have been 'freely and rapidly divided'.[70] By contrast

Figure 8.2

Three ways of holding the scalpel, with the surgeon's cuffs turned back. Figure 4 'combines more elegance, freedom and firmness of movement' than other grips: from Robert Liston's <u>Elements of Surgery</u>.

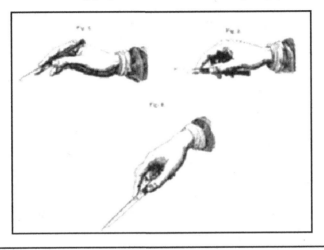

Abernethy himself, though a reluctant operator, took pride in the precision of his incisions and dissection. 'Well,' he told his students, 'you ought as much to expect a draftsman to draw a line in a direction he did not intend ... as to expect that a surgeon would cut fibres if he did not intend it.'[71] Samuel Cooper described the dilemma of a surgeon trying to excise a tumour, cutting out 'first a few fibres on one side; then on another ... a complete specimen of surgical awkwardness'.[72]

Surgical authorities freely and unselfconsciously employed terms seemingly more appropriate to art than to medicine. William Fergusson recommended a grip on the scalpel as conducive to 'elegance' as well as dexterity but conceded that each anatomist and surgeon exercised 'a taste of his own in these matters'.[73] Fergusson, although as hard-headed an operator as any, commended in his lectures a slightly different 'address' in operating (the golfing term perhaps an early connection between doctors and the game). The result, a more neatly-formed flap, was not the only advantage. 'The operation,' Fergusson wrote, 'will look somewhat more elegant' although he did have the decency to wonder 'if the term be applicable to such a proceeding'.[74] Astley Cooper worked with 'elegance ... without affectation', exhibiting the 'graceful efforts of an artist'.[75] According to Sir Charles Bell, Roux operated 'with grace without affectation'.[76] Most incongruous was Charles Aston Key's style which an admirer described as the 'poetry of surgery'.[77]

Others, however, worked with what John Bell denounced as 'affected and cruel deliberation'.[78] 'Brilliancy was the chief object' said a surgeon trained in the period.[79] The trend to elegance had its limits. Frederic Skey when told by a 'medical friend' that he had just witnessed a 'beautiful operation', retorted 'Sir, I do not comprehend what a "beautiful operation" means'. But if Skey had 'never seen the operation to which the term beautiful could apply' he nevertheless recognised and advocated the cultivation of style.[80] Comparing the use of the scalpel to 'penmanship' he urged his students to prefer light pressure to hard: 'firm, but light and graceful'.[81]

Surgery, we must conclude, was an intensely personal challenge. George Macilwain reflected that he had seen 'a very bungling operator' perform an operation extremely well and the 'very worst operation we ever saw' performed by a man famed for his dexterity.[82] The conclusion is that each operation demanded anew the application of technical skill and moral courage and that even the best surgeons and operators could never for a minute assume that their record would be enough to sustain them in each fresh case. In contrast to the econiums to 'graceful' surgery, Thomas Alcock brought his colleagues up short by telling them bluntly that the 'most free from reproach is merely the least awkward'.[83] John Bell had held out the ideal of the 'good surgeon' at the century's outset. He entertained neither vain nor selfish ambitions, shunning 'masterly turns of his knife' to seek applause. He should suppress all thoughts except those relating to his patients' safety, conscious that he inflicted cruelties which may with prudence heal.[84]

'Time to wink': speed in surgery

Perhaps the most persistent impression of painful surgery is that it occurred rapidly. Exactly how rapidly – and what rapidity meant – remains open to question. Frederic Skey boasted of being able to remove a limb at the upper arm or thigh in thirty seconds.[85] There is considerable doubt however that this time related to the entire operation. Rather, it described only 'the cutting part'. Contemporaries recorded a great variety of times for the conduct of operations, many of which omitted the time-consuming suturing and dressing. The times taken to conclude the cutting part are indeed astonishing. In amputating at the shoulder, with the patient properly placed and secured, Liston undertook that the arm 'may be on the floor in twelve or fifteen seconds'.[86] William Fergusson reckoned on no more than twenty seconds for an amputation at the hip on the dead subject and not much more on the living.[87] Fergusson kept his fingers – of the left hand – supple by playing the violin and making his own instruments and was among the most nimble of a generation of rapid operators.[88] The cultivation of the mystique of speed contributed to the developing image of the surgeon in the first quarter of the century. It was exemplified by Astley Cooper: 'You should see Sir Astley,' students would say knowingly, 'he doesn't give you time to wink'.[89]

All the same, in practice longer times are recorded for the cutting part alone, especially for operations involving excision and dissection. James Miller decried the 'absurd idea' that dexterity could be commensurate with rapidity. Despite admiration for speed text after text emphasised the need to work slowly when necessary and the fact that in many procedures rapidity was simply incompatible with effective surgery. Experienced surgeons regarded speed as often inconsistent with the avoidance of pain. Charles Bell recommended that a lithotomy incision be made 'slowly and deliberately'.[90] George Guthrie, who had honed his skill in the hospitals of the Peninsula, advised that eye surgery must be done 'very gently, very tenderly, and without giving pain'.[91] Charles Bell recommended that in amputating, the extremities of nerves should be 'buried deep in the flesh'. If they appeared to project they should be 'drawn out and divided higher up'.[92] Likewise, William Hey described how the large crural nerve could be found on the inner surface of the flap. Not only did he urge that it should always be dissected out but advised that 'when gently extended, should be divided near the extremity of the stump'.[93] This was not a procedure that could be completed at speed. Certainly surgeons could ignore the nerves: when Thomas Eshelby amputated Nelson's arm (by the light of a lantern on a heaving sea) he accidentally tied a nerve in a suture causing months of agony. On the other hand, operative surgeons working in hospitals under the scrutiny of their colleagues operated under the dual impulse of combining rapidity with care. In contrast to the picture of the surgeon working swiftly, John Bell depicted a more realistic image of a surgeon 'cutting rapidly and dexterously' when all was safe and 'slowly and cautiously' when there was danger.[94] It is therefore not surprising to find references to surgeons stopping to confer with colleagues or to ensure the propriety of their next action. When Charles Bell, newly arrived in London, was asked to assist William Lynn at the Westminster Lynn 'stopt' in mid-operation for so long that it 'gave me opportunities of sketching'.[95]

Samuel Cooper's *Dictionary* alerts us to the complexity which could arise in virtually any operation that involved severing a large artery. If such an artery were inadvertently punctured – a common accident given the struggles of many patients – Cooper suggested a remedial procedure. If compressing the artery did no good Cooper advised exposing the artery (which could involve careful dissection). Then he recommended a double ligature be prepared and passed under it using an eye-probe. Once the ligature could be tied above and below the puncture the operation could safely proceed.[96] How could operations have been terminated so swiftly when detailed and painstaking procedures such as this formed a part of so many? Cooper's caution explains George Guthrie's advice that arteries should be secured 'without reference to time'.[97]

The speed at which a surgeon operated was not, curiously, necessarily an index of the duration of an operation. Because surgery entailed much more than cutting and sawing operations even by famously quick surgeons could still take longer than we might suppose. The duration of an operation depended, of course, on its nature and the skill and attitude of the surgeon. Lithotomies were the most uniformly quick operations followed by the simpler amputations. Ironically as excisions and re-sections gradually superseded amputations so the length of operations increased. While the cutting part in the amputation of an arm might be over in ninety seconds the excision of an elbow joint could take fifteen minutes.[98] The more unusual the procedure the longer it would have taken. We have seen how early aneurism operations took hours rather than minutes. Tumours too enforced care in preparation and dissection. In 1832 John Sensire, a 58-year-old 'free black' of St Thomas in the West Indies, consented to have an 'enormous tumour' removed from his jaw. Tying the artery to enable the operation to proceed took the surgeon, George Stedman, fifty five minutes while cutting out the tumour itself took a further forty eight, a business 'embarrassed' by further bleeding. Although held down by three men John Sensire displayed 'amazing fortitude' scarcely uttering a groan throughout the ordeal.[99]

Nor would the ordeal end with the conclusion of the 'cutting part'. The tying of the arteries and closure of what surgeons called 'the wound' – contemporaries favoured the brutal term over the more refined, modern equivalent 'incision' – was often regarded as the more painful part and was certainly the more protracted. Joseph Pancoast regarded it as 'frequently more difficult ... than the operation itself'. In removing a leg at the calf six arteries had to be tied, two of which needed to be dissected from adjoining tissue.[100] James Miller, in an account of painful surgery intended to persuade recalcitrant colleagues of the merit of chloroform, reminded them of the pain of 'doing up'. As dressers wiped a sponge over the raw surface 'perhaps studded by the truncated ends of large nerves,' patients would twitch and gasp. At each 'catch of the forceps and noosing of the ligature' the patient might shriek. Miller acknowledged that, anxious to conclude the operation, operators were always tempted by 'unwise expedition'. 'Imprudent haste' could result in arteries being tied insecurely only to bleed beneath the bandages.[101]

Doing up might, however, follow the initial incision by hours rather than minutes. The patients of surgeons subscribing to the delayed dressing of wounds – including Astley Cooper, Lizars and Syme – might lie for hours waiting for the surgeon to pronounce that the would had 'granulated' sufficiently to allow them to bring the flaps together. Coster recommended an hour's delay in closing the flaps of a mastectomy incision.[102] James Syme, who first advocated the policy of delayed closure in 1825, recommended waiting up to twelve hours 'until after the bloody and serious oozing shall have ceased'.[103]

Dressing the wound would likewise vary between surgeons over time. English and Scottish surgeons increasingly deprecated the 'thick' or 'heavy' dressings favoured by their predecessors and by French colleagues still. British surgeons in general opposed 'loading the stump' with the yards of bandages formerly applied. Robert Liston criticised the 'filthy and very disgusting practice' of applying of layers of bandages often soaked in oil or ointment. Opponents of heavy dressings advocated simply bathing the wound in water (cold in summer, warm in winter).[104] Only after the cutting part would a patient receive relief for pain. Opium could at last be administered – perhaps thirty drops after a mastectomy or the removal of a large tumour. Exhausted, but also often relieved by the removal of infected limbs or painful joints, patients would often sleep for hours.

'Surgical ethics': indifference and empathy

The cutting part was indeed as colleagues described Guthrie's operation for popliteal aneurism, 'painful, difficult, bloody, tedious and dangerous'. In all these aspects, however, surgery differed from the current, conventional view. It was of course painful but perhaps not as painful as it might have been. Many surgeons attempted by technique, timing and mechanical assistance to ameliorate the pain they could not avoid inflicting. It was more difficult, more complex, more varied and more subtle than historians have allowed. It was bloody but perhaps less routinely bloody than we might have imagined because surgeons took the trouble to avoid or suppress bleeding. It was tedious – taking much longer on the whole than we have wanted to believe. It was dangerous with surgical mortality a fearful hazard to be contemplated by surgeons proposing operations and by patients pondering whether to submit. In all this the cutting part could often be brutal and distressing for all concerned: but if we can look past the blood and the cries we may yet see, as many surgeons saw, a noble calling, one which truly and increasingly prevented as well as inflicted suffering.

The growing publicity which surgeons attracted contributed to the strain under which they worked. In 1828 James Lambert published an account in the *Lancet* of a lithotomy performed by Bransby Cooper that went badly wrong.[105] The patient, Samuel Pollard, a 53-year-old labourer from Sussex, married with six children, had come to London reportedly asking to be operated upon by 'the Nevey of the great Sir Arstley'. Bound upon the table and watched by Guy's students he was operated upon by Bransby Cooper with the assistance of Thomas Calloway. At first matters went as expected but after enlarging the incision (using 'my uncle's knife'), inserting forceps and then a finger Cooper exclaimed that 'I can't reach the bladder with my finger'. After more cutting and introducing various other instruments Cooper's anxiety became apparent. The dialogue recorded by Lambert – whom it has to be said was no friend of Cooper – suggests the desperate straits in which he found himself.:

> I really can't conceive the difficulty – Hush! hush! Don't you hear the stone? – Dodd [the demonstrator] ... have you a long finger? Give me another instrument – Now I have it! Good God! ... the forceps wont [sic] touch it. – O dear! O dear!

Sensing Cooper's difficulties, the spectators had stilled by this time. The only sound they could hear was 'the horrible squash, squash,' of the forceps in the perineum. 'Oh! let it go – pray let it keep in!' the patient cried. After fifty minutes of an operation that usually took less than five Cooper at last grasped the stone. Holding the forceps aloft he turned triumphantly to the students to discuss the cause of the difficulty. The following day the exhausted patient

Figure 8.3

A caricature lampooning the reaction of Bransby Cooper (1792-1853) to the Lancet's strictures over the botched lithotomy he performed on Samuel Pollard in 1828. At right a figure representing Thomas Wakley claims that 'A Lancet is far superior to Cooper's Adz ... it will perform a Scientific Operation with Expedition'.

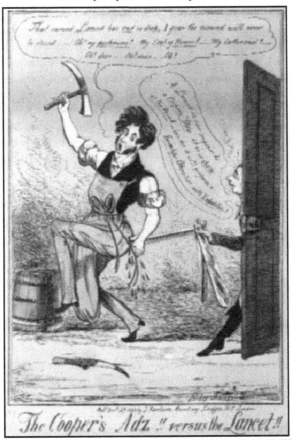

died. A post-mortem (in which Astley Cooper's adversary Thomas Hodgkin participated) found that the man did not have a 'deep perineum' nor was the stone especially large. The dissemination of the post-mortem's findings sparked 'squibs and epigrams' denigrating Cooper who felt he had no alternative but to sue for libel. Despite compelling evidence tendered by an independent, qualified witness he won the case but received derisory damages.[106]

Publicly humiliated, Bransby Cooper had to return to the same theatre to perform another lithotomy under the eyes of his colleagues and students. So notorious had the case become that *The Times* had a correspondent attend. He recognised that 'any difficulty, any delay ... would have been his ruin'. Forgetting the patient the reporter felt that Cooper needed 'iron nerves' to carry him through 'the ordeal'. Cooper responded to the challenge operating with a coolness and self-possession the reporter regarded as 'admirable'. His manner was calm, his hand steady despite the 'trembling anxiety' of his friends. To the end the patient, from whom Cooper removed a large calculus, remained unknown.[107] Although surviving this test and remaining popular with students Bransby never recovered his reputation or his equilibrium becoming 'unduly emotional' thereafter.[108]

So deficient is the evidence and what there is so ambiguous that it is almost impossible to discern the subtleties of those about the operating table. It is possible that the indifference which many surgeons displayed not only concealed a feeling for those who suffered, but also that the patients were, in a way, able to draw strength from it. A colleague said Charles Aston Key was 'if anything, too cold and unemotional'. This seeming indifference fuelled the 'calm power' a contemporary described as 'striking'. Evident at the bedside, it 'gave instant confidence to the patient and his friends'.[109] It is also possible that concentration appeared as indifference in many men. George Mayo, a pupil of Charles Bell at the Middlesex Hospital, became a prominent surgeon in South Australia. After performing an amputation by transfixion in the Adelaide Hospital he remarked 'How quiet the patient has been!' A colleague, startled at his absorption, retorted 'Why, man, he was screaming all the time'.[110]

Some surgeons believed that to feel for patients would diminish their capacity to act as operators. Others disagreed. In 1820 James Gregory reassured his colleagues that they could 'feel whatever is amiable in pity, without suffering it to enervate or unman them.' The balance would have been difficult to reach: elsewhere in his book intended to correct deficiencies in practitioners' relationship with their patients, Gregory counselled that an 'excess of sympathy' could 'cloud his understanding' and prevent him acting with vigour.[111]

Astley Cooper said of himself that he 'felt too much before he began [operating] ever to make a perfect operator'.[112] This does not gainsay the existence of clumsy or heartless operators. Indeed, the medical press denounced both. Surgeons could forgive clumsiness knowing that every operation confronted them with problems of identifying structures and tissues and that even a cool and skilled operator could be confused or rattled by emergencies or the unexpected. Less excusable were those who, in Samuel Cooper's graphic words, went 'wading through blood to reputation': men who saw in the attention which this path opened, a route to standing in their profession.[113] John Bell wrote that some hospital surgeons lose no occasion of charming his assemblage of spectators'.[114] It was a temptation he recognised and perhaps shared, a 'selfish and dangerous passion, which every ingenuous man must confess he feels lurking within his own breast'. In 1801 Bell had warned his students that 'boldness is a seducing word' and cautioned them against 'the passion of acquiring character in operations'. 'Should not ... the present suffering of the patient', he asked, 'and above all the trust that is reposed in him, occupy the surgeon's mind too much to leave room for vain or selfish thoughts?'[115] Bell counselled in vain. In 1846 – the year in which ether anaesthesia was first introduced – Benjamin Brodie of St George's Hospital had attacked what he sarcastically called the 'accomplished operator'. Brodie condemned the surgeon who 'looks at his watch to see in how short a space of time an operation may be completed'. He castigated those who 'during an operation, put[s] himself in the situation of those who are looking on, considering what they will say, and anxious to appear dexterous in their eyes'.[116]

Many surgeons were unreflective men. Even so, the exceptions offer startling and often moving insights into the effects of their calling upon them. There is evidence that surgeons observed and remarked upon the tensions which confronted those obliged to inflict suffering in surgery. That they lived in an age and a society that countenanced the open expression of emotion among men sharpened rather than eased the tension. Science imposed a duty to objectivity: to surrender to the emotions would be to betray scientific surgery. In a lecture on the 'Conduct and Duties' of medical practitioners Benjamin Brodie urged his colleagues to subject their emotions to 'the domination of the intellect'.[117] Others worried at the implications of their work. Frederic Skey asked in a lecture whether there was 'no medium?':'Is harshness or indifference,' he wondered, 'the sole alternative to ... failure in decision' caused by undue sympathy with the patient's sufferings?'[118] The evidence of how surgeons coped with deaths they may have prevented and suffering they may have caused remains intractable and elusive. That Henry Mayhew decided, with implausible exactitude, that one in 68 of London's medical practitioners were above the average in drunkenness (more than brewers or shopkeepers but less than sweeps or smiths) is merely a reminder that some must have sought to block the memory of suffering with alcohol.[119]

Philibert Roux, who was admired by British surgeons, acknowledged that in being 'so continually brought into contact with death, ... our sensibilities become blunted' and that suffering made 'but a slight and transient impression upon ourselves'.[120] How this could be so might appear obvious but it is clear that many surgeons struggled to remain aware of their patients' sufferings while continuing their work. Again instances of honest self-criticism can be found. William Sands Cox, for example, surgeon to the Queen's Hospital in Birmingham, became an authority on amputation. His clinical triumph occurred in 1844 when he successfully amputated the leg of a young woman, Elizabeth Powis, at the hip joint. The operation was novel, dangerous and difficult, inflicting an immense wound and threatening Miss Powis's life from shock during the operation and from sepsis after. Cox recorded his triumph in a monograph devoted to Miss Powis's case (complete with a lithograph of her displaying a huge scar) and accepted the adulation of his peers. Even Cox, though, confessed to having pondered the probity of proceeding, asking his colleagues to 'weigh well the consequences against the vanity of having to say "I have done it".[121] Vanity and indifference alike could subject patients to pain to no purpose.

Terrible scenes were enacted in the operating rooms. Sights, sounds and sensations which would appear to us as nightmarish accompanied operations which we might regard today as routine, even minor. A surgeon complained in the *Lancet* in 1844 that 'The public do not understand us', accusing surgeons of 'want of feeling'.[122] The charge was unjust. It is evident that many surgeons felt: but they also had to cut. Therein lay the essential, inescapable tension of their calling.

Notes

1. Frederic Skey, *Operative Surgery* (London: John Churchill, 1850), 9.
2. *Lancet*, 1835–36, Vol. I, 736.
3. Charles Bell, *Illustrations of the Great Operations of Surgery* (London: Longman, 1821), 1–3.
4. John Erichsen, *The Science and Art of Surgery* (London: Walton & Maberly, 1853), 49.
5. Bell, *op. cit.* (note 3), 1–3.
6. J.W. Chelius, (trans. and ed. J.F. South), *A System of Surgery*, 2 vols (London: Henry Renshaw, 1847), Vol. II, 855 .
7. *Lancet*, 1835–36, Vol. I, 152.

8. Samuel Cooper, *A Dictionary of Practical Surgery* (London: Longman, Hurst, Rees, Orme & Brown, 1829), 68.

9. Benjamin Bell, *A System of Surgery*, 3 vols (Edinburgh: Bell & Bradfute, 1801), Vol. III, 475.

10. Philip Crampton, *Cases of the Excision of Carious Joints* (Dublin: Hodges & McArthur, 1827), 204.

11. *Edinburgh Medical & Surgical Journal*, 1827, Vol. 27, 45–49.

12. Norman Moore & Stephen Paget, *The Royal Medical and Chirurgical Society of London, 1805-1905* (Aberdeen: Aberdeen University Press, 1905), 49.

13. Nathan Smith, *Medical and Surgical Memoirs* (Baltimore: William A. Francis, 1831), 35.

14. Robert Liston, *Lectures on the Operations of Surgery* (Philadeliphia: Lea & Blanchard, 1846), 191.

15. William Gibson, *Institutes and Practice of Surgery* (Philadelphia: J. Kay, Jnr & Brother, 1841), 504; Benjamin Brodie, *Clinical Lectures on Surgery* (Philadelphia: Lea & Blanchard, 1846), 35; William Fergusson, *A System of Practical Surgery* (London: John Churchill, 1846), 38.

16. J. Coster, *Manual of Surgical Operations* (Philadelphia: H.C. Carey & I Lea, 1825), 38.

17. 'Sir Everard Home's lectures', c. 1811, f3,334, RCSEng.

18. Skey, *op. cit.* (note 1), 6, 9.

19. Victor Plarr, *Lives of the Fellows of the Royal College of Surgeons*, 2 vols (London: Simpkin, Marshall Ltd, 1930), Vol. I, 399.

20. Erichsen, *op. cit.* (note 4), 49.

21. Anthony Carlisle, Lecture III, 'Surgical ethics', 42.f.28, RCSEng.

22. Liston, *op. cit.* (note 14), 393.

23. *Lancet*, 1831–32, Vol. II, 31.

24. Erichsen, *op. cit.* (note 4), 49.

25. Gibson, *op. cit.* (note 15), 504.

26. Skey, *op. cit.* (note 1), 7.

27. Henry Jacob Bigelow, *An Introductory Lecture delivered at Massachusetts Medical College* (Boston: David Clapp, 1850), 10.

28. John Abernethy, *Lectures on Anatomy, Surgery and Pathology* (London: James Bullock, 1828), 521.

29. Skey, *op. cit.* (note 1), 29.

30. Agatha Young, *Scalpel: Men who made Surgery* (London: Robert Hale, 1957), 132. The story is apocryphal but recurs, sometimes adding a patient's testicle to the collateral damage, sometimes erroneously connected to a particular surgeon, often Robert Liston.

31. Cooper, *op. cit.* (note 8), 49.

32. Forbes Winslow, *Physic and Physicians: A Medical Sketch Book*, 2 vols (London: Longman, Orme, Brown, 1839), 32; Charles Bell, *Institutes of Surgery*, 2 vols (Edinburgh: Longmans & Co., 1838), Vol. I, 324.

33. John Flint South, *Memorials of John Flint South* (Fontwell: Centaur Press, 1970), 52 .

34. Bransby Cooper, *The Life of Sir Astley Cooper, Bart.*, 2 vols (London: John Parker, 1843), Vol. I, 302.

35. South, *op. cit.* (note 33), 52–53.

36. H.G. Cameron, *Mr Guy's Hospital 1726–1948* (London: Longman, Green & Co., 1954), 104.

37. James Miller, *Surgical Experience of Chloroform* (Edinburgh: Sutherland & Knox, 1848), 30.

38. Chelius, *op. cit.* (note 6), Vol. II, 853–54.

39. Anthony Carlisle, Lecture III, 'Surgical ethics', 42.f.28, RCSEng.

40. James Paget, *Studies of Old Case Books* (London: Longmans & Co., 1891), 156–57.

41. *Lancet*, 1835–36, Vol. I, 282.

42. George Guthrie, *Commentaries on the Surgery of the War in Portugal, Spain, France, and the Netherlands* (London: Renshaw, 1853), 14.

43. Samuel Warren, *Passages from the Diary of a Late Physician*, 2 vols (Edinburgh: William Blackwood, 1834), 42.

44. *The Times*, 18 May 1839, 7c.

45. Miller, *op. cit.* (note 37), 26.

46. Brodie, *op. cit.* (note 15), 37.

47. William Fergusson, *op. cit.* (note 15), 33; Skey, *op. cit.* (note 1), 37.

48. *Lancet*, 1834–5, Vol. I, 105.

49. Benjamin Bell, *A System of Operative Surgery* (London: Longman, Hurst, Rees, Orme & Brown, 1814), Vol. III, 530.

50. Liston, *op. cit.* (note 14), 19. He repeated the advice with variations several times, on p. 391 specifically referring to amputation.

51. Bell, *op. cit.* (note 32), Vol. II, 35.

52. Robert Druitt, *The Surgeon's Vade Mecum* (London: Henry Renshaw, John Churchill, 1851), 385 .

53. Miller, *op. cit.* (note 37), 30.

54. *Lancet*, 1835–36, Vol. II, 135.

55. Astley Cooper & Frederick Tyrrell, *The Lectures of Sir Astley Cooper, Bart.* ... (London: Thomas Tegg, 1824), 152–53.

56. 'Pain and Anaesthetics', in William Hammond, *Military Medical and Surgical Essays* (Philadelphia: J.B. Lippincott, 1864), 390.

57. James Moore, *A Method of Preventing or Diminishing Pain in Several Operations of Surgery* (London: T. Cadell, 1784); James Latta, *A Practical System of Surgery*, 3 vols (Edinburgh: G. Mudie, A. Guthrie

& J. Fairbairn, 1795), Vol. II, 533.

58. Cooper, *op. cit.* (note 8), 68.

59. James Arnott, *On Neuralgic, Rheumatic, and Other Painful Afflictions* (London: 1851), 18–21.

60. *Lancet,* 1823, Vol. I, 14.

61. William Griffin, *An Essay on the Nature of Pain* (Edinburgh: J. Moir, 1826), 41.

62. Cooper, *op. cit.* (note 8), 219.

63. John Bell, *The Principles of Surgery,* 2 vols (Edinburgh: T. Cadell & W. Davies, 1801), Vol. I, 142.

64. Charles Bell, *Surgical Observations* (London: Longmans & Co. 1816), 233.

65. Miller, *op. cit.* (note 37), 32.

66. Fergusson, *op. cit.* (note 15), 165.

67. *Ibid.,* 164.

68. Charles Bell, *Practical Essays* (Edinburgh: Maclachlan, Stewart & Co., 1841), 4.

69. George Macilwain, *Memoirs of John Abernethy,* 2 vols (London: Hurst & Blackett, 1854), Vol. II, 204.

70. Skey, *op. cit.* (note 1), 4.

71. Abernethy, *op. cit.* (note 28), 502.

72. Cooper, *op. cit.* (note 8), 855.

73. Fergusson, *op. cit.* (note 66), 20.

74. *Ibid.,* 381.

75. William White, *Great Doctors of the Nineteenth Century* (London: Edwin Arnold, 1935), 38.

76. Thomas Pettigrew, *Biographical Memoirs of the Most Celebrated Physicians, Surgeons, etc., etc.,* 3 vols (London: Fisher, Son & Co., 1839–40), Vol. III, 2. Bell was so taken with the praise that he told his brother George of it: letter 2 Feb 1816.

77. J.F. Clarke, *Autobiographical Recollections* (London: J. & A. Churchill, 1874), 73.

78. Bell, *op. cit.* (note 63), Vol. I, 12.

79. *Transactions of the Intercolonial Medical Congress of Australiasia* (Adelaide, 1887), 123 .

80. Skey, *op. cit.* (note 1), x.

81. *Ibid.,* 6, 4.

82. Macilwain, *op: cit.* (note 69), Vol. II, 204.

83. Thomas Alcock, 'An Essay on the Education and Duties of the General Practitioner in Medicine and Surgery' in *Transactions of the Associated Apothecaries and Surgeon Apothecaries of England and Wales* (London: the Society, 1823), 53.

84. Bell, *op. cit.* (note 63), Vol. II, xxvii.

85. Skey, *op. cit.* (note 1), 322.

86. Liston, *op. cit.* (note 14), 411.

87. Fergusson, *op. cit.* (note 66), 395.

88. Isobel Rae, *Knox: the Anatomist* (Edinburgh: Oliver & Boyd, 1964), 111.

89. Ella Hill Burton Rodger, *Aberdeen Doctors at Home and Abroad* (Edinburgh: W. Blackwood, 1893), 117.

90. Bell, *op. cit.* (note 32), Vol. II, 59.

91. George Guthrie, *On the ... Operation for the Extraction of a Cataract* (London: W. Sams, 1834), 10.

92. Bell, *op. cit.* (note 3), 32.

93. William Hey, *Practical Observations in Surgery* (London: T. Cadell Jnr & W. Davies, [1803; 1814]), 545.

94. Bell, *op. cit.* (note 63), Vol. I, 12.

95. Charles Bell to George Bell, 13 December 1804, George Jospeh Bell, (ed.), *Letters of Sir George Bell* (London: John Murray, 1870), 24.

96. Cooper, *op. cit.* (note 8), 635.

97. Guthrie, *op. cit.* (note 42), 72.

98. *Lancet*, 1830–31, Vol. I, 269; *Edinburgh Medical & Surgical Journal*, 1829, Vol. 31, 264–65.

99. 'Dr Stedman's Contributions to Operative Surgery', *Edinburgh Medical & Surgical Journal*, 1832, Vol. 37, 21–25.

100. Joseph Pancoast, *A Treatise on Operative Surgery* (Philadelphia: Carey & Hart, 1852), 167–68.

101. Miller, *op. cit.* (note 37), 32.

102. Coster, *op. cit.* (note 16), 39; 81.

103. James Syme, *Principles of Surgery* (Edinburgh: Sutherland & Knox, 1842), 41.

104. Liston, *op. cit.* (note 14), 66–67.

105. Lambert's report appeared in the *Lancet* on 29 March 1828. It is reproduced with a commentary in Clarke *op. cit.* (note 77), 29–33.

106. Detailed accounts of the trial can be found in S. Squire Sprigge, *The Life and Times of Thomas Wakley* (London: Longmans, 1899) and Plarr, *op. cit.* (note 19), Vol. II, 151–53.

107. *The Times*, 19 January 1829, 4e.

108. Plarr, *op. cit.* (note 19), Vol. I, 269.

109. Clarke *op. cit.* (note 77), 74.

110. Plarr, *op. cit.* (note 19), Vol. II, 49.

111. James Gregory, *On the Duties and Qualifications of a Physician* (London: W. Creech, 1805), 19; 11.

112. Cooper, *op. cit.* (note 34), Vol. II, 474.

113. Cooper, *op. cit.* (note 8), 1071.
114. Bell, *op. cit.* (note 63), Vol. I, xxvi.
115. *Ibid.,* 12.
116. Brodie, *op. cit.* (note 15), 32.
117. *The Times*, 10 October 1829, 4a.
118. *Lancet*, 1835–36, Vol. I, 72.
119. Henry Mayhew, *London Characters* (London: Chatto & Windus, 1881), 405.
120. William Hey (jun), *The Retrospective Address in Surgery* (Worcester: Deighton, 1843), 89–90.
121. William Sands Cox, *A Memoir on Amputation of the Thigh, at the Hip-Joint* (London: Reeve & J. Churchill, 1845), 17.
122. *Lancet*, 1845, Vol. I, 615.

9

'Our little patient':
Surgeons and Children

Astley Cooper, the most celebrated operating surgeon of his time, is recorded to have lost control of his emotions only once. A Quaker friend brought him his grandchild, a toddler, to ascertain whether Cooper could cut off a naevus – a birthmark. The child smiled so sweetly at Cooper that he turned away and burst into tears.[1] Cooper's reaction, while uncharacteristic of both him and his colleagues, is understandable. And yet, both Cooper and other surgeons did, of course, operate upon children. Painful surgery performed on children is the most distressing aspect of the subject for modern readers: as it was for contemporaries.

'Dreadful consequences': children and the realities of life

Children were highly visible in early-Victorian Britain, with a third of the population under fourteen. Their health and lives were even more precarious than those of their mothers and fathers. Charles Kingsley, in his fairy tale, *The Water-Babies*, reflected on how dangerous life was for children. His character Tom pondered the misfortunes to which children were subject. Most died 'by fever, and cholera, and measles, and scarlatina, and nasty complaints' but he also thought of those who 'come to grief by ill-usage or ignorance or neglect', who are 'let to drink out of hot kettles, or to fall into the fire'.[2] Children were subject to the great range of accidents and mishaps that surgeons were called upon to treat, victims of the accidents common in workshops, streets and factories, although most accidents then, as now, occurred in children's homes. 'The life of a parent', Sydney Smith wrote in 1803, 'is the life of a gambler'.[3]

Coroners' reports make grim reading. In 1844 Thomas Wakley held thirteen inquests on children burned to death in 'the past few days'; the following year another coroner heard five such cases in one day.[4] As Kingsley observed, among the most common accidents were children rolling or falling into fires and drinking from the spouts of boiling kettles. The impact of the industrial revolution added to the domestic accidents reported in newspapers under the heading 'fatal and melancholy accident'. In 1816, for example, nearly half of

Manchester's cotton operatives were aged under 18 and the employment of children as young as ten had increased during the French wars.[5] Indeed, in that year Charles Bell detailed the case of a ten-year-old boy who on the third day after starting work in a 'manufactory where a steam engine was in use, had his hand drawn into the machine and mangled'.[6] The overwhelming causes of children's deaths were, however, medical rather than surgical. While surgical consequences of such accidents were relatively uncommon the affected families experienced a particular trauma.

Sickness and injury was dreaded because it so often led to death. Mortality among children horrified even contemporaries. In 1799 London's Bills of Mortality disclosed that 42 per cent of the capital's 18,134 deaths were of children under ten.[7] In 1843 the proportion of the dead under fifteen was 47 per cent.[8] Across the period as a whole a fifth would die within a year of birth; one in three before reaching their fifth birthday.[9] Children often fell ill and each time there was a good chance that 'it' would die. The indifference seemingly conveyed by the customary impersonal pronoun is misleading. Although widespread, the grief inflicted by this scale of loss was felt individually and was no less profound for being common. William Logan's *Words of Comfort for Bereaved Parents* appeared in numerous editions in mid-century.[10] It retains its power not so much from the homilies offering pious consolation as through the poems which permit empathy with loss. Parents who had lost children offered comfort to those facing bereavement. 'Thus,' wrote Rev. Alexander Beith, 'in the space of six short weeks we were called upon to part with four of our darlings'. Wordsworth's 'We are seven' might seem to be darkly satirical doggerel to an age which generally does not have to watch children lying in agony:

> The first that died was sister Jane;
> In bed she moaning lay,
> Till God released her from her pain;
> And then she went away.

At a time in which the suffering and death of children was a reality verses describing 'Our First Taken' or how 'Wee Katie's Gane' suggest the unavoidable extent of childhood loss.

Early Victorian Britain represented a period of transition in the understanding of childhood and the treatment of children. Casual violence and accepted abuse coexisted alongside loving family care. Beatings and birching were sanctioned by law – about 1813 Henry

Figure 9.1

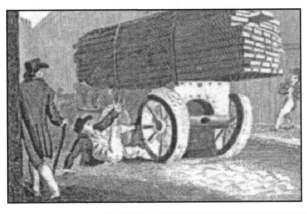

'*The Danger of the Streets' from <u>Profitable Amusement for Children</u>, a cautionary tale from 1802 which described explicitly the surgical consequences of childish 'giddiness and folly' for little George Manly.*

Ricketts at Winchester recorded how he received 'an uncommon flogging this morning. The blood ran through my shirt into my britches.'[11] Prevailing medical theories resulted in a hearty approach to children's health. Popular opinion held that those most exposed to cold grew up hardy, leading 'many parents to expose their children thinly clad to all the severities of weather'.[12] William Dewees met a woman who, although having lost several children to croup, continued to believe that 'exposure to all kinds of weather' would 'protect and harden' them. Children were subjected to the same robust treatment as adults. John Coley advocated 'bleeding to syncope' and 'the most violent purgatives' for even 'the youngest infants'.[13] James Kennedey advised blistering 'in young children' until the skin became 'uniformly reddened'.[14] Clearly the cause of much illness was poverty combined with prevailing standards of hygiene and the existence of endemic disease: diphtheria, measles and ignorance of and indifference to their causes.

Books published to provide *Examples for Youth* reveal how children, at least those of better-off families, confronted the realities of contemporary life through improving literature. 'Mrs F.', in a domestic parable 'Presence of Mind', bids her daughter to watch her be bled by a surgeon. 'Dear Mamma!' her daughter Eliza exclaims, 'I can never bear to see you bled'. Her mother replies, 'O if I can bear to feel it surely you may to see it ...'. She avers that 'it will do you good to be accustomed to such sights'.[15] This story sets the tone of a genre of juvenile instructional literature imparting an awareness of life's dangers and consequences. *Profitable Amusement for Children*, a book read by at least two generations of children in a family during the first quarter of the century offers many stern examples. It includes stories of children 'burned to death', 'buried alive', 'shockingly cut', drowned, stung and concussed from falls. One, 'The Danger of the Streets', describes George and 'the dreadful consequences of his giddiness and folly'. Little George slips and falls under a loaded wagon shattering his leg 'in a most shocking manner'. 'Mangled and wracked with pain' he is carried home on a window-shutter 'crying and lamenting all the way'. A surgeon, finding the leg beyond relief declares that he must 'cut it off entirely at the knee'. George 'roared worse than ever' but 'as nothing could be done [he] ... was forced to submit'. The surgeon 'took out his instruments, cut the flesh all around with a sharp knife, [and] cut through the bone with a saw'. Hardly surprisingly then as another story puts it, that 'the other children in the neighbourhood were so shocked ... that they too were afraid to expose themselves to ... danger'.[16]

During the period, however, a change is discernable in the way children were regarded and treated. What Dewees called 'the Eutopian notions of Jean Jacques Rousseau' became gradually diffused.[17] 'I do not approve of shutting the little offender in a closet' wrote Mrs Child in *The Mother's Book* in 1834.[18] In literature, children became, for the first time, the characters and subjects of verse and novels. Blake's 'The Chimney Sweeper' and Wordsworth's 'Ode on the Intimations of Immortality from Recollections of early Childhood' conveyed with a startling immediacy that a child's perspective was different from an adult's. Novels – *Oliver Twist, Jane Eyre, Alton Lock* and *Little Dorrit* – enabled adult readers to imagine a child's experience and to appreciate, however imperfectly, that childhood manifested special characteristics. At the same time, the employment of children became the subject of official investigation, such as the Commission on the Employment of Young Persons and Children of 1842 which both reflected a new philanthropy and accelerated its acceptance. While for the remainder of the century children continued to work in houses, farms, workshops and factories, from the 1840s legislation was introduced to restrict child labour: for example from 1842 women and children were forbidden to work underground.

Even so, especially early in the century, surgeons did not invariably treat children with the institutionalised solicitude which we have since come to expect. In 1824 Astley Cooper operated on a child on a Monday and learned on the Tuesday morning that the child had vomited and lay in a stupor. Rather than attend immediately, he told the father to administer calomel and bathe the infant. When he finally visited that evening he found the child dead. Although sententiously remarking that 'the danger of the infantile period is considerable' Cooper appeared not to have altered his routine accordingly.[19] Nor was he unusual. One of his 'subordinates', R.J. Taynton, reported to him how he had been summoned to examine a two-year-old girl in 1831. He found her 'breathing with great difficulty, the skin ... of a livid hue, the eyes ... fixed ... in short ... dying'. Taynton told the girl's parents 'that it was too late to do anything for its relief'. She died within the hour. Taynton, seemingly more interested in the child dead than alive, dissected her corpse.[20] His purpose of course was to understand the causes of her death, reflecting the greater interest children aroused among the medical community.

'Disorders peculiar to themselves': children's complaints

Children had remained for the most part invisible in medical literature if not in practice. In a review of a pioneering French text on the diseases of children a contributor to the *Lancet* in 1833 acknowledged that despite the progress of medicine generally, children's diseases generally had been neglected. They had been attributed to teething, worms or vaguely to 'growth'.[21] Paediatric medicine as a specialism developed only in the second half of the century. However, surgeons increasingly recognised a number of conditions exclusive to or common among children, described in a series of texts published between 1815 and 1850. John Clarke, one of the earliest authorities to attempt to describe them, observed that children were 'liable to many disorders ... peculiar to themselves'.[22] These included malfunctions and deformities able to be treated surgically such as wry neck, curvature of the spine, birthmarks, cleft palate, hare lip and club foot. In the course of the period all came under the treatment of surgeons.

Limited by contemporary understanding, many conditions were treated in ways which later generations of doctors would regard as cruelly ineffective. The spinal tumour, spina bifida, although regarded as 'inevitably ... fatal' still attracted surgical experiment. Samuel Cooper described four 'trials' to which infants suffering from spinal tumours were subjected. Astley Cooper's theory was that compressing the swelling could relieve the condition.[23] He had attempted to puncture tumours with a 'minute needle' after which he pressed them 'firmly'. He claimed to have succeeded but James Hamilton discouragingly warned that 'any attempts for its cure or alleviation' were 'quite unavailing'.[24] Paralysis (the result of 'derangement of the brain from pressure or inflammation') could have been treated by applying blisters or 'stimulating embrocations' to the back, seeking to maintain discharges in accordance with the prevailing doctrine of counter-irritation.[25]

The most common congenital malformations were 'deformities in the lower extremities, styled CLUB-FEET'.[26] Though some surgeons resorted to amputation others advised the use of 'mechanical contrivances' to shape the bones. James Hamilton urged parents always to seek the advice of a 'regular practitioner' rather than a glib irregular. Even the young Byron was treated by the Nottingham Hospital's truss-maker before being referred to Matthew Baillie in London.[27] Surgeons attempted to correct club foot by forcing the limb into wooden, metal or pasteboard splints or moulds inflicting much pain on children without necessarily rectifying the condition. Surgical alleviation of the condition came from Germany to Britain in the late 1830s, an example of the profession's international outlook. In 1816 and 1823 Jacques Delpech in Paris, correctly identifying its cause in the tendons rather than the bones, attempted to correct the deformity by cutting the tendons. The procedure failed, probably from post-operative infection. In 1830, however, Georg Stromeyer of Hanover devised a subcutaneous operation. It involved making a small incision and the cutting of tendons by touch. A British student, William Little, who himself suffered from club foot, witnessed and submitted to Stromeyer's operation. Relieved of the deformity Little returned to Britain to promote the treatment of club foot at the Orthopaedic Institution he founded in London.[28] The procedure, involving a small incision and relatively little pain, relieved children not only of the condition but also of long, uncomfortable and useless months in braces and splints.

The correction of the congenital defect of the division of the soft palate had rarely been attempted before 1825 when Philibert Roux published his account of a successful operation upon the Canadian medical student John Stephenson.[29] Although difficult, because it occurred in a small, slippery space, the operation for cleft palate was not regarded either as a major procedure or a particularly painful one. William Fergusson who performed over two hundred cleft palate operations with a mortality rate of one in a hundred, is said to have done so without anaesthetic after it was available.[30]

Hare-lip was supposed by 'philosophical anatomists' to have been caused by the foetus remaining in a lower form of evolution in the womb, proof of the ontological theory they espoused, to the scandal of conservative physiologists, who had no explanation at all.[31] Astley Cooper regarded the condition as a 'disgusting deformity' and urged that it be corrected using pins and ligatures inserted through the upper lip.[32] Originally deferred until patients turned five, 'after various trials' John Bell recommended operating on infants as young as six months old.[33] Samuel Cooper explained why: older children showed 'a thousand times more dread of the pain' than did infants.[34] It too was regarded as a minor procedure. First the surgeon marked the lines of incision on the child's upper lip and cut using a knife or scissors. The wound was then brought together. 'Having introduced the needle', Liston explained, 'you make two points of suture, secure them by a thick twisted thread, and cut off the ends of the pins'. Despite French practice no complex instruments were needed. He urged 'fingers are the best forceps'. Liston once found a family of four boys – John, Charles, James and Toby – all with hare lip. He brought them into the theatre one after another, alternating with capital operations: the sight of the theatre must surely have unnerved them.[35] Operations to correct hare-lip caused children 'acute suffering' not only during mercifully brief operation but also for hours afterwards. James Miller recalled the 'constant sob and tear, and the occasional scream' in the wards after children had undergone these operations.[36] William Fergusson was proud of his ability to insert the pins twenty seconds after making the initial incision and so quickly that 'scarcely any blood is lost'.[37]

Birthmarks were explained by even the gruff John Abernethy as 'a consequence of some Fantasy of the Mother'. Surgeons could chose between three methods for removing birthmarks, operations effectively constituting cosmetic surgery. They could be burned off by the application of caustics, cut off with a knife or excised by the use of ligatures. The first two were of course painful either for a few minutes or for several weeks or months. Abernethy described an operation he had performed to remove a growth the size of a half-crown from the forehead of a little girl. He worked as quickly as possible, in under a minute, but described the bleeding as 'frightful'.[38]

Understandably many parents and presumably surgeons favoured the ligature because 'the operation was bloodless'. In 1832 John Scott at the London Hospital performed the operation using the ligature on a girl aged about eighteen months who had a naevus about an inch in diameter on her forehead. Scott pushed two pins through it and drew a strong ligature around it cutting off the blood supply and allowing him to cut it off. The child the *Lancet's* reporter believed 'did not appear to suffer very great pain' during the operation because 'its cries ceased almost directly it was restored to its mother's arms'. Within a fortnight a healthy scar had formed and, presumably because she was not kept in hospital, there was little chance of post-operative infection occurring.[39]

Stuttering, a psychological rather than a physiological condition, was particularly susceptible to the claims of 'scientific' surgeons seeking novelty and notoriety. In the early 1840s British surgeons learned of operations performed in Germany and France that promised to cure the affliction. Innovative and ambitious British colleagues were moved to tackle the condition using different techniques. James Yearsley MRCS, proprietor of the Sackville Street Ear Institution, contended that stuttering was caused by defects in the uvula which restricted the egress of air in speech. Yearsley proudly proclaimed that he was the first surgeon to perform an operation based on his idiosyncratic diagnosis. He promised a 'safe and almost painless operation', offering for inspection two boys, John Topliss aged nine and William Russell aged eleven, who had undergone his operation two months before. Colleagues may have expressed scepticism as well as interest. A week later Yearsley assembled 26 patients, operating on them one after the other before a 'numerous body of scientific men'. Yearsley's rooms must have resembled an abattoir as one after another he excised the patients' uvula and tonsils. *The Times's* reporter conceded that the procedure had been executed skilfully, and that it had given the patients 'instantaneous' relief. Patients previously 'scarcely able to articulate half a dozen words' became able to speak 'with a wonderful degree of fluency'.[40]

'Big merciless hands': children and surgeons

The parents of children like these often faced a terrible choice. They confronted the dilemma of having to decide whether to agree to inflict pain upon their children by consenting to treatment. Many naturally hesitated and refused. A correspondent to the *Edinburgh Medical and Surgical Journal* complained how parents 'could never bring their minds to consent to an operation until his life was despaired of' – by which time it was often too late.[41] Instead they might be obliged to watch their son or daughter suffer from inflammation or exhaustion unable to consent to the infliction of pain.

If surgeons alarmed adults, how much more did they terrify children. Nothing exposes the pity of painful surgery like the experience of children subjected to it, or the surgeon's burden in having to operate upon children. Contemporary medical treatment, even if it did not involve surgery, unavoidably involved pain and for reasons children would not have understood. They would, however, have remembered those responsible for its infliction and sensitive surgeons knew it. Charles Bell once encountered a boy sent to collect medicine for his sister. Bell noticed that he had a squint and learned that he saw double despite having had two operations for its correction. The boy, 'though a little fellow', made clear that he 'by no means congratulates himself on having fallen into the hands of the surgeons'.[42] Alfred, Lord Tennyson (born in 1809) surely evoked childhood memories in sketching the surgeon in his poem 'In The Children's Hospital', who:

> Sent a chill to my heart when I saw him come in at the door,
> Fresh from the surgery-schools of France and of other lands
> Harsh red hair, big voice, big chest, big merciless hands ...[43]

Little wonder that John Elliotson remembered meeting a nine-year-old boy who burst into tears at his approach 'thinking that I should give him loads of physic to swallow, and blister him, as others had done'.[44]

Surgeons faced many obstacles in identifying and treating these conditions, not least their ignorance of children. 'Gentlemen', Charles West told his classes at the Middlesex Hospital in the late 1840s, 'children will form at least a third of all your patients'. Then, as now, young doctors faced obstacles in examining them. 'You cannot question your patient' West explained. 'It' might be too young to speak, or might be tongue-tied, 'from fear'. Doctors needed to gather information from a child's expression or demeanour, again not always an easy matter. 'The child is fretful and will not be looked at, you endeavour to feel his pulse, he struggles in alarm: you try to auscultate his chest, and he breaks out in a violent fit of crying.' Some young men, unfamiliar with children and accustomed to a more robust regime, never learned to understand their young patients. West urged them to persevere. Although a baby could not talk 'yet it has a language of its own, and that language must be your object to learn'.[45]

Thomas Goldie Scott sought his father's advice while practising as a new cantonment surgeon in Bombay having to treat the families of colonial officials and soldiers. William Scott summarised contemporary ideas which added up to relatively little. 'In all infantile disease,' he advised, 'careful attention should be given to the head'. In contrast to current notions for adults he urged Thomas to avoid emetics, and warned that children 'do not stand much bleeding'. 'Many are destroyed by leeching' he cautioned. If Thomas was obliged to prescribe something ('either to satisfy yourself or the parents') he recommended milk of magnesia. It did no harm but kept 'the bowels open and the skin moist'.[46] Indeed most childhood illnesses were treated either by mothers at home – hence the titles of works '*Intended Chiefly for the Use of Parents*' – or by apothecaries. Operating surgeons saw only the most extreme cases, usually of injury.[47] Even in the years 1857-64 only 47 of the Royal Edinburgh Infirmary's 3,651 surgical patients were children under ten.[48]

That surgeons must have appeared 'merciless' is understandable and many struggled with the responsibility. James Miller confessed that 'many and many a time' he had felt 'sorely beset' in treating hip and joint injuries 'especially in children'. Miller, himself a father, recalled as an advocate of anaesthesia how there was 'nothing so painful to the operating surgeon ... as being compelled ... to inflict tortures on young children'.[49] It is possible that younger surgeons' advocacy of excision rather than amputation was motivated partly by a desire to save children from the more serious, dangerous and maiming operation: certainly Benjamin Travers prevailed over Joseph Green to excise dead bone rather than amputate a seven-year-old boy's arm in 1837.[50] Frederic Skey counselled his colleagues only to perform operations to which they 'would unhesitatingly subject his own child'.[51] Some surgeons refused to treat children or did so reluctantly. Rowland Fawcett's commonplace book includes three poems he had copied dealing with the deaths of infants while his case books for 1823-27 disclose that he did not treat children under ten.[52] While many surgeons entertained a reluctance to operate on children others were not so fastidious. Convinced of their ability and impatient of parents' misgivings, some surgeons believed that they were empowered to act in place in parents, able to decide in the best interests of the child. Charles Bell recalled with distaste a colleague who, denied the unprecedented opportunity to amputate the leg of a child at the hip, 'actually tore his hair and exhibited the appearance of the deepest distress'.[53]

Many surgeons adopted, perhaps deliberately, a distance from the children on whom they operated. For example, George Ballingall, the military surgeon turned Professor of Military Surgery at Edinburgh, continued to treat patients at the Royal Infirmary. In 1826 he examined David Meek, a 'delicate looking boy' aged six. David had had difficulty urinating and suffered from pain, often clutching at his genitals, the classic symptom of bladder stone. After sounding the boy Ballingall decided to operate. Before five hundred observers in the Infirmary's operating theatre he performed the 'high' operation of lithotomy finding, after an unusually long operation in which he had to widen and extend the incision, two large stones. The spectators gasped together when with a 'moderate degree of force' he extracted two stones, each two inches across. David Meek gradually sank, insensible even to his mother, for whom he nevertheless called repeatedly and after 32 hours eventually died. Ballingall's account of his operation, ... *in which Unusual Difficulty was experienced in the Extraction of the Stone*, contains few sympathetic references to 'the little patient' and barely any indication of Ballingall's own feelings toward the infliction of pain or regret at its outcome.[54]

A satirical attack on George Guthrie's emphatic lecturing style suggests not only the virulence of feuds within the surgical community, but also, perhaps, the carapace of indifference with which Guthrie, himself a loving father, assumed in operating:

> The child whose *thigh* I have just cut off is eleven years old ... His mother or his aunt brought him here last week, for the purpose of having it amputated. I *did* this by making a flap on each side, so that you might have an opportunity of seeing the different methods of operating (*Expressions of wonder*) ... operations ... occur much too infrequently in our hospitals – (*shudders among the audience*) – I mean, gentlemen, too seldom for the advantages of instruction ('*Oh,*' '*oh,*') – although quite frequently enough for the sake of the sufferers. (*Hear, hear.*)[55]

Though likely unfair to Guthrie (at fifty he had become a figure of fun among irreverent students) the satire illuminates the growing awareness that children demanded a special consideration.

'Dear mamma, ... they must have hurt me a little': operating on children

Until the mid-nineteenth century Britain had neither institutions nor wards specifically for children. In Paris the Hospital des Enfants

Malades made available five hundred beds for children from three to ten years old. Here, naturally, only children with the most serious conditions presented. Characteristically, the place offered curious French pathologists unrivalled opportunities, and despite its frightful mortality it contributed to the recognition and treatment of conditions peculiar to children. British hospitals for children developed later. John Bunnell Davis's Royal Universal Dispensary for Children, established in London in 1816, treated nearly 175,000 children in its first thirty years, but all as out-patients at 'stations' south of the Thames, none as in-patients.[56] Guy's Hospital reportedly set aside a ward for children in the 1830s, but for the most part children, when they were admitted at all, were placed in adult wards.[57] Even if they enjoyed the special attention of nurses or their parents' care, the sights and sounds to which they would have been exposed, from swearing to surgery, appalls a modern sensibility. Relatively few were admitted and then, presumably, only cases requiring surgery or prolonged treatment. Dispensaries for children opened in Liverpool, Manchester and London, but all treated children as out-patients. Charles West's Children's Infirmary in Lambeth treated about 14,000 children in the period 1839-47, mainly as out-patients.[58] Bunnell Davis had believed that children were best treated at home; Charles West found that they died there. He sought to remove acutely ill children from dirty or hungry homes and urged the establishment of hospitals for children. His Great Ormond Street hospital opened in 1852, pre-empted by the Liverpool Institution for the Diseases of Children a year earlier. Hospitals specifically for children proliferated: in Manchester in 1856, Leeds in 1857 and Edinburgh in 1860. In the following decade they were established all over the empire and the world.

Before the foundation of children's hospitals they must have been terrifying places. An evangelical author – a hospital visitor – recalled a 'poor blind girl' she had seen in a ward. 'I feel very lonely', she said, 'I have been here two months and I have no one to speak to'.[59] Children were, as ever, vulnerable. Florence Nightingale, in her influential *Notes on Hospitals* of 1863, set out the first rules to guide the operation of hospitals devoted to children. Dedicated to the acceptance of women as hospital nurses, her rules included ensuring that 'women must be in undisputed charge of a child's hospital', and that 'no male attendants must ever be attached to children's wards'. Sadly but realistically she urged that 'reverent decency, so much neglected in England, is particularly desirable in children's hospitals'.[60]

In the meantime, children continued to be operated upon by surgeons in the major hospitals. Unable to find the fortitude which adults were able to display, children often made 'restless and noisy' patients. Robert Liston complained that 'they will not open their mouths'.[61] George Ballingall observed bad-temperedly that the 'extreme irritability' of children made them 'upon the whole rather unfavourable to capital operations'.[62] Their reactions under examination aggravated the difficulties of surgery: 'Stoneless' lithotomies became the inevitable outcome of the difficulties of sounding patients who could neither be still nor silent under a procedure requiring both. At the same time, remarkably, many surgeons testified that children, though 'more susceptible of pain than men' could, as William Griffin noted, 'surpass them in fortitude'.[63] A number of accounts substantiate Griffin's observation.

William Fergusson in 1842 enhanced his reputation with a 'formidable' operation, excising a tumour the size of an orange from the face of a twelve-year-old girl. The half-hour operation, conducted before two hundred spectators in the theatre at King's College Hospital, was, like Earle's excision of Mrs Cave's tumour a decade before, reported in detail in *The Times*, a further indication of the willingness of the public to confront the reality of surgery. Fergusson gained immense prestige from the operation, in which he 'never once lost his presence of mind' though all about turned pale at the 'frightful excisions' he was obliged to make. His unnamed patient at first 'cried piteously', but then 'exhibited great moral courage'.[64] Though unidentified, she was granted the dignity of forbearance which the watching society valued so highly. If Fergusson emerged as the heroic surgeon, his patient represented the heroic sufferer, one whom contemporaries so much admired.

Extraordinary though it may seem, children were apparently able to bear serious operations with the same fortitude as adults. Surgical texts refer to many examples. In the 1840s, for example, a surgeon recalled a case at St George's about 1811. A boy of 6 or 7 who was to undergo lithotomy promised that if his nurse were present he would not cry. Blind-folded on the table, he was unable to hold the nurse's hand, but spoke to her throughout the operation '*in his usual tone*' – 'Nurse, are you there?' 'Yes, my dear', and 'no cry, no groan, not a murmur escaped his lips!' The impression lingered of 'simple nature at its most guileless age'.[65]

John Abernethy offered two instances of the fortitude of children in a postscript to his 1819 Hunterian Oration.[66] As a young surgeon, Abernethy had seen a senior cut a five-year-old boy for stone. The boy struggled as the sound was inserted in his penis. The old surgeon patted the child on the cheek and said, 'You know, … I would not hurt you if I could help it'. 'I know it, Sir,' the boy is said to have replied, 'and I will cry no more'. Throughout the lithotomy, Abernethy said, his teeth remained clenched, his lips working, but he remained silent. A few weeks before delivering the oration, Abernethy had himself treated a seven-year-old boy for a diseased knee joint, at last reluctantly deciding that he must amputate at the thigh. Abernethy – who did not know what his family had told the boy – said 'I suppose, my little fellow, that you would not mind having this knee removed, which pained you so much and made you so very ill'? 'Oh, no', the boy is said to have replied, 'for mammy has told me that I ought'. During the amputation he displayed 'neither hesitation nor opposition', and remained also quiet. While the dialogue is stilted – and while the perspective is the surgeon's – Abernethy was speaking to an audience whose members had operated on hundreds of children between them. There is no reason to disbelieve his account that children could maintain their composure during such an ordeal. The courage of children in operations such as this has never been recognised. One of Liston's friends told the story of an un-named little girl who, hawking up some blood after losing her tonsils, said simply, 'Dear mamma, I think they must have hurt me a little'.[67]

'One of my proudest days': saving children

Many surgeons – perhaps most – increasingly saw children as patients demanding particular care. Many accordingly adopted treatments that would relieve suffering with minimal pain and if possible obviate the need to operate. The case book of William Hey senior illustrates how he was able to do so. In September 1785 the Rev. Mr Eyre and his wife brought their four-month-old daughter – who was nowhere named – because of a tumour on her neck. The child's maid had noticed a growth – about the size of a pigeon's egg – as she washed the baby. Soft and blue, it evidently did not pain her. No one could think of a reason for its appearance, except that some weeks before the child had suddenly screamed while being dressed. Hey decided that it was a varicose distention of the neck, caused by the child's screaming fit, and remained content to watch it, hoping that 'a little of time,' might cure it. A week later a worried Rev. Eyre wrote informing him that the tumour had grown alarmingly, and that they would be returning to Leeds. It had grown to four times its original size, reaching from the clavicle to the jaw bone.[68] Hey wondered whether he needed to take up (that is, ligate) a ruptured blood vessel, but rather than opening the child's neck to find out, he decided on pricking the growth to establish its contents. After consulting a local physician and an apothecary (nicely demonstrating their mutual dependence irrespective of the machinations of the metropolitan colleges) he decided to puncture the tumour with a large needle. Three times he punctured the growth, collecting a quantity of dark blood and observing it grow no larger. 'We now entertained hopes', he recorded, 'that this formidable disease would give us no further trouble'. Hey and his colleagues – and of course the child's parents – saw to their dismay that it grew again. Waiting for an anxious week, Hey punctured it again, this time seeing bright arterial blood flow. For reasons Hey did not disclose, he regarded the blood as a hopeful sign. 'Our little patient' was taken home and, indeed, the tumour slowly subsided. It gave Hey (and all concerned) 'great pleasure to see this alarming disease subdued by such gentle means'.

Surgeons approached child patients from a range of emotions and motives, however, an ambivalence apparent from the story of the baby of Elgin. In September 1833 the parents of a baby boy aged seven weeks brought the child to the Elgin Hospital, in north-east Scotland. The baby – who was also nowhere named in the report published in the *Lancet* – suffered from a swelling of the right leg.[69] The hospital's surgeon, John Paul, diagnosed fungus haematodes. The customary response in an adult would have been amputation, but, fearful of the effect on an infant, Paul advised the parents to simply await developments. After ten days the swelling burst. The bleeding almost killed the child, but he rallied after two days and entered the hospital, his leg swollen and ulcerated. Paul, realising that the boy would die if untreated, evidently persuaded the parents that amputation offered his only hope. On 4 October, assisted by colleagues and a student, he amputated the child's right leg above the knee. The baby was perhaps the youngest person on whom amputation had until then been attempted, and Paul's report claimed due credit.

The baby suffered no depression (unlike adults, conscious of the trauma before and after the operation) and accepted his mother's breast soon after. He improved daily and gained weight, while the stump healed rapidly at the first intention. A fortnight after the operation, though, he became fretful and in pain, the stump 'glistening'. Paul recognised erysipelas and prescribed poultices and quinine, with port wine and water to fortify him, to little avail.

Within a few days the child's scrotum became distended and later ulcerated, while the inflammation spread across his back and abdomen. Though by this time the stump had virtually healed, the baby sank into a fever. He refused the breast, developed diarrhoea and on 2 November at last died.

John Paul naturally wondered whether he had been right to attempt so serious an operation on a baby not quite ten weeks old. He had, he mused, no experience to draw on, but knew that without surgery death would have been imminent. Paul espoused a curious compound of pragmatism and philanthropy, believing that 'if a surgeon will undertake nothing under this guidance, it is evident that surgery must remain stationary, in place of being progressive'. Conceding that 'the life of an infant ... is not equal to that of an adult', he nevertheless argued that 'no one will contend that an infant ... [ought] to be consigned to inevitable death, if the smallest prospect of saving its life can be held out'. The result, he acknowledged had not been what he had 'ardently wished for', but he contended that 'in a surgical point of view the result is of the same high importance'. He had clearly hoped to be able to report a clinical triumph, a record for the youngest patient to survive a major amputation, and almost succeeded. 'No stump', he wistfully reported, 'did better for the first fortnight'. Had it not been for erysipelas he would have been able to claim to contribute to bringing surgery to 'a still higher degree of perfection'. Tragically, he discovered only after the baby's death that one of the hospital's nurses had erysipelas and was herself confined to bed. The baby's mother had 'not only been in the habit of going into the ward, ... but of actually sitting on the side of her bed, and of allowing her to have the child in her arms'. Paul's triumph had unwittingly been undone by the endemic infection of the wards. The infant's leg, he recorded, 'I have presented to my friend Mr Liston, and it may be seen in his museum'.

And yet, children suffered and died for want of surgery, as well as because of it. An account of one operation, a lithotomy, performed on a small child by Henry Spry, offers an insight into both the tension of operating but also into the reasons why surgeons could countenance the suffering they inflicted upon children.[70] Spry was surgeon in India to the 3rd Bengal Light Cavalry, stationed at Meerut in 1830. He described to his brother, also a surgeon, the operation he had performed on a child three-and-a-half years old. It was, he wrote 'the most perfect success ... one of my proudest days'. Without practising on a 'dead subject' – presumably because of the urgency of the case and the impossibility of locating a cadaver, Spry 'unhesitatingly' began to operate on 'the little sufferer', his hand 'steady as a rock'. Despite much bleeding, he extracted the stone in about five minutes. Nursing the child in his own house, after three weeks 'the little fellow was quite well', his mother 'showering a thousand blessings on my head'. The child had been 'tormented' for a year and she had trekked from cantonment to cantonment seeking a surgeon willing to operate. The operation which Henry Spry performed upon this unnamed 'little sufferer' subjected the child to five minutes of trauma and intense pain, an ordeal which none of us would willingly witness, much less inflict. Spry reflected on none of this. He felt pride – surely justifiable – in successfully completing a difficult operation. His capacity to operate, however, derived as much, perhaps, from seeing the child's sufferings, and knowing that without surgical intervention they would continue and become worse until he died, worn out by chronic pain.

Of all patients who entered the hospitals of the early nineteenth century, perhaps the most poignant is the child. William Henley, who as a young man in the early 1870s had spent months in the Edinburgh Royal Infirmary with tubercular bones, evoked in his verses 'In Hospital'

A small, strange child – so age'd yet so young! –
Her little arm besplinted and beslung
Precedes me gingerly to the waiting room ... [71]

Notes

1. R.C. Brock, *The Life and Work of Astley Cooper* (Edinburgh: E. & S. Livingstone, 1952), 154–55.
2. Charles Kingsley, *The Water Babies: A Fairy Tale for a Land-Baby* (London: Macmillan, 1863), 199.
3. Smith to Francis Jeffrey, [Dec 1803], Nowell Smith, (ed.), *The Letters of Sydney Smith* (Oxford: OUP, 1953), Vol. I, 92.
4. *Illustrated London News*, 21 December 1844; 29 March 1845.
5. D. Arnold & A.D. Harvey, *Collision of Empires: Britain in Three World Wars* (London: Phoenix, 1994), 48.
6. Charles Bell, *Surgical Observations* (London: Longmans & Co. 1816), 305–06.
7. John Clarke, *Commentaries on Some of the Most Important Diseases of Children* (London: Longman, Hurst, Rees, Orme & Brown, 1815), 5.

8. *London Medical Gazette*, 16 February 1844.
9. Charles West, *Lectures on the Diseases of Infancy and Childhood* (London: Longman, Brown, Green & Longmans, 1852), 1.
10. William Logan, (ed.), *Words of Comfort for Bereaved Parents* (London: Religious Tract Society, 1877).
11. James Walvin, *A Child's World: A Social History of English Childhood, 1800–1914* (Harmondsworth: Penguin, 1984), 48.
12. Clarke, *op. cit.* (note 7), 9.
13. Review of Coley's *A Practical Treatise on the Diseases of Children*, *London Medical Gazette*, 16 October 1846.
14. James Kennedey, *Instructions to Mothers and Nurses on the Management of Children* ... (Glasgow: R. Griffin, 1825), 201.
15. 'Dr Aiken & Mrs Barbauld', *Evenings at Home; or, the Juvenile Budget Opened* (London: William Milner, 1844), 245–46.
16. Anon, *Profitable Amusement for Children; or Puerile Tales Uniting Instruction with Entertainment* (London: Verno & Hood; J.Harris, 1802). The British Library's copy was given to Mary Evans ('the gift of her Papa') in 1808 and passed to Jessy Ellen Evans in 1829.
17. William Dewees, *Treatise on the Physical and Medical Treatment of Children* (London: John Miller, 1826), xi.
18. Lydia Child, *The Mother's Book* (Glasgow: T.T. & J. Tegg, 1834), 21.
19. Astley Cooper & Frederick Tyrrell, *The Lectures of Sir Astley Cooper, Bart.* ... (London: Thomas Tegg, 1824), Vol. II, 396.
20. R.J. Taynton to Astley Cooper, April 1831, Astley Cooper papers, RCSEng.
21. *Lancet*, 1833–34, Vol. I, 367.
22. Clarke, *op. cit.* (note 7), 19.
23. Samuel Cooper, *A Dictionary of Practical Surgery* (London: Longman, Hurst, Rees, Orme & Brown, 1829), 1040–41.
24. James Hamilton, *Hints for the Treatment of the Principal Diseases of Infancy and Childhood adapted to the Use of Parents* (Edinburgh: Peter Hill, 1824), 14–15.
25. Clarke, *op. cit.* (note 7), 189.
26. Hamilton, *op. cit.* (note 24), 13–14.
27. Leslie Marchand, *Byron: A Biography* (London: John Murray, 1957), 54–55.
28. Frederick F. Cartwright, *The Development of Modern Surgery* (London: Arthur Barker, 1967), 148–50.
29. Francis, 'Repair of Cleft Palate by Philibert Roux in 1819', *Journal of the History of Medicine and Allied Sciences*, 1963, 210–19.
30. Bruce, 'The Footprints of Scottish Paediatric Surgery', *Journal of the Royal College of Surgeons of Edinburgh*, 1976, 136.

31. Adrian Desmond, *The Politics of Evolution: Morphology, Medicine, and Reform in Radical London* (Chicago: University of Chicago Press, 1989), 86.

32. Cooper & Tyrrell, *op. cit.* (note 19), Vol. II, 396.

33. Guenter Risse, *Hospital Life in Enlightenment Scotland: Care and Teaching at the Royal Infirmary of Edinburgh* (Cambridge: CUP, 1986), 170.

34. Cooper, *op. cit.* (note 23), 594.

35. Robert Liston, *Lectures on the Operations of Surgery* (Philadeliphia: Lea & Blanchard, 1846), 187–89.

36. James Miller, *Surgical Experience of Chloroform* (Edinburgh: Sutherland & Knox, 1848), 36.

37. John Snow, *On Chloroform and Other Anaesthetics* (London: John Churchill, 1858), 292–93.

38. Abernethy, 'Report of his lectures on Surgery', 42.b.16, RCSEng.

39. *Lancet*, 1831–32, Vol. II, 288.

40. *The Times*, 5 March 1841, 3f; 10 March 1841, 5b.

41. 'Mr Chrichton on Lithotomy', *Edinburgh Medical & Surgical Journal*, 1828, Vol. 29, 232.

42. Charles Bell, *Practical Essays* (Edinburgh: Maclachlan, Stewart & Co., 1841), 80.

43. Tennyson, 'In the Children's Hospital'.

44. [William Lang], *Mesmerism: its History, Phenomena, and Practice* (Edinburgh: Fraser & Co., 1843), 51.

45. West, *op. cit.* (note 9), 1–3.

46. William Scott to Thomas Goldie Scott, 31 Aug 1844, Acc. 9266/1, NLS.

47. Andrew Combe, *The Management of Infancy ... Intended Chiefly for the Use of Parents* (Edinburgh: Machlachlan & Stewart, [1840], 1890).

48. Roberts, 'The Origins of Paediatric Surgery in Edinburgh', *Journal of the Royal College of Surgeons of Edinburgh*, 1969, 299–315.

49. Miller, *op. cit.* (note 36), 51; 24.

50. Travers papers, Glass Case 333, RCSEng.

51. Frederic Skey, *Operative Surgery* (London: John Churchill, 1850), 14.

52. Fawcett case book, 1823-27 Add. MS 155; Commonplace book, Add Ms 155, RCSEng.

53. Charles Bell, *Observations on Injuries of the Spine and of the Thigh Bone* (London: Thomas Tegg, 1824), 39.

54. George Ballingall, *Case of the High Operation of Lithotomy , in which Unusual Difficulty was experienced in the Extraction of the Stone*

(Edinburgh: Medico-Chirurgical Society of Edinburgh, 1826).

55. *Lancet*, 1835-36, Vol. II, 567.

56. A. White Franklin, 'Children's Hospitals' in F.N.L. Poynter (ed.), *The Evolution of Hospitals in Britain* (London: Pitman Medical, 1964), 107–08.

57. H.G. Cameron, *Mr Guy's Hospital 1726–1948* (London: Longman, Green & Co., 1954), 116.

58. West, *op. cit.* (note 9), 1.

59. Anon, [Mary Stanley], *Hospitals and Sisterhoods* (London: 1854), 2.

60. Florence Nightingale, *Notes on Hospitals* (London: John Parker & Sons, 1863), 131–32.

61. *Lancet*, 1844, Vol. II, 66.

62. George Ballingall, *A Clinical Lecture delivered to the Students of Surgery in the Royal Infirmary of Edinburgh* (Edinburgh: A. Balfour, 1827), 12.

63. William Griffin, *An Essay on the Nature of Pain* (Edinburgh: J. Moir, 1826), 42.

64. *The Times*, 3 February 1842, 4f.

65. Ross Leitch, *Mesmerism in 1845* (Edinburgh, 1845), 38.

66. John Abernethy, *Introductory Lectures Exhibiting Some of Mr Hunter's Opinions Respecting Life Diseases* (London: Longman, Hurst, Rees, Orme & Brown, 1819), 62n.

67. *Lancet*, 1844, Vol. II, 66.

68. William Hey, *Practical Observations in Surgery* (London: T. Cadell Jnr & W. Davies, [1803; 1814]), 488–93.

69. *Lancet*, 1833–34, Vol. I, 439–41.

70. Henry Spry to E.J. Spry, 5 May 1830, Photo.Eur 308, OIOC, BL.

71. William Ernest Henley, *A Book of Verses* (London: David Nutt, 1888), 3.

10

'Fortitude':
The Patient's Experience of Surgery

The dominant voices in this as well as virtually all previous accounts of surgery have been those of surgeons and, to a lesser extent, their students. Their patients' voices are faint and elusive. It is possible to devise a 'celebrity ward', assembling operations from the great figures of the period: Lord Nelson's arm, the Earl of Uxbridge's leg, Sir Walter Scott's gallstones, Princess Charlotte Augusta's fatal confinement, King George IV's steatoma, Fanny Burney's breast. This would have offered insights into the nature of surgery, the suffering it involved and the qualities demanded to survive it. Moving beyond these well-known figures, however, it is possible to recover new or refreshed accounts of surgery which will explore the patient's experience in two ways. First, by attempting to recover the words of patients during surgery and second, by considering individuals whose testimonies allow us insights into the experience of surgery.

'The hardest day's work': patients' voices

Surgery was an intense experience and patients sometimes described it vividly.* A tailor in a Highland regiment described an operation for aneurism comparing it 'with the thrusting of a red hot iron into his heart'.[1] A patient told James Esdaile that the operation for hydrocele, a testicular condition, felt 'like a coir rope, round my loins, being pulled at each end by some persons as hard as they could'. Not surprisingly the sweat ran from his head 'as if some one was sprinkling water on my hair'.[2] Another patient described a lithotomy as 'not worse than being shaved with a blunt razor'.[3] As a student in

---

* Elaine Scarry's *The Body in Pain* builds an important argument about the capacity of intense pain to destroy language. This appears true for the victims of torture whom she studied. Without gainsaying that many surgical patients experienced the phenomenon, many examples of articulate patients suggest that the effects of the pain of involuntary and unnecessary torture differ from those of surgery undertaken for medical reasons and often voluntarily.

261

Paris in the 1880s John Bland-Sutton witnessed an iridectomy – excision of the iris. The patient recalled that 'when the knife entered my eye it seemed like a flash of lightning'.[4] These impressions, though revealing the diversity of experience, also relate only to sensation: they do not illuminate surgery as a joint undertaking between patients and operators.

An account of the first English amputation at the hip by Astley Cooper in 1824 hints at this hidden dimension of the operating room. Acting impulsively, Cooper decided to attempt amputation at the hip on a man suffering from necrosis of the bone in the stump of a thigh he had lost some years before. At several hours notice he consented to an operation which had never been attempted in London before. Cooper took twenty minutes to remove the limb and a further fifteen to secure the arteries and dress the immense wound. The patient, a man about forty, felt faint during the operation, but bore it with 'extraordinary fortitude'. As Cooper finished he said to the surgeon that 'that was the hardest day's work he had ever gone through'. Cooper replied that 'it was almost the hardest he ever had'. Surgeon and patient recognised how they had shared in the ordeal, a partnership of suffering and its relief. After six months in hospital the patient recovered, convalescing at Cooper's country house.[5]

The pain of surgery affected patients in many different ways. Some sat or lay immobile throughout the most severe operations. Some, said John Elliotson, 'keep their jaws firmly closed, some sing, whistle, chatter, laugh, or smoke'.[6] Others struggled, writhed, 'uncontrollably turbulent' perhaps obliging the surgeon to desist lest a slip of the knife cause a fatal haemorrhage.[7] Some surgeons might summon porters or dressers to compel them to be still; some were gagged and blindfolded. Other operators, in a response suggesting that restraints were less general than we may suppose might, like Charles Bell, acquiesce to a patient rolling about during a lithotomy. He explained that he 'thought it cruel to withdraw the knife and leave the operation unfinished'.[8] Perhaps the majority shrieked or cried uncontrollably, inarticulate except in conveying their torment. Others – and we will never know how many – found the resource to speak. Patients' words while on the table convey immense power: 'Oh, you hurt me, Sir!' a woman undergoing a Caesarian delivery called out, 'are you going to do it *again?*'[9]

One of the most poignant accounts of a patient's attempts to communicate during surgery comes from the travails of a thirty-year-old Chinese labourer named Hoo Loo. Travelling at the expense of the East India Company in China he came to London in 1831 from

262

a village near Canton expressly to have a London surgeon remove an enormous tumour in his groin.[10] A man of 'cheerful disposition' Hoo Loo quickly became popular among the staff and nurses of Guy's Hospital for his gentle manners. An exotic object of curiosity, he was soon 'absolutely besieged' by medical gentlemen eager to be associated with a challenging operation, one whose completion ensured popular acclaim: if it succeeded. So many wished to watch Aston Key remove the tumour that the operation had to be moved from Guy's operating theatre to the larger anatomy theatre. Almost a thousand spectators thronged the room. At one o'clock, laughing and in the high spirits that had made him so popular, Hoo Loo was ushered into the theatre, secured by straps and had a handkerchief placed over his face. Key, assisted by four other surgeons including Bransby Cooper, secured the veins surrounding the tumour as he went. At the outset Key had decided to preserve the man's genitals but, realising that this would prolong the operation, 'decided to sacrifice them'. Hoo Loo lost sixteen ounces of blood and became weaker. He felt faint, was fanned and given brandy as assistants chafed his feet and chest. A medical student volunteered to transfuse blood and eight ounces were injected but to no avail. Hoo Loo sank further and died on the table after being in theatre for nearly an hour and three-quarters. The tumour weighed fifty-six pounds and measured four feet in circumference.[11]

The nurses and patients of his ward cried on learning of Hoo Loo's death which the surgeons attributed to loss of blood. Later that week letters appeared in the press casting further light on the operation. 'T.C.' suggested that the many spectators in the hall had 'heated and contaminated' the air and counselled that however much the benefit of science demanded that professional gentlemen observe, the patient's 'well-doing' should have been paramount. During the operation spectators could hear but not understand his exclamations although a witness detected 'plaintive acknowledgment of the hopelessness of his case'.[12] The following day a witness wrote to describe what probably he alone had understood. The only person present to understand Chinese, he was able to translate what Hoo Loo had called out during the operation. 'Unloose me, unloose me!' he had called. 'Water! Help! Water! Let me go!' His last words had been 'Let it be – let it remain! I can bear no more! Unloose me!'[13]

Hoo Loo's is an unusually well-documented case. The contemporary record, often distant from the tension of the moment, usually gives a very imperfect impression of what was said and how. The words jotted down by students, visitors and the *Lancet's* often clandestine reporters nevertheless suggest the great diversity of reaction. Patients' voices come to us in fragments, snippets overheard because a surgeon or a student thought to record a remark or an exchange. We must recognise that we make inferences based on these shards of dialogue. We must also acknowledge that some patients spoke no words and that the words of others do not necessarily reflect their real feelings. In 1834 a fifty-year-old ropemaker 'W.P.', lying in the London Hospital with a compound fracture of the left leg, replied to all enquiries as to how he was doing with 'quite nicely'. Although his wound was oozing blood and discharging matter, he refused to consent to amputation. His breezy reply, surgeons thought, 'probably arises from his dread of losing the limb'. He died without surgery after three weeks.[14] Sometimes patients' exclamations bespeak bravado. Abernethy recalled a man on whom he operated for lithotomy who spent the entire operation – three minutes – 'hallooing all the time'. 'What are you at, my boys?' he cried, 'Pull away, pull away, my hearties; go on pull away'.[15] Other patients bore pain with the fortitude that all admired. 'A woman who survived one of Charles Clay's ovariotomies in 1842 which involved an incision reaching 24 inches across her abdomen, claimed that she had endured more severe pain in childbirth.[16]

We may be astonished at what patients might bear but surgeons expressed no surprise that patients would endure without comment or complaint what we would now regard as major ordeals. In detailing eye surgery William Mackenzie described how 'labouring people' would 'not infrequently tie up their eye with a handkerchief and ... resume their usual employments'.[17] Accustomed to operations, surgeons and students often failed to appreciate the gravity of the experience from the patient's perspective. The spirit patients could display is truly remarkable. In 1832 at St George's Hospital a young woman with necrosis of the bone suffered the leg being opened and the dead bone excised with bone pliers, a procedure the *Lancet's* correspondent described as 'trivial'. Rather than scream inarticulately, she 'lavished' 'hysterical endearments' on the operators which 'frequently convulsed the whole theatre'. 'Oh, when will you have done with me, my dear?' the woman asked. An exasperated pupil replied 'Here, take and bite this towel'.[18] Others, however, responded appreciatively to displays of spirit. In 1832 John Scott at the London Hospital removed a bony growth from the upper jaw of a forty-five-year-old man in an operation taking three-quarters of an hour. After displaying 'the most stoical fortitude' throughout the operation, at its conclusion Mr Scott asked him whether he had suffered much. The man smiled, saying 'Oh, I'll tell you another time', and then insisted on walking to his bed, to the cheers of the spectators.[19]

While acknowledging that many patients were the unwilling subjects of surgery, we also need to consider the likelihood that others participated in the operation by exercising choice over their actions to assist their own recovery. Those who submitted without complaint were particularly commended. Innumerable accounts describe patients bearing the pain of capital operations with a resolve noted and admired by contemporaries. A man who had lost a leg by Astley Cooper consulted him with continuing pain (possibly from 'phantom' pain or perhaps an incorrectly tied nerve) which 'incommoded him very much'. He asked Cooper to amputate part of the stump. Cooper tried to dissuade him but the patient remained obdurate. He sat in the chair for the operation, refusing to be strapped in 'saying he knew well what the pain was' and in the event did not move a muscle.[20] Brodie told the story of a young man who consulted a succession of doctors for a swelling on his right leg until Brodie proposed amputation. The young man bore the operation with the 'utmost fortitude'. 'A bystander', Brodie wrote, 'could not have supposed that he suffered the smallest pain'. Sadly, the patient suffered haemorrhage, fever and shock, and died soon after.[21]. The courage of patients competed with the skill of the surgical celebrity as an explanation for the triumphs of modern surgery. In 1827 the *Times* carried an account of a half-hour-long operation by Robert Liston to restore the nose of a young man whose resolve had been 'screwed up to the cutting point'. Indeed, *The Times's* correspondent found it 'difficult to say whether the dexterity of the operator or the fortitude of the patient were most to be admired'.[22]

Few patients possessed the will or the resources to record their experience of surgery in detail. Considering several surviving accounts, however, allows us to understand what they underwent from their perspective. Their recollections are often vivid. Patients under the knife often observed their surroundings with an unusual clarity and experienced time as passing with literally excruciating slowness. A man who lost a testicle to Robert Keate saw one of Keate's dressers pause during the operation to wipe a spot of blood from his white trousers (in itself further evidence that operations were not expected to be unduly bloody). Afterwards the patient rounded on Keate saying that he had intended to give the man twenty guineas but 'as he regarded the purity of his trousers more important than my sufferings, I will not give him a farthing'.[23] A few patients, however, were able to record their reactions to surgery. The following accounts begin with a reminder of the persistent background pain which virtually all people endured before and often after 1850. They increase in intensity to deal with several surgical operations. Collectively these accounts suggest something of the ordeal and the qualities which surgery evoked in those who submitted to it.

'Tolerable health': Mary Thomas's infections

Among the first British settlers in the colony of South Australia was the sixteen-year-old Mary Thomas. In December 1839 Mary's mother called a doctor to treat her throat, which he found to be 'full of ulcers'. The diagnosis began five years of an intermittent and largely ineffectual battle with a series of intractable infections and associated conditions. Mary detailed her complaints and her stoic endurance of a range of treatments in her diary. Although relatively minor, Mary Thomas's complaints demonstrate not only the nature of surgical treatment of minor illnesses in accord with the doctrine of counter-irritation but also the fortitude expected and demonstrated by even a young patient.[24]

Four months after diagnosing the ulcers her doctor decided that parts of Mary's throat had fused and separated the tissues with the handle of a tablespoon. After months of gargling with 'a black liquid' the condition eased somewhat. Although her throat remained quiescent for several years she suffered from a 'gathering' on her eyeball which a Mr Charles lanced. Mary's only objection to the procedure was that it should not be performed at the surgeon's house. Early in 1842 Mary's throat complaint recurred. She was again given a gargle, this time a 'caustic', and by April her ulcers had to be 'touched' with caustic applied on a rag tied on the end of a stick. In June she was 'taken ill', an attack blamed by another doctor on the caustic prescribed earlier. Mary's mother herself 'cauterised' her throat but without success and in August another surgeon cut the growths in it 'in two places with large scissors'. This did little good and in September another doctor applied blisters to Mary's throat. By October the blisters were joined by more cauterisation and cabbage leaves were applied to draw out the infection. In November a convention of medical men argued over Mary's throat. Some wanted to cut the growths out but a Mr W objected strenuously fearing that if an artery were accidentally pierced she could bleed to death.

In 1843 Mary suffered from an intermittent fever which was treated by daily shower baths, leeches (which she was declared 'too weak to bear'), cupping and shaving of her hair. No sooner had she recovered than she was bitten by a dog and suffered pain 'so violent I cannot even read Shakespeare'. Three months later she was 'attacked with toothache' and in extracting the tooth Dr W broke it off at the root. Despite inflamed gums he reassured her that she 'will not suffer any inconvenience'. An attempt to remove the root from the gum was deferred due to excessively windy weather. Mr Charles, though hesitant to 'extract pieses', enjoyed a splendid dinner at the Thomas's and then 'took out remnants of tooth' in Mary's laconic summary. Dr W was delighted at his colleague's work but a fortnight later Mr Charles discovered 'an obstinate piece' still in the gum. Removing this entailed a further operation. He used a lancet to expose the bone, found yet another piece of tooth and attempted unsuccessfully to draw both using a hook and pincers. He told Mary candidly that 'nothing but punching will ever do it any good'. Later that spring Mary suffered from a sore arm which took months to heal.

Early in 1846 Mary's throat trouble recurred and Dr Charles applied more caustic and performed a series of operations on the ulcers, again using Mrs Thomas's scissors. By September Mary recorded to her (and our) relief she was in 'tolerable health'. Mary's troubles did not require what she or her doctors would have regarded as serious surgery: and yet she spent many months in aggravating pain, her throat cut half a dozen times with scissors and treated often with caustic. Her experience reminds us of the background of suffering which patients brought with them to the operating room.

'A sad business': the death of William De Lancey

In such a cataclysmic battle as Waterloo the individual can all too readily be subsumed by the mass. It is through the experience of one of Waterloo's wounded – perhaps the only one to be nursed by his wife – that the impact can be seen. Colonel Sir William De Lancey and Magdalene Hall had married in Scotland in April 1815. Magdalene and William, Wellington's Quartermaster General (his chief staff officer), had honeymooned in Brussels, then crowded with the Allied army assembling against the threat of the restored Napoleon. The De Lanceys rarely went abroad, venturing out when other English gentry were at dinner. The couple's idyll ended on 16 June when Wellington learned of the French advance into Belgium. William went with the Duke's headquarters while Magdalene remained with the English civilians in Antwerp. On the afternoon of 18 June she heard the sound of battle 'rolling like the sea at a distance'.[25]

One of the explosions she heard had fired a ball that struck her husband. William had remained by the Duke throughout the long bloody afternoon of the battle. At about four, near the centre of the British line, he was hit in the back by a cannon ball. Falling from his horse he was carried to a cottage near the village of Waterloo. Prey to the rumours washing back from the battle, Magdalene first heard that he had been desperately wounded, then that he had been killed; then that he was wounded. Against the advice of concerned friends she set out for Waterloo passing the hideous columns of wounded straggling toward Brussels. At last she reached Waterloo and the cottage in which William lay. 'Come, Magdalene', he said, 'this is a sad business, is it not?'

For a week Magdalene, helped by her maid Emma nursed her husband. Dr Hume, Wellington's own surgeon, told her that William's wound was grave and was expected to be mortal. The ball which had struck him had forced eight ribs from the spine, and one rib at least had punctured the lungs. There was little that could be done and William knew it. 'Pray tell them', he begged Magdalene', 'to leave me and let me die in peace'. He ate little – a few morsels of toast – but drank tea and lemonade. Magdalene sat with him, bathing him, but powerless to arrest the inflammation of his lungs or ease the terrible pain of breathing. Dr Hume and other surgeons came by occasionally. Surprised that he had not succumbed, they attempted remedies. 'It does no harm', they reasoned, 'to be trying something', putting a blister on his chest and leeches after. 'Was it not a great pity to torment him?' Magdalene asked herself in the narrative of William's last days that she later wrote.

Several days later Lieutenant William Hay, who had been sent back to Brussels to find his regiment's wounded and stragglers as Wellington's army advanced into France, found the 'little wretched cottage' in which Magdalene nursed her husband. Hay had known the couple during their recent engagement and was naturally shocked to learn of De Lancey's wound. He found Magdalene, 'an amiable, kind and beautiful young woman' sitting on a broken chair – the cottage's only furniture – and 'plunged in the deepest distress'. She pointed to William lying under his coat with 'just a spark of life left' and ushered Hay out. Rallying, she then offered Hay wine in a broken teacup (the only one in the house) and he left the couple in silence together.[26]

William grew weaker. One night later in the week they lay together on William's rough bed and slept for a few hours. William woke at three and lay uneasily through the rest of the night. That afternoon, the ninth day after the battle, the surgeons came again but there was little they could do. William gave 'a little gulp' as if something was in his throat' and died. Charlotte Eaton, who saw Magdalene soon after, described how she endured 'her irreparable loss with astonishing firmness'.[27]

'Perfect blessedness': Mr X's lithotomy

On the last day of 1811 Henry Cline junior and his dressers drove to the London home of a gentleman of about forty. Cline described the man as possessing the advantages of 'a liberal education ..., an uncommon share of cheerfulness and a firmness of mind' which he retained 'under the most trying circumstances'. The patient had agreed to submit to lithotomy:'my mind was made up' he recorded. Those who could avoid entering hospital did so and Cline treated the man privately.[28]

After Cline and his assistants had assembled the patient asked leave to retire for a moment and knelt in prayer for a while. Returning to the waiting surgeon he showed them to the room where the operation was to be conducted. Taking off his breeches and underclothes he climbed onto the table and allowed the dressers to restrain him in the usual manner with his hands bound to his feet. The man had prepared himself for a 'shock of pain of extreme violence', so much so that he had over-rated it and he found the first incision 'did not even make me wince'.

He had evidently discussed the operation with Cline who had advised him not to stifle his cries because the effort of restraint 'could only lead to additional exhaustion'. Soon after the initial incision, therefore, he began to cry out. The 'first real pain' he felt came from the insertion of the staff, the metal rod inserted in the urethra as a guide to the delicate penetration of the perineum. His pain intensified as Cline inserted the gorget but eased with the gush of urine from the bladder. Cline now took up the forceps and inserted them into the bladder to feel for the stone. After several unavailing attempts to grasp it the patient heard Cline whisper to an assistant 'it is a little awkward ... give me the curved forceps'. Every movement of the forceps increased the patient's pain until at last Cline said 'I have got it'. The patient by this time had imagined that the worst was over. Now, though, Cline withdrew the forceps while grasping the stone. The patient recollected that the sensation was 'such that I cannot find words to describe' adding that besides the 'positive pain', there was 'something most peculiar in the feel'. The duration of this was short and he heard one of the operators say 'now sir, it is all over!' 'Thank

God! thank God' the man exclaimed. He professed to be 'quite unable' to describe his feelings at that moment but struggled to convey 'the most captivating vision ... the most enchanting harmony'. He felt 'a combination of everything that is calculated to delight the senses' and the 'perfect blessedness of my situation'. Pondering the chronic pain of the stone and the acute agony of the operation he decided that if he should be afflicted with stone again he would unhesitatingly submit to surgery again: provided Cline or an operator as skilful could be found.

'Emmie': taken from life

Alfred Lord Tennyson was born in 1809 and lived in the era of painful surgery. His 'dramatic poem' 'In the Children's Hospital' was composed in 1880 but, as George Orwell pointed out, it derives from and speaks of the era before 1850. Tennyson is reputed to have based the tale on a story he had 'taken from life' but it is infused by an awareness of the horror of surgery performed on children, in itself a sign of the changing sensibility in the hospitals of the mid-nineteenth century. The poem is narrated by a nurse, Annie, who describes the last days of a child in hospital.[29] It opens by establishing the orientations of the main characters, contrasting the piety of the nurse against the innocence of the children and the hard rationalism of the surgeon. The red-haired, loud-voiced doctor the nurse describes was 'happier using the knife than trying to save the limb': an excusable appeal to prejudice in the circumstances. Examining a boy 'caught in a mill and crushed', he 'handled him gently enough' but 'his voice and his face were not kind'. Hearing the doctor pronounce the boy 'a hopeless case' the nurse replies that she will pray for him. 'Can prayer set a broken bone?' he retorts with the scepticism of the modern surgeon, 'the good Lord Jesus has had his day'. Shocked, the nurse affirms her faith, 'O how could I serve in the wards' she asks, 'with the sights and the loathsome smells of disease ... if the hope of the world were a lie?'

The nurse and the surgeon pass on to the ward where the younger children lie. An empty cot reminds her of the loss of orphan Emmie, 'patient of pain though as quick as a sensitive plant to the touch'. Emmie had been examined by another doctor who had said, thinking that she was asleep, that he would operate the next day 'though she'll never live through it'. Emmie overhears and asks Annie what she should do and the nurse counsels her to call upon the Saviour who said 'suffer the little children to come unto me'. Emmie wonders how Jesus would recognise her in a ward of sick children and the nurse advises her to pray and tell Jesus that she will lay with her arms outside the blankets. The nurse had sat by Emmie for three nights. Exhausted, she slept, dreaming that 'in the gray of the morning ... she stood by me and smiled'. At dawn the doctor comes with his 'ghastly tools'. Emmie lies seemingly asleep with her arms outside the blankets. 'The Lord of the children had heard her, and Emmie had passed away.' Tennyson's ballad is sentimental and pious but, like John Brown's story of Allie, it conveys powerfully and sensitively the dread of operations performed on children.

Dr A, Charles Dickens and Macvey Napier's fistulas

It is important to acknowledge that patients could experience and recall similar operations very differently. The repair of anal fistula, one of surgery's minor procedures, could prompt strikingly diverse reactions. Three patients' accounts exemplify the possible reactions.

'Dr A', a Scottish physician, wrote to James Syme around 1860 recording his memory of an operation for anal fistula which Syme had performed about twenty years before.[30] Dr A remembered how he had 'suffered intensely' from the pain and discomfort of the fistula, 'unfit for anything'. He could not work and found it uncomfortable to be in society 'on account of my extreme <u>unrest</u>'. Conscious of faeces leaking onto his underclothes, 'I was constantly fidgeting about ...' while 'my suffering at stool' was for months unbearable. He frequently sat bathed in sweat as he felt 'pure lancinating pain ... mixed with intense itching' persisting for hours at a time. 'I was always miserable' he concluded. Syme's operation worked wonders: 'You ... cured it as if by magic' Dr A proclaimed. 'Of course I could not see what you did' but Syme explained that he had performed the procedure as described in his *Principles of Surgery* which involved cutting the sinus to connect it with the sphincter. Dr A wrote that he had felt 'little or no pain ... indeed, the sensation caused by the knife was comparatively pleasant'. Twenty years on Syme remained anxious to convince even medical colleagues of the operation's ease and effectiveness. Told by a visiting English doctor that the operation was 'too dreadful for human endurance' he persuaded him that it could be remedied by 'an incision so trivial that the patient was not aware of its performance'.

Late in 1841 Charles Dickens also felt the symptoms of fistula. He believed that the complaint had been caused by 'too much sitting at my desk'. On the morning of Friday 8 October, as he told a friend, he was 'obliged to submit to a cruel operation', one devoted to the 'cutting out root and branch' of a condition which had been

271

'gathering for some years'. On the evening of the operation his close friend Macready called round, only to be regaled by Dickens and his wife with an account of the operation. Like many Macready understandably did not wish to know the surgical details – and 'suffered agonies' as they described the procedure. Four days later Dickens was still confined to a sofa, so unwell as to have to dictate his correspondence to his wife. A fortnight later he had regained his 'usual appetite and spirits' and was at last able to drive out in his carriage. The operation had been performed by Frederick Salmon, formerly of the Aldersgate Dispensary, to whom Dickens presented copies of *The Pickwick Papers, Nicholas Nickleby* and *Oliver Twist* in a 'spontaneous and most heartfelt emotion ... of gratitude'. However, a month after the operation, 'having stood too long, finishing Barnaby', Dickens wrote to tell Salmon that he had felt 'all manner of queer pains' in his calves, legs, feet and 'shooting through that region which you have made as tender as my heart'. Following Salmon's instructions, Dickens 'parboiled' his feet in hot salt water and had his back rubbed with camphor ointment.[31]

As he sat gingerly upon cushions Dickens received a letter from his friend Macvey Napier, Professor of Conveyancing at the University of Edinburgh and editor of the *Edinburgh Review*. Napier's experience suggests how great an impact surgery and its consequences had on patients. He offered his sympathies. 'Three times' he had submitted to operations for the same complaint, operations 'bungled by the Edinburgh surgeons'. Not until he travelled to London to place himself in the 'skilful hands' of Sir Benjamin Brodie did he find relief. Napier looked back on his operations with horror: 'my flesh yet creeps', he remembered, 'though it is now over five years ... since Sir Benjamin did the job'. Even so, owing to 'a still more cruel complaint' – a chronic stricture 'under which I underwent the operation of burning out ... by caustic' – his health had never recovered. Napier urged Dickens to take his advice. 'Use your sofa for a long time to come' he advised. 'I beseech you,' he said, 'not to sit during your whole after life, upon either stone or turf' and to resort to 'careful ablution' with cold water at least twice a day. 'Avoid cold as you would the great enemy of mankind', urging Dickens not to embark upon a sea voyage 'so soon after undergoing a cruel operation'.[32] Dickens, however, felt stronger and early in 1842 embarked for America. Surmounting fistula demanded 'bottom' in every sense.

•

'A factory cripple': William Dodd's arm

In 1841 a 37-year-old one-armed man wrote to Lord Ashley (later Lord Shaftesbury) to describe 'the experience and sufferings of ... a factory cripple'.[33] William Dodd's narrative is a measured exposé of the effects of perhaps the worst period of the industrial revolution on those harmed by it. He represents the many patients who came to surgery after years of suffering. For Dodd the pain of surgery, awful though it of course was, still represented only a more intense form of the recurrent pain he had long endured as a consequence of his occupation. Dodd, of Kendal, Westmoreland, was sent to work in a local woollen mill at the age of five, around 1809, and for nearly thirty years he worked in mills as a piecer, a spinner and overseer. His narrative appeared as part of his book *The Factory System Illustrated* which described conditions in the industrial north revealing the toll of injuries and the less spectacular but more insidious wastage from long hours, poor nutrition and, above all, the impositions and hardships of the work itself. As a piecer young William's hands became chapped and bloody each day from the friction of the rough wrappings of the wool cardings he fed into the spinning machine. For weeks at a time his fingers would bleed by day, heal overnight and break out anew each morning, ravages aggravated by the swelling from the greasy, cold wool and the whale oil and animal fat saturating everything. The piecers, wearing clothes as wet and greasy as the wool they spun, had to stand in a position next to the machine they fed that placed a continual strain on their developing frames. Over time their knees and feet became deformed – he recalled that on Monday mornings his joints creaked 'like so many rusty hinges'. Before reaching ten he worked long hours – twelve hours a day – for two shillings a week, often abused and struck for failing to maintain the pace set by the spinners for whom he worked. Later, factory regulations prevented children younger than nine from doing the work: William Dodd was a victim of the earlier, unregulated period.

Dodd was unusual in that a mill master, seeing him tracing letters in chalk on a discarded board, taught him to read and write. Becoming a member of a Mechanics' Institute he anticipated the injunctions of Smilesean 'self-help', read and attended 'lectures on various subjects' and became an office-bearer in the Society of Odd Fellows. The deformities which factory work wrought on growing bodies like Dodd's eventually brought him to the operating room. 'If the bones go wrong,' he wrote, 'the blood vessels must go wrong also'. In 'us poor factory cripples', he believed, the blood lodged 'as it were, in little pools, in crannies and corners'. The consequence was, so medical men told him, that the marrow in the bones dried up. 'The bones then decay ... amputation is resorted to, or life is lost'. By 1840, spurned by respectable women because of his deformed body and rejecting the less choosy mill girls who would have been glad to escape the factory by marrying him, Dodd moved to London. Denied the opportunity of training as a teacher in a school ('in consequence of being a cripple') he tramped the south in search of work and found a situation as a clerk. In the spring of 1840, however, the pain he had often felt in his wrists and joints intensified, resisting the liniment and warm flannel he had customarily applied. Consulting 'some of the most eminent medical practitioners' he failed to obtain a cure. Now workless, he was obliged to enter St Thomas's Hospital. Here he remained for six months with the wrist swelling to a circumference of twelve inches as he wasted to 'a mere skeleton, unable to sleep ... generally starting up from pain'. Surgeons told Dodd that he must lose his hand or his life. On 18 July 1840 he submitted to the amputation. Afterwards he was told the bone of his forearm presented a 'very curious appearance' resembling an empty honeycomb. This, he felt, explained the weakness and pain he had felt for years and he ascribed the cause of his sufferings to the 'factory system'.

William Dodd was discharged late in November. He must have retained some favour with the hospital's governors – perhaps through the intercession of Odd Fellows – to have extended his ticket to six months. Mutilated, discharged in winter, far from home and with only eight shillings in his pocket, he faced penury and the workhouse. Instead within a year he had penned (or rather dictated) his book describing and denouncing the factory system. Dodd's experience reminds us that for many surgery was merely a stage in a long process of bodily abuse and degeneration, of chronic and continued pain, placing the relatively brief agony of amputation in perspective. Dodd resolved to accept amputation to save his life: others, as we have seen, either chose not to submit or could not decide and paid the price.

'Cannot be expressed in words': George Wilson's foot

Towards the end of 1842 Dr George Wilson, Professor of Chemistry at the University of Edinburgh, lay desperately ill. In constant pain, he only slept with the help of opiates. Exhausted by a pulmonary affliction he suffered from an extensive mortification of his left ankle caused, it was supposed, by disease aggravated by a pedestrian tour of the Highlands. George lay in pain, unable to walk. He composed a hymn expressing his distress:

> As I lay upon my bed,
> Weeping and complaining,
> Turning my weary head,
> Hope and help disdaining.

James Syme was called to attend him. Syme realised that the conventional treatment for mortification, amputation below the knee, would likely be fatal. He explained to Wilson that he felt justified in attempting the novel course of amputating at the ankle itself. Wilson, aware of his situation, readily consented asking only that the operation be deferred for a week. He did not hope that the mortification might subside but, anticipating that he could die, wished to prepare for death and order his affairs. He was unusual not only in submitting to a difficult and almost experimental operation but in recording an account of it almost unique among those who underwent painful surgery.[34] George Wilson, one of the most articulate witnesses of the experience of painful surgery, was uniquely qualified. He had commenced medical studies at Edinburgh in 1832 at the age of fourteen and had witnessed operations performed by Syme. Although he obtained his degree, he was disillusioned as much by the 'drudgery' of medical study as by the 'immoral companionships' it encouraged. He turned instead to lecturing on chemistry and later became Professor of Technology and Director of the Scottish Industrial Museum. George Wilson was well known and admired in Edinburgh's cultural life. 'Amiable, talented, and popular', he was remembered as 'a very attractive man, gentle and persuasive, learned and imaginative'.[35]

The intervening week passed both so slowly and too quickly. Wilson prepared for the ordeal regarding it as 'a dreadful necessity from which there was no escape'. He slept badly, troubled by the pain of his mortifying foot, awaking each morning to consider whether he ought to consent, but resolving each day to proceed. Aware of his family's disquiet he strove to conceal his foreboding from them. At last the morning of the operation dawned. Wilson, attempting to reassure his loved ones that his courage remained firm, took particular care shaving, taking comfort in signs that his ploy had succeeded. He took two cups of tea and a little toast and awaited Syme's arrival. He later compared waiting for the surgeon to 'a condemned criminal preparing for execution'. He counted the days before the appointed day; the hours to the appointed hour. He listened for the sound of the surgeon's carriage, the sound of the doorbell, his foot on the stair, as the surgeon and his assistants arrived. Then, 'revolting at the necessity', Wilson gave himself up to be bound and held and Syme, after speaking 'a few grave words', commenced the operation.

Although the new procedure would leave him with a more useful stump it obliged him to suffer a 'more tedious' operation. It did not involve, he stressed, 'a few swift strokes of the knife': the myth of rapidity was of contemporary origin. Instead it entailed 'cruel cutting through inflamed and morbidly sensitive parts'. It may not have been more painful than most severe operations, he conceded, but he asked his readers to accept that it was not less painful either.

Wilson had no words to describe the agony to which the operation subjected him: 'suffering so great' he believed 'cannot be expressed in words'. We must recognise that at the extremities of human experience we can only observe a decent silence. However, he could recollect the 'black whirlwind of emotion' he felt, 'the horror of great darkness, and the sense of desertion by God or man, bordering close upon despair' that consumed him. Throughout the operation, Wilson remembered, his sense remained 'preternaturally acute' as he had been told was general in surgery – in itself one of the most valuable insights into this experience. Presumably sitting, he was able to see Syme at work, watching with 'fascinated intensity'. He still recalled vividly 'the spreading out of the instruments; the twisting of the tourniquet [and] the first incision'. He remembered 'the fingering of the sawed bone; the sponge pressed on the flap; the tying of the blood-vessels; the stitching of the skin; and the bloody dismembered limb lying on the floor'. These, he concluded, 'are not pleasant remembrances ... easily brought back, and ... never welcome'. Throughout the operation George's family waited in an adjoining room, listening helplessly to 'irrepressible cries of anguish'. Nearly twenty years later his sister Jessie described how 'the scene is as vividly before the eyes of the survivors, and the cries ring as loudly through their hearts'.[36] As his family bribed bagpipers and street-organists to stay away from the house, George's stump healed. He still faced 'many weary, wretched, sleepless hours' but after six weeks a healthy scar had formed, leaving only a tiny aperture which continued to weep until the following June. After that Wilson experienced no pain or uneasy sensations and rarely the phenomenon of feeling the phantom limb. Writing to Syme in 1846 he described, fittingly for a future Professor of Technology, how he sometimes wore a cleverly contrived light, wooden foot fitted into a boot but often padded about his house in a stump sock. George Wilson died in 1859 and was widely mourned.

'I write to bid you farewell': Tina Malcolm's breast

Lady Clementina Malcolm was the daughter of the great Scottish Tory family, the Elphinstones, who produced a succession of admirals, generals and Governors General to serve Georgian and Victorian Britain. Born in 1775, she had married at the unusually advanced age of 34 a rising naval officer, Sir Pulteney Malcolm. She was known as 'Tina' to her family, whose papers reveal her to have been a lively woman with a wide circle of friends. Her future sister-in-law, Maria, wrote to her brother commending his choice of bride observing that 'her mind' was 'of a superior cast'.[37] After Napoleon's exile to St Helena Pulteney commanded the island's naval squadron and Clementina beat the Emperor at chess. He was also amused by her 'quickness'.[38] Three years after her marriage Clementina gave birth to a son, George. A week later, writing to Pulteney, who was serving at sea she described her pleasure in her 'Boy' but confessed that she felt 'cheated' because she was unable to suckle him, a wet nurse having been obtained. Like many a new mother she felt 'doubt that if I should have had enough [milk] for him'. Did she, sixteen years later, wonder whether not breast-feeding her sons might have contributed to the breast cancer she developed early in 1830?

Between early May and mid-July of that year Tina Malcolm kept a journal of her condition.[39] She charted her symptoms daily in detail, the remedies prescribed and the inexorable progress of a disease that her physicians could not arrest. 'Burning, stinging pain,' she described, 'like pins pressing in ... cutting pain under the arm'. She records a succession of pills, bark and baths, the efficacy of which she doubted. 'I dislike Mr W.'s medicines' she wrote of her physician's prescriptions. 'I cannot perceive any of them act as he says'. The aperients did not ease her bowels; the tonic and pills only disordered her digestion. And all the while the tumour in her breast became more painful and uncomfortable: the 'discharge is considerable and very offensive', she noted. Although able to go out in her carriage she could not walk because the motion shook her breast and caused her pain. The pain of her cancer permeates her journal:

Wednesday[;] ... Mr W. took off the plaster and left me a sort of bark to make a Poultice[.] He said I sh[ould] find [it] very soothing. I had a better night but not free from pain ... Thursday[;] the tumour very painful and looked more red ...

Clementina's journal ends pessimistically: 'very doubtful' and her stoicism eventually led her to decline Mr W.'s medicines. Her physician must privately have shared her opinion. A text published soon before she fell ill admitted candidly 'we have no medicines that can cure this disease'.[40] Mr W., however, persisted. In an undated and unsigned note to her he admonished her: 'I cannot understand,' he chastised, 'why you should not try the efficacy of a small opium pill [during] severe attacks of pain'.[41]

Lady Clementina's diary is not that of a hypochondriac relishing informing friends and family of the minor fluctuations of symptoms. The salient point is that she endured her disease alone deliberately striving to keep at bay those to whom she was closest. Her boys were sent to school, she appears to have avoided her family, her husband was far away in blissful ignorance. In 1828 Pulteney had been appointed Commander-in-Chief in the Mediterranean, a command expected to last three years. Despite his entreaties ('I do wish you were here') Clementina remained in Britain in her house in Harley Street, London or at East Lodge, Enfield, outside the capital. Pulteney was a prolific correspondent writing long, chatty letters full of naval and diplomatic gossip, sending gifts of fruit and sculpture and advice about their boys' education and prospects. He was puzzled to receive brief or uninformative replies: 'I wish you could give me better accounts of yourself' he complained. Although enjoying his post, cruising between Gibraltar and the Dardanelles in command of a powerful fleet, Pulteney wanted to be home. 'I wish that my time was nearer a close,' he wrote, 'I do not want it extended an hour'.

Clementina, observing the progress of a condition against which her physicians remained powerless, sensed that her time was close. At last, probably in the late summer of 1830, she consented to undergo an operation to excise the cancer from her breast and later agreed to a second. 'My dearest George', she wrote to her son on black-edged paper, I write in case I do not survive the operation ...'. 'My dearest Willy, I am obliged to submit to an Operation, and lest it does not end so well as the first, I write to bid you farewell ...' Because they were performed privately no details of the operations survive.

Only then did she inform her husband of the gravity of her condition. 'My Dearest Pult' she began. 'I have been mistaken in supposing that this sad Disease eradicated and lest I do not survive it I write to you to bid you farewell ... to you I owe the Happiness of my Life ...'[42] Pulteney received the letter in late September. From his flagship at Naples he wrote to the First Lord of the Admiralty, Lord

Melville, 'grieved' to inform him that his wife 'is threatened with a Cancer on her breast'.[43] Even then, Clementina diminished the gravity of her condition ('she is not sure of the danger of her situation, nor is it probable that the Disease will increase for some months ...'). Tina extracted a promise from him not to give up his command. After alerting his superior to his wife's condition all Pulteney sought was permission to leave for home at the end of his tenure, in June 1831. Pulteney's letter to Melville reached the Admiralty on 1 December. By then his wife had already been dead for eleven days. Major newspapers in Scotland and England did not publish obituaries and only one brief notice appeared. Tina Malcolm offers an extraordinary example of individual courage in the face of an incurable disease and intense suffering.

Notes.

1. 'Case of a Dissecting Aneurism of the Aorta', *Glasgow Medical Journal*, (NS), Vol. I, No. 1, 1.
2. James Esdaile, *Mesmerism in India and its Practical Application in Surgery and Medicine* (London: Longman, Brown, Green & Longmans, 1846), 80.
3. Cock, 'Anecdota Listoniensia', *University College Hospital Magazine*, 1911, No. 2, 58.
4. John Bland-Sutton, *The Story of a Surgeon* (London: Methuen, 1930), 70.
5. *Lancet*, 1823–24, Vol. II, 424–28.
6. John Elliotson, *Numerous Cases of Surgical Operations Without Pain* (London: H. Ballière, 1843), 16.
7. James Miller, *Surgical Experience of Chloroform* (Edinburgh: Sutherland & Knox, 1848), 28 .
8. Charles Bell, *Illustrations of the Great Operations of Surgery* (London: Longman, 1821), 119–20.
9. *Lancet*, 1832-33, Vol. I, 538–59.
10. Undated paper, Astley Cooper papers, RCSEng.
11. *The Times*, 11 April 1831, 2f; Samuel Wilks & G.T. Bettany, *A Biographical History of Guy's Hospital* (London: Ward & Lock, London, 1892), 332–33; *Glasgow Medical Journal*, Vol.IV, No. XIV, May 1831, 209–12. The sources disagree on details.
12. *Glasgow Medical Journal*, Vol.IV, No. XIV, May 1831, 211.
13. *The Times*, 18 April 1831, 6b; 19 April 1831, 3c.
14. *Lancet*, 1833–34, Vol. II, 174–75.
15. John Abernethy, *Lectures on Anatomy, Surgery and Pathology* (London: James Bullock, 1828), 557.

16. John Shepherd, *Spencer Wells: the Life and Work of a Victorian Surgeon* (Edinburgh: E. & S. Livingstone, 1965), 43.

17. William Mackenzie, *The Cure of Strabismus by Surgical Operation* (London: Longmans, Orme, Brown, Green & Longmans, 1841), 21.

18. *Lancet*, 1832–33, Vol. I, 112–13.

19. *Lancet*, 1831–32, Vol. II, 604.

20. *The Times*, 18 May 1839, 7c.

21. Benjamin Brodie, *Clinical Lectures on Surgery* (Philadelphia: Lea & Blanchard, 1846), 48.

22. *The Times*, 19 April 1827, 2c.

23. J.F. Clarke, *Autobiographical Recollections* (London: J. & A. Churchill, 1874), 380–81.

24. Mary Thomas's diary is in the Mortlock Library of South Australiana at PRG 1160/6. The medical aspects of it were published in Margaret McNair, *Nursing in South Australia: First Hundred Years 1837–1937* (Adelaide: Nurses' Memorial Foundation of South Australia, 1938), 18–19.

25. B.R. Ward, (ed.), *A Week at Waterloo: Lady De Lancey's Narrative* (London: John Murray, 1906).

26. William Hay, (ed. S.C.I. Wood), *Reminiscences 1808–1815 Under Wellington* (London: Simpkin, Marshall & Co., 1901), 203–04.

27. [Charlotte Eaton], *Narrative of a Residence in Belgium During the Campaign of 1815* (London: John Murray, 1817) Four years later Magdalene married Captain Henry Harvey of the Madras Army, bore him two children and died in 1823.

28. Marcet, 'History of a Case of Nephritis Calculosa ... and an Account of the Operation of Lithotomy Given by the Patient Himself', *Transactions of the Medico-Chirurgical Society*, 1819, 147–60 .

29. Tennyson, 'In the Children's Hospital'.

30. James Syme, *Observations in Clinical Surgery* (Edinburgh: Edmonston & Douglas, 1861), 68–70.

31. The letters between Dickens and Thomas Beard, Macvey Napier and Frederick Salmon in October and November 1841 can be found in M. House & G. Storey (eds), *The Letters of Charles Dickens*, 7 vols, (Oxford: Clarendon Press, 1965-99), Vol. 2, 1840–1841, 401–19.

32. Macvey Napier to Charles Dickens, 26 October 1841, HM 18561, Huntington Library.

33. William Dodd, *The Factory System Illustrated*, [1842] (London: Frank Cass, 1968).

34. Prof. Wilson's accounts of the operation can be found in Syme, *op. cit.* (note 30) 41–44, and in J. Duns, *Memoir of Sir James Y. Simpson*,

Bart.. (Edinburgh: Edmonston & Douglas, 1873), 262–70.

35. Robert Chambers, *A Biographical Dictionary of Eminent Scotsmen*, 2 vols (Edinburgh: Blackie & Son, 1875), 537–42; James Crichton-Browne, *Victorian Jottings from an Old Commonplace Book* (London: Etchells & Macdonald, 1926), 46.

36. Jessie Aitken Wilson, *Memoir of George Wilson*, (Edinburgh: Edmonston & Douglas, 1860), 296–97.

37. Maria Malcolm to Pulteney Malcolm, 25 December 1808, Malcolm Papers, Acc. 8391, NLS.

38. Arthur Wilson & Muriel Kent (eds), *A Diary of St Helena: the Journal of Lady Malcolm* (London: Allen & Unwin, 1929), 24; 131.

39. Malcolm Papers, 'Medical journal of Lady Clementina Malcolm', Acc. 9756, NLS.

40. Thomas Castle (ed.), *A Manual of Modern Surgery ...* (London: E. Cox & Son, 1828), 110.

41. Malcolm Papers, [Miscellaneous papers, 1701–1845], Acc. 9756, NLS.

42. Malcolm papers, Acc. 8391, NLS.

43. Malcolm to Viscount Melville, 25 September 1830, Melville Papers, GD51/2/1087, SRO.

11

'The rights of pain':
The Acceptance of Anaesthesia

Despite 'progress' in 'modern surgery' the essential experience of surgical illness and treatment until the middle decade of the nineteenth century remained one of unrelieved and often unbearable pain. Joseph Wilde, who had spent so many dark months in the Devon and Exeter Hospital, recorded his memory of the sleepless nights he had spent in pain. 'O Pain!,' he began, 'thou worst of evils here below'. Wilde recalled how

> In total darkness, dreadful shapes present
> To his bewilder'd fancy: horrid gulphs,
> On gulphs more horrid, op'ning without end;
> And, in the lower deep, a lower deep,
> On his appall'd imagination, yawns.[1]

Wilde recalled the relief when he received laudanum:

> O blest narcotic! sovereign remedy!
> Thou richest gift that heaven e'er sent down.

'A change in the earth': anaesthesia envisaged

As we have seen, a few unavailing attempts were made before 1800 to alleviate surgical pain. Ironically, in their eagerness to explore the possibilities opened by John Hunter's anatomical enquiries, surgeons seem to have forgotten his determination that surgery should inflict as little pain as possible. An apprentice once asked him how he should treat an old lady dying of a bleeding, malignant breast tumour. 'Give her opium' Hunter replied. The apprentice explained that he administered a pill three and four times a night: what should he do then? 'Give her more opium', Hunter replied emphatically, 'Opium, Opium, Opium'. 'Sir,' Hunter went on, 'the Almighty would have fallen far short of his acknowledged mercy, if He had not furnished us with Opium when He gave us pain'.[2] Charles Bell argued in his *Anatomy and Philosophy of Expression* in 1806 that pain was 'necessary to our existence'. 'To imagine the absence of pain,' he wrote, 'is not only to imagine a new state of being, but a change in

283

Figure 11.1

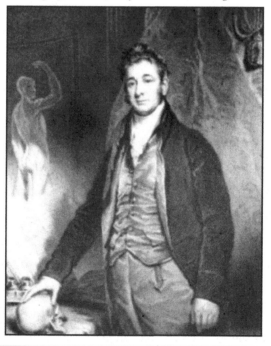

Sir Anthony Carlisle (1768-1840), who in a lecture to the Royal College of Surgeons of England in 1818 proposed that 'the time is arrived for ... the introduction of moral influence to mitigate or arrest the sufferings of surgical patients'. Carlisle's pose captures the dignity with which he faced dismissive colleagues.

the earth and all upon it'.[3]

In 1818 Anthony Carlisle, in a lecture delivered soon after his humiliation over the oysters, declared that 'the time is arrived' for an 'addition to our humane resources' and to consider ways of 'abating the sum of pain' in 'violent operations'. Carlisle ineffectually canvassed iced water as an anaesthetic but looked to the mood of the operating room as the best way to ameliorate suffering. He advised his colleagues to create a mood of 'easy cheerfulness' in the theatre urging them to use 'animated conversation' and 'humourous stories' to divert patients. Carlisle himself claimed to have found 'interrogations about remote concerns' and 'argumentative disputes most efficacious' to the point that patients had asked 'is this all!' as he put his instruments away.[4] Despite Carlisle's reputation for genial ineffectiveness his colleagues listened without demur.

The 'change in the earth' that Bell, Carlisle and others sought became theoretically possible from about 1800 but was to be practically impossible until the mid-1840s. Despite awful reminders every time they cut a patient few surgeons imagined that pain might be relieved. Indeed so fundamental was pain to surgery that attempts to introduce drugs or techniques to lessen it failed. Shakespearean allusions to mandrake and henbane hinted at possibilities from herbal antiquity but almost no-one seriously pursued alternatives to suffering pain. In the early nineteenth century, however, several possibilities arose. The term 'anaesthesia' seems to have been first used in 1833 when the *Lancet* published a translation of a French article discussing the condition of 'diminution, or total loss, of bodily sensation' with a view, ironically, to its cure.[5] It is possible that, in the manner of scientific surgeons, describing and naming the phenomenon in nature led to them becoming open to the possibility of inducing it by design.

The most obvious routes to oblivion – opium and alcohol – need to be dealt with firmly. As we have seen, opium was a valuable aid to relieving post-operative pain but could not alleviate acute pain. 'The strongest dose we dare venture', James Moore explained, 'has little or no effect in mitigating the sufferings of the patient during the operation'.[6] A large dose produced nausea rather than insensibility. Many people, rich and poor, used it to relieve chronic pain and as a route to cheap oblivion.[7] Samuel Taylor Coleridge, with his addiction to Kendal Black Drop, was only one notable opium user. Others included Gladstone's sister Helen and Tennyson's brothers.[8] One of its disadvantages was, of course, that it was addictive: as an apprentice William Hey indulged in what his biographer called the 'delightful illusions' of opium.[9] Sometimes 'a tepid solution of opium' would be applied 'topically', or directly, to relieve extreme pain.[10] Astley Cooper did this to the stump of a child whose leg he had removed observing 'more immediate relief than I ever remember to have witnessed'.[11] Why he and his colleagues did not do so more often is unknown. The explanation may be that 'as a general rule' surgeons were wary of relieving pain because of its value in diagnosis.[12]

It is still a common misconception that patients were sedated by drinking rum or brandy before operating: the question was asked in every seminar or talk presented in the course of researching and writing this book. There is virtually no evidence that surgeons used alcohol in any form to suppress surgical pain. When administered, in

Figure 11.2

Charles Bell (1774-1842),
notable as a physiologist as well as an operator who was tortured by the
memory of the operations he performed. As early as 1806 Bell
imagined in his <u>Anatomy and Philosophy of Expression</u> 'the absence of
pain' as 'a change in the earth and all upon it'.

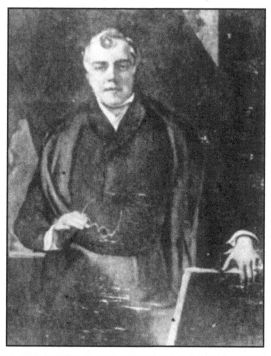

the navy or in almost every operating room, it was either to fortify patients to enable them to bear the ordeal or to revive them in the event of fainting. In any case the clinical effects of alcohol made it a doubtful ally in surgery. In small quantities a stimulant, in larger doses it acts as a depressant, its capacity to dilate blood vessels making haemorrhage more likely.

The substances which were to be used as chemical anaesthetics had all been discovered, described and even used well before the 1840s. Joseph Priestley had described nitrous oxide in 1772 and in 1800 Astley Cooper is supposed to have attended a demonstration of its effects at Guy's.[13] Henry Hickman's failure to interest the Royal Society in carbon dioxide is well known. John Morgan of Guy's had used it in 1834 to relieve a young man suffering from tetanus although no one seems to have made the connection between the insensibility it induced and the relief of pain in surgery. (Morgan, a 'plodding' and dull man was paradoxically famous as a rapid operator.)[14]

Ether had been known for half a century before its anaesthetic properties were employed. It was used to treat burns, credited as early as 1801 with restoring the sight of a labouring man whose eyes were splashed with oil of vitriol.[15] Michael Faraday had described in the *Quarterly Journal of Sciences* in 1818 how ether acted like nitrous oxide.[16] In 1847 a correspondent to the *Edinburgh Medical and Surgical Journal* wrote – after news of ether's use arrived from Boston – that it had 'long been known' as a powerful antispasmodic and narcotic and its effects 'abundantly observed by many'. The author cited a case from 1817 in which a woman had swallowed a hare's jaw which had been removed from her throat with the assistance of ether. (The article's tone might have been more humble, one might have thought, since these 'many' observers had failed to make the connection until 1846.)[17] One who seems to have done so was Robert Collyer, a graduate of University College, who knew the properties of ether. He went to the United States and returned in 1843 to practise using a combination of ether and mesmerism in Liverpool. It seems that neither Collyer nor his professional acquaintances made anything of his knowledge.[18]

Chloroform had first been discovered and described in the early 1830s (clearly not very comprehensively because its soporific effects remained unrealised) and had been used only as an 'antispasmodic' in the treatment of asthma. Morphia had likewise been available since the beginning of the century. Derived from opium in 1803, it had been ignored for over forty years by the time of chemical anaesthesia's acceptance. In 1826 it had been recommended for the treatment of obstinate vomiting, severe colic and neuralgia or rheumatic headache.[19] Six years later, however, Dr Robertson lamented that few British colleagues had followed the advice.[20] Morphine was, however, used by invalids seeking a tranquilliser. Elizabeth Barrett Browning called it 'my elixir'. In combination with ether she wrote it 'quiets my mind, calms my pulse – warms my feet – spirits away any stray headache [and] gives me an appetite'.[21]

It has been argued that these unavailing pioneering efforts eventually alerted surgeons to the possibility of painless surgery. In popular accounts this occurred late in 1846 with the demonstration of ether in the Massachusetts General Hospital in Boston and its subsequent rapid adoption in Britain. The conventional interpretation is that surgeons embraced ether enthusiastically as soon as it became available. There are two difficulties with this view. First, it is odd that most surgeons had refused to accept the feasibility of anaesthesia through mesmerism. Second, many did not accept chemical anaesthesia for several years after its introduction. Both objections derived from their belief that pain, far from being undesirable, was natural and beneficial. Medical practitioners – and their patients – accepted the existence or necessity of pain. Harriet Martineau, whose devotion to invalidism led her to write a meditation on *Life in the Sick Room*, expressed the ' supposition – indispensable and, I believe, universal, – that pain is ... ordained for, or instrumental to good'. No stranger to chronic pain she also believed that even acute pain (when 'occasional and not extremely protracted') was 'vivifying and cheering'.[22] Its very absence, a surgeon asserted, was itself 'a symptom of disease'.[23] Unable to relieve pain except by opium, and then imperfectly, hospitals encouraged a stoicism of which the bossy demeanour of the old-fashioned nurse is perhaps the last faint echo. Patients could read devotional works offering, for example, *Motives and Encouragements to Bear Afflictions Patiently* which suggested 'the more Pains ... 'the greater Glory'.[24] Doubts over these views were first expressed in the 1840s when mesmerism demonstrated that pain could be suppressed in surgery.

'No pain at all': mesmerism demonstrated and derided

Mesmerism, the somnambulist state first induced by Anton Mesmer, offered the most important and first viable alternative to painful surgery. Despite its clear capacity to suppress pain mesmerism claimed only a few adherents and many opponents. To those of a scientific persuasion mesmerists' explanations for the phenomenon remained unconvincing. Mesmer claimed 'Animal Magnetism' to be 'a fluid universally diffused ... the medium of a mutual influence between the heavenly bodies'.[25] A profession which had spent half a century in rigorous anatomising could find no sign of the vessels by which such fluids were conveyed and remained sceptical.

Mesmer's 'magnetical state', adapted and promoted by followers such as the Marquis de Puysegur, became the basis of a parlour and fairground diversion which swept Europe, Britain and later North America in the last decade of the eighteenth century. Individual enthusiasts revived interest in its medical uses and in 1829 the French surgeon Jules Cloquet removed a cancerous breast using 'hypnotic analgesia'. Stimulated by an investigation by the Academie de

Medicine in 1831 mesmerism underwent a revival in the 1830s and '40s. By the time it was applied to surgery in the 1840s it had become a symbol among the scientific and medical community of gullibility and fakery. Mesmerism meant 'spirit-rapping & Table-turning' and those who advocated it were regarded as fools or charlatans.[26]

John Elliotson, Professor of the Theory and Practice of Medicine at the University College Hospital, had, in accordance with the responsibilities of his chair, taken an interest in phrenology and in mesmerism. Intrigued by the Okey (or O'Key) sisters, Elizabeth and Jane, he conducted many seances at which they demonstrated their powers of clairvoyance, some of which were in the wards of the hospital. Thomas Wakley encouraged Elliotson to demonstrate the Okeys' powers and exposed them as a sham. Benjamin Brodie exemplified opposition to mesmerism, reminding subscribers to the *Lancet* of how 'the girls who are magnetised deceive and cheat. They pretend to read with the back of their head, and prophecy all sorts of stuff'.[27] Elliotson's dabbling with mesmerism's mysticism aroused the ire of his more conventional colleagues, who complained to the College's Medical Committee. Although the College authorities refused to witness the Okeys' demonstrations they censured Elliotson who nevertheless continued his experiments. Representations to the College's mentor Lord Brougham and objections by Samuel Cooper led to Elliotson resigning in 1838 despite a vote in his favour by the College's students with whom he was a popular lecturer.* By 1842 Elliotson was widely regarded as unsound – 'a tom-fool' – and a liability in advocating the medical and surgical uses of mesmerism.[28] In a reply to the College's Medical Committee he retorted that 'these phenomena I know to be real ... independent of imagination ... of the most interesting, most extraordinary & important character'.[29]

While doubtful of its ostensible physiological explanation contemporaries read accounts of mesmeric trances during which surgery was performed which could not be so readily dismissed. 'There are more truths involved in it than many may feel at first disposed to admit' acknowledged an otherwise sceptical commentator.[30] Another, deprecating the jargon it spawned, accepted the fact of mesmerism while admitting his inability to explain it. He described it as 'a pyramid of error inverted on an apex of truth'.[31] By the end of 1842 many accounts had been published of operations

---

* Ironically, Elliotson had praised University College in 1832 for its 'toleration and forbearance towards those of other creeds and doctrines' in a commencement address to medical students.

conducted painlessly; too many to be dismissed easily as imposture. In Chatham in May 1842, for instance, a nurse employed by an army officer had had decayed teeth and 'spicula' of bone projecting through the gums removed. To the 'astonishment' of medical observers and the patients' incredulity, she felt no pain during the operation.[32] Other reports arrived from Leicester, Portsmouth and Sheffield along with accounts from Paris and Jamaica. The mesmerist organ, the *Zoist*, published upwards of 300 reports.[33] The critics' scepticism might be justified except that compelling evidence exists of many cases in which mesmerism was used successfully to eliminate pain in major surgery.

In 1842 William Topham, a London barrister, and W. Squire Ward, a Nottinghamshire surgeon, performed and described an operation, the most documented and debated of many using mesmerism. It both demonstrated mesmerism's viability and, by precipitating opposition among conventional surgeons, exposed and entrenched the positions of the respective camps. James Wombell, a farm labourer aged 42, was obliged to lose his leg. Topham's account of the operation provoked a 'violent discussion' at a meeting of the Royal Medical and Chirurgical Society in November 1842.[34] Ward, who had trained at Bart's, admitted that he was 'by no means sanguine of success'. Still, as Topham maintained Wombell's trance, he took up the catlin. After looking earnestly at Wombell Ward 'slowly plunged' his knife into his thigh drawing it around to cut into the muscle down to the bone. 'The stillness', recorded an observer, 'was something awful'. 'I saw', Topham concluded, 'and was convinced' of mesmerism's effects. Wombell slept throughout the operation moaning quietly at times. 'There can be few,' Ward proclaimed, 'even of the most bigoted objectors', who will ... deny its powers'.[35]

The assembled London medical men had great difficulty in accepting the provincial surgeon's account however.[36] They did not believe that it was possible for pain to be eliminated but they had seen patients bear surgery without flinching. Mr Coulson, 'anxious to distinguish himself as the leader of the opposition to mesmerism' rose first, to express his conviction that 'the man had been trained to it!' 'What d___d stuff' he exclaimed. Rutherford Alcock said that he had often seen patients bear severe operations without manifesting the slightest pain. This reaction diverted the meeting for a time. Elliotson, who reminded the gathering that he had trained under Astley Cooper and had seen many severe operations, pointed out that while patients may not have spoken or screamed they had always shown signs of suppressing pain. He recalled how a sailor had once astonished Cooper by not uttering a sound as his leg was amputated: even so the man had folded his arms and compressed his lips. Elliotson pointed out that Wombell had been in 'a sound and beautiful sleep' throughout the operation. He had declared that he had felt 'no pain at all'. Robert Liston scoffed at mesmerism as 'humbug' echoing Thomas Wakley in the *Lancet* the month before who had decried mesmerism as 'too gross a humbug' and had urged that 'quacks and imposters be hooted out of professional society'. Benjamin Brodie, remarking on a case of imposture in 1706, observed unconvincingly and irrelevantly that 'some people really do not seem susceptible of pain'. Bransby Cooper, although unwilling to contradict his uncle and patron, nevertheless asked that the opponents of mesmerism not have it their own way. Dr Mayo agreed, saying that the subject was 'one of the greatest importance' and urged his colleagues not to ridicule it but the mood of the gathering was against giving Topham and Ward a hearing. The meeting ended in dispute and confusion with the 'disbelieving and ignorant' unconvinced of the fact much less the merit of mesmerism.

A week later the Society met again. Members censured Topham for having published the paper (which he had disgustedly withdrawn from the Society). A visitor who spoke in his favour was rudely silenced by Caesar Hawkins. The visitor retorted that a few days before he had seen Hawkins amputate the leg of 'a poor young woman' amid 'agonizing shrieks'. She had been consumptive and had died on the day of the meeting. Elliotson sat silently through this charade. Most of those present remained unconvinced, the wavering Bransby declaring with the majority. 'No men ever had a more complete beating' Elliotson wrote despondently. The meetings reflected the balance of medical opinion. Thomas Wakley, a force for reform in medical politics, advised that nineteen out of twenty letters to the *Lancet* on mesmerism opposed it. Elliotson simply pointed out that 'nineteen persons, of course, purchase more Lancets than one'.

The practicality of mesmerism, however, was demonstrated on a larger scale by James Esdaile, a Scot and a surgeon at a 'native hospital' in Hooghly near Calcutta. Esdaile noticed two medical curiosities of India; the prevalence of massive disfiguring tumours, and Hindu practices of hypnosis. He used the latter to treat the former, in combination with western surgery. In the early-1840s he used mesmeric techniques to conduct over 950 operations including amputations of the arm, breast and penis and 200 cases of scrotal tumours.[37] Esdaile described numerous cases and obtained endorsements from witnesses including army officers and surgeons, missionaries and distinguished visitors. It is clear that he achieved remarkable success, performing bloody and demanding operations gently and slowly that would otherwise have involved struggles and suffering. 'Wah! brother', Bengalis exclaimed, 'what a soft man the doctor Sahib is!' Esdaile's successes became known to Europeans in Bengal and to colleagues in Britain. 'Dr Esdaile', Major Corfield of the 20th Bengal Native Infantry wrote to the Calcutta newspaper the *Englishman*, 'is destined to be a blessing to mankind and an honour to his profession'.[38]

Unfortunately, accounts of Esdaile's operations, published in the *Calcutta Medical Journal* in April 1845, reached England in the aftermath of the Wombell case and he was subjected to conventional doctors' disdain. His later accounts coincided with news of ether and were disregarded in favour of 'an agent which requires neither selected cases, darkened rooms, ... nor any mystery in its employment'.[39] Retiring to Scotland in 1851 he found fewer of his compatriots susceptible to hypnosis or persuaded by his publications. Esdaile was influenced by the mysticism prevailing in mesmeric circles – his title *Natural and Mesmeric Clairvoyance* gave no encouragement to sceptics – and he offered scientific sceptics no explanation for his success. But he did document the opposition of mesmerism's critics, who described it as 'an odious fraud' or a collection of 'bold assertions, half-observed facts and multifarious inventions'. 'Wherever there are clever girls, philosophic Bohemians, weak women [and] weaker men' mesmerism would succeed, sneered the *Lancet*.[40] The critics variously comprised those sceptical of mesmerism's claims and those like Dr Copeland who decried the need to eliminate pain at all. It was, he asserted, 'a wise provision of nature ... patients ought to suffer pain ... they are all the better for it'.[41] Despite the encouragement of James Simpson, the *Edinburgh Journal of Medical Science* declined Esdaile's 1852 paper. Although a Mesmeric Hospital opened in Calcutta supported briefly by official funding, he never saw the realisation of his dream, the *Introduction of Mesmerism into the Public Hospitals of London*.

And yet the endeavours of the mesmerists confronted those unconvinced by the dream of painless surgery with the possibility of Charles Bell's 'change in the earth and all upon it'. William Lang, an advocate of mesmerism, sadly described his colleagues as 'a stubborn and stiff-necked generation'.[42] Their dilemma is exemplified by Robert Liston. In the early-1840s Liston was at the height of his power and fame. After declaring Ward and Topham's account of the amputation of James Wombell's leg to be 'humbug', he had risen again at the meeting of the Royal Medical and Chirurgical Society. This time he made a poor joke. Leaning forward pugnaciously, he asked sarcastically whether Wombell had been able to 'read with the back of his neck or with his belly' since the operation. The support or even the toleration of one of the most heroic surgeons could have made a difference. As it was no one smiled at his clumsy sally and many shifted in embarrassment. In alluding to mesmerism's clairvoyant fringe, Liston expressed the dilemma of the conventional surgeon. As scientific men they could neither understand nor accept a practice fundamentally tainted with mysticism, one whose advocates could not explain in rational terms. They saw on operating days the horrible effects of surgery. Mesmerism offered them an opportunity to embrace humanity but at the cost of surrendering their faith in science.

So deeply did the scientific spirit imbue the profession fifty years after Hunter's death most surgeons simply could not make the leap. Despite his reputation for boldness it is arguable that Liston increasingly felt the strain of painful surgery in the early 1840s. His daughter had noticed how he was 'very silent and absorbed' driving to the hospital on operating days.[43] Shortly before, he had confessed to his close friend James Miller how he was 'overwhelmed with operations' and 'sick of the work'.[44] It is conceivable, then, that in the early 1840s his willingness to operate diminished despite his technical prowess and reputation. Perhaps, like 'surgeons of experience' before him – John Abernethy and Charles Bell – he wished to 'refuse to do those feats which they were eager to perform in their younger days'.[45] A prisoner of his own reputation, perhaps he was unable to stop operating and as a prisoner of the prevailing scientific paradigm he was unable to accept the solution offered by mesmerism.

Mesmerism was an imperfect solution to surgical pain. It did not work with every patient and its administration demanded personal qualities the opposite of those required by operating surgeons. Many of the qualities which made a good surgeon – assertion, courage, willpower – militated against those demanded of a hypnotist. Nor were crowded and noisy operating theatres amenable to inducing trances. Even those willing to try it did not always succeed: James Simpson had attempted it before realising that it required both a gift on the part of the operator or a receptivity on the part of the patient.[46] Still, the fact is that it was possible for British surgeons to operate without inflicting pain at least five years before 1846 and that mesmerism eliminated not only the pain of surgery but also post-operative pain. The opposition to mesmerism expressed by Liston and others became the orthodox view and it still dominates anaesthetic history in which the 'invention' or 'discovery' of anaesthesia dates from 1846 and not from the first successful use of mesmerism. How much agony persisted because of the 'stubborn, stiff-necked generation'?

'This Yankee dodge': ether in Britain

The knowledge that painless surgery was at least possible, however, arguably fostered a tension in the minds of some surgeons. Unable to embrace mesmerism they were all the more amenable to the next alternative on offer which came to Britain when the steamship *Acadia* docked at Liverpool in December 1846 bearing news of the use of ether in Boston.

Soon after *The Times* published a letter from Dr John Ware of Boston describing 'A New Means of Rendering Surgical Operations Painless': 'new' meaning newer than mesmerism. *The Times*, which had devoted much space to detailed accounts of painful and mesmeric operations, presumably recognised the wide interest the letter would attract. Ware described the amputation of a thigh, the extirpation of a breast and the drawing of teeth all without patients suffering pain. Nevertheless, he outlined the reservations expressed by Bostonian operators. 'One of our best operative surgeons' – presumably Warren – had told him that ether was most suitable to large and painful operations which were performed rapidly. Puzzlingly, for longer 'more delicate operations' he preferred to 'have the patient in his usual state'. Even so, Ware hesitated to say what limits might be imposed upon the new anaesthetic.[47]

The first surgical operation to be conducted in Britain under chemical anaesthesia was not, contrary to persistent belief, Robert Liston's amputation of Frederick Churchill's leg at University College Hospital on 22 December 1846. Rather it was William Scott's operation at the Dumfries and Galloway Royal Infirmary two days before.[48] Liston's operation was the more significant however because it was performed by a prominent surgeon in a major metropolitan hospital. The real significance of Liston's immediate adoption of ether was, as he said at its conclusion, was that 'this Yankee dodge beats mesmerism hollow'. Liston embraced ether not only because it conquered pain but also because it offered a viable alternative to mesmerism. 'Hurrah! Rejoice!', he crowed, 'Mesmerism and its professors have met with a heavy blow'.[49]

News of ether spread rapidly albeit from London not Dumfries. On 23 December, the day after Liston's first London operation, James Miller stood before a class in his lecture room at Edinburgh and read a hasty letter from Liston 'announcing in enthusiastic terms, that a new light had burst on Surgery'.[50] Its ability to banish pain, as Miller recalled, 'surprised, excited, [and] charmed' the medical profession. In London early in 1847 not only surgeons but also curious celebrities visited operating rooms to view the miracle. Prince Jerome Bonaparte visited the Westminster Ophthalmic Hospital to watch Charles Guthrie (George Guthrie's son) remove a bladder stone and then St George's to watch an amputation. A report of an operation at the Westminster Hospital in January for the excision of a tumour on a young woman, read like a stray from the social columns. The spectators included Lords Walsingham and Merton, Viscount Falkland, Sir Henry Mildmay, Sir George Wombwell, Admiral Sir Charles Napier and, among 'many distinguished foreigners', the ubiquitous Prince Jerome.[51] The excitement spread generally. In Edinburgh members of respectable society entered an operating room for the first time, feeling apprehensive perhaps but also hopeful. 'A considerable number' crowded into the operating room of the Royal Infirmary to witness the phenomenon. (Their presence, Miller reassured, 'did not interfere with the business of the place'). Although doubtless queasy at the 'bloody and severe' operations they witnessed they were able to remain composed 'feeling little,' Miller remarked, 'because the patient felt not at all'.[52]

Surgeons beyond London quickly adopted the innovation. Within a month a Liverpool vet had used ether to remove a tumour from a Newfoundland dog.[53] In Bristol, using ether produced by a 'well known analytical chymist', a surgeon at the General Hospital amputated a man's leg above the knee. The patient, who had suffered from a 'white swelling' of the knee for three months may have been prepared to suffer indefinitely had it not been for ether.[54] From Poole in Dorset came a report of a 17-year-old Scottish sailor, landed with frostbite in both feet and ankles. A local dentist administered ether and the sailor's legs were amputated in two operations ten days apart. On one occasion the young man inhaled for three minutes before rising from the table and muttering 'wild incoherent expressions' before losing sensibility after a further five minutes. Asked how he felt on awakening, he replied 'How con a drunken mon tell?'[55] News of ether spread around the world carried by copies of newspapers aboard merchant vessels. By mid-1847 it had reached Australasia. The first public demonstrations of ether in Australia were made simultaneously in Sydney and Launceston, Van Diemen's Land (Tasmania), on 7 June. The first operation under ether in New Zealand occurred in Wellington on 26 September.[56]

Reports of operations detailed the varied effects of the drug. Some patients awoke claiming to have enjoyed 'a beautiful dream' or with 'apprehension, wonder and delight'. A journalist from *The Times* expressed his wonder that a surgical operation should have become 'an enjoyment too quickly passed away'.[57] Surgeons and students were amused by, as a Bart's student of the 1850s recalled, a clergymen who uttered oaths and a 'foul-mouthed' butcher who sang Watts's hymns.[58] Others saw less positive sights. Ether was difficult to administer and remained unpredictable in its effects and not all operations in which it was used went as hoped. Liston himself experienced problems. Early in the New Year he had a woman inhale for twenty minutes without producing any effect and proceeded to remove a tumour in her breast 'with the usual accompaniment of severe pain'. A few days later he gave up attempting to induce anaesthesia after ten minutes and amputated a man's arm with 'the usual amount of pain'.[59] At St George's Hospital patients not only could not be anaesthetised but resisted the inhaler. Caesar Hawkins abandoned an operation to remove the toe of a young man because 'what with fright and what with coughing' he could not be made unconscious. Another young man resisted the mouthpiece so forcefully that bystanders wondered whether 'ether was as bad as the operation or worse'.[60] James Simpson later pointed out that the best effects were obtained by having the patient keep still 'and preventing all noise and talking'.[61] How this was to achieved in the crowded, noisy operating theatres with students and spectators eagerly watching for and discussing the new drug helps to explain ether's initially uneven effects. Well into 1847 operators were reporting failures to induce painless surgery: it seemed, like mesmerism, to be unreliable.

Other observers saw conscious patients undergo operations sometimes at their own request. At King's College Hospital on 5 January William Fergusson offered a woman ether when about to repair lacerations of the perineum (presumably the result of a difficult labour). She refused because it would render her insensible and she preferred to know what the surgeon was doing. Fergusson, who had been operating without anaesthesia for two decades, complied.[62] Other operators at first used ether as an aid to ease the most painful parts of an operation rather than inducing unconsciousness throughout. In January 1847 Frederic Skey performed a Caesarean on a 27-year-old unmarried dressmaker who was just over four feet tall with a deformed pelvis. The unfortunate woman had become pregnant when, 'under a temporary excitement, she had connexion with a young man', her lodger. Discovering her condition at seven months she was referred to Skey at Bart's. Skey made an incision eight inches long in her abdomen and closed the wound with eleven sutures using ether only for the initial incision.[63] As they gained experience in its administration operators even found they could use ether, if imperfectly, for operations on the mouth. In November 1847 Henry Johnson of St George's attempted 'one of the most difficult and dangerous' operations excising a fungoid tumour from the face of a youth of 19. Although unable to maintain the supply of ether through an inhaler to achieve complete insensibility Johnson was able to add to the young man's 'ease and composure'. The Council of the London college took the unusual step of specially commending Johnson.[64] What the 'several non-professional men' who witnessed the operation felt was not recorded.[65]

'Agreeable, fragrant, fruit-like': chloroform

A year after the introduction of ether to Britain the Edinburgh obstetrician, James Simpson, discovered the anaesthetic effects of chloroform at the celebrated evening in his house in Queen Street early in November 1847. A few days later Liston's friend, James Miller, performed the first operation under chloroform in the Royal Infirmary on a young child. Miller gripped the little boy's arm, skilfully closing on the arteries with his left hand and making a rapid incision with the scalpel in his right. The boy lay still, gently breathing. Miller continued cutting an H-shaped incision, exposing a diseased elbow joint which he cut away before closing the wound. The operation took a few minutes, the surgeon looking up to ensure that his patient made no sound. Porters carried the still sleeping boy back to the ward.[66] The patient, a fearful 4 or 5-year-old Gaelic speaking boy who had not understood what the doctors were about apparently survived, returning to his Highland croft and obscurity.

Although American surgeons favoured ether, British operators soon showed a preference for chloroform. It was more rapid in its effect, less liable to cause nausea and could be used in operations around the mouth that ether, with its clumsy mouthpiece precluded. (Chloroform also attracted abuse almost immediately: George Keith, who had been present at Simpson's celebrated discovery of chloroform later admitted that within six months he had taken chloroform three hundred times. 'I had such a craving', he confessed, 'that I sometimes broke through all rules of propriety in attempts to get possession of it'.[67]) A significant reason for chloroform's adoption, Alison Winter argues persuasively in *Mesmerized,* was that ether's characteristics and effects were very similar to those of mesmerism. It did not work on all patients, seems to have required a 'rapport' for effective anaesthesia and induced a partial state of insensibility in which patients talked, moaned or sang. A chemical anaesthetic inducing a deeper insensibility enabled 'etherists' to distance anaesthesia from the 'mesmerists'. Chloroform, however, put patients into a profound sleep: sometimes so profound that they did not waken. Those doubtful of anaesthesia had had only three months to wait before reports began to appear of deaths of patients on the table under ether. 'A Surgeon' wrote to *The Times* appealing against undue suspicion. Pointing out that five hundred operations had been conducted under ether over the preceding several months, he urged that a single fatal case could not be 'construed into an argument' and suggested a committee of inquiry into a boon he described as 'the weightiest ... for a century'.[68] These deaths under anaesthesia focused and mobilised those suspicious of or opposed to it, a debate which intensified after the discovery of the addictive properties of chloroform.

The death of Hannah Greener in Newcastle in January 1848 suggests how complex was the attribution of the cause of deaths of patients under chloroform. Hannah, a 15-year-old 'bastard child ..., much thrust about' by her family, suffered from an ingrown toenail. The flesh about the nails had gone 'rotten' and Mr T.N. Meggson had decided to remove the nail. Hannah may have been troubled by a similar complaint, perhaps in the other foot, because she had already had an operation under anaesthesia, probably ether. However this had left her with 'a heaviness in her head'. Her step-father had said 'she had better suffer a bit of pain for a moment' than have her head 'made bad again' but Hannah was adamant, saying that 'she would not have her nail taken off without it'. It is possible that she had lost a nail before without anaesthesia and knew, as Liston had said, that the removal of a nail was among the most painful procedures. As the surgeon arrived she began sobbing. Hannah's wishes prevailed and Mr Meggson removed the nail under chloroform, kneeling before the fire with Hannah's uncle holding her foot. As Meggson completed this minor operation Hannah collapsed. He bled her and administered brandy but she sank. Just as at the time it remains impossible to say what had caused Hannah Greener's death and whether chloroform played any part in it. Still, deaths such as hers served to alarm conservative surgeons. They remained doubtful about an agent which had saved a patient from the pain of what they regarded as a trifling operation but at the cost of her life.[69]

'Pain for ever': anaesthesia opposed

Some doctors responded warily to ether and chloroform. While Australian surgeons tried ether as soon as they learned of the Boston and London operations others remained doubtful. Isaac Aaron, the editor and proprietor of the *Australian Medical Journal*, warned within days of the first Australian operations of 'a FASHION … the RAGE just now' for ether. Aaron counselled his readers against hastily adopting anaesthesia, a mistrust persisting at least until his journal folded later in 1847.[70]

Like Aaron, the sceptical or timid preferred to wait until the safety of the novelty had been proved beyond doubt. A 'leading professional man' wrote to James Simpson from Dublin to explain his quandary. He dare not try it on the rich 'for my own sake' – a death under chloroform would ruin him – and he was loath to experiment upon the poor, for theirs'.[71] Simpson was perturbed to find, a year after ether became available, that only a handful of London physicians had used it in obstetric cases and none of Dublin's had even tried it until November 1847.[72] The innovation 'jostled and disturbed … settled notions'. Miller described how they 'closed their ears, shut their eyes, and folded their hands'. Pain, they argued, was a necessary evil which must be endured.[73] The author of the article in the *Edinburgh Medical and Surgical Journal* which had carried the account of the Boston operation, himself expressed doubt of the value of the innovation. Pain was 'not the worst thing' in operations, he claimed. He had observed that patients who suffered severe pain often made good recoveries while those able to 'suppress the external indications … often make bad recoveries or die soon after'. He advised caution in adopting 'the present mania for etherism' and questioned whether anaesthesia could meet the expectations held out for it.

This faction asserted what James Miller called 'the rights of pain'. Dr William Gull ('ominous name', quipped Miller) questioned ether's use. Gull, a sarcastic but influential physician, argued that it was dangerous to abolish pain and that in any case ether was a poison. Surgeons who heard him address the South London Medical Society early in 1847 generally agreed. Benjamin Travers junior said that he believed that ether was a 'dangerous remedy' while Bransby Cooper (forgetting his willingness to give mesmerism a hearing) was now 'convinced that ether was a poison'.[74] Dr Radford saw 'nothing but evil' in anaesthesia.[75] Authoritative contributions came from Britain and France: Dr Nunn could not see 'how surgeons or surgery were to get on without [pain]'; Mr Cole regarded chloroform as a 'highly pernicious agent': François Magendie's discouraging cry became 'pain for ever'.[76] Although these men were clearly on a losing wicket it is nevertheless worth examining their objections. Those doubtful about or opposed to the use of anaesthetics advanced several arguments: medical, scriptural and philosophical, many of which they had rehearsed against mesmerism several years before.

'We had always understood,' wrote the author of an anonymous pamphlet, 'that pain was given us as a blessing'.[77] It was a view to which many older or conservative surgeons subscribed. Opponents argued that anaesthesia encouraged haemorrhage, presumably because of the relaxation and dilation of blood vessels. Advocates of anaesthesia contested this view reminding them of how a patient's struggles could displace a tourniquet and of how difficult it was to suture the arteries of a moving patient. Dr James Pickford, a Brighton general practitioner, wrote to the *Edinburgh Medical and Surgical Journal* to alert his colleagues to the 'Injurious Effects of Inhalation of Aether'. Suspicious of anaesthesia's 'sudden and violent effect' he alleged that it must alter the circulation, producing 'black vitiated blood' similar to that found in 'putrid and malignant fevers'. He feared haemorrhage, unhealthy discharges and flabby and gangrenous stumps. Dr Pickford claimed that pain was desirable and that its annihilation would be 'hazardous to the patient'. He may have been the first to quote publicly the verse from Genesis that exemplified the acceptance of pain: 'in sorrow shall she bring forth children'.[78] Conservatives also argued – as late as 1865 – that union by first intention was less likely with anaesthesia, that patients died of asphyxia, coma, spitting of blood, convulsions or pneumonia, and even from explosions of the ether.[79] These claims, it transpired, were based on neither logic nor evidence.

Philosophically inclined opponents argued that sensation of any kind was natural and that to seek to suspend it was to 'set at naught the ordinances of nature'. Drawing on Biblical authority they believed that 'man is born to suffering'.[80] A Dr Meiggs expressed the more crude view that anaesthesia represented 'a questionable attempt to abrogate one of the general conditions of man'. Simpson retorted contemptuously that 'riding and railway travelling abrogate[d]' such 'general conditions' as well.[81] A 'London divine' put the more substantial objection that he did not regard the alleviation of pain as a problem, rather it was 'the destruction of consciousness'. 'The Surgical mind,' Simpson later observed, 'is a very curious piece of metaphysics'.[82] He countered by pointing out simply that all consented to the destruction of consciousness every night at bedtime.[83] There was also a moral qualm. A 'Dr G.' wrote to Simpson early in 1848 objecting that chloroform might be used as a 'means of debauching innocent women'.[84]

Perhaps the crux of the opposition lay in the remark by one of its most articulate representatives, Frank Hamilton, who claimed that with anaesthetics available 'patients will no longer submit to operations without them': anaesthesia diminished the surgeon's authority over his patient. Correspondingly, as one of James Simpson's numerous correspondents put it, 'Chloroform will make its own way – but it will be through the patients'.[85] Indeed it is possible that surgeons adopted it into the 1850s because patients expected or demanded chloroform and that in a free market they would patronise surgeons prepared to use it: Catherine Dickens's surgeon only used it for her eighth confinement early in 1849 because Charles insisted on it.

Advocates of anaesthesia contested these views. James Simpson wrote prophetically that surgeons would look with horror upon those who countenanced painful surgery as 'insignificant', 'proper' or 'desirable'.[86] Deeply committed to chloroform's acceptance and constitutionally pugnacious, Simpson embarked on a sustained campaign of scholarly lobbying. He collected statistics from several dozen hospitals tabulating the mortality of amputations before and after the introduction of anaesthesia. He was able to show a substantial difference between deaths for identical operations in a large number of hospitals. For the most formidable of the operations he canvassed, amputation at the thigh, the mortality was about 1 in 2. With anaesthesia, despite the continuing hazards of infection, it was 1 in 4. Anaesthesia made the most serious operations half as dangerous: it not only preserved patients from pain but saved many of them from death.[87] By 1850 surgeons at Bart's had used chloroform on nine thousand patients without notable adverse effects.[88] During the 1850s opposition to anaesthesia diminished markedly and a succession of surgical authorities pronounced in its favour albeit with qualifications. James Syme administered it 'if the patient has a great dread of pain'.[89] John Erichsen used it 'almost invariably' by 1850.[90] George Guthrie accepted its use 'in all cases of great suffering'.[91] George Ballingall expressed grudging approval: in the 1855 edition of *Outlines of Military Surgery* he was 'inclined to think favourably of it'.[92] Within a few years ether and chloroform had gained widespread acceptance, as Miller had predicted, over Europe, America, Australia and even – reflecting Edinburgh's traditional disdain – 'over the greater part of London'.[93]

'The shock of the knife': painful surgery continues

We may assume that the blessing of anaesthesia relieved grateful surgeons from ever again having to directly inflict pain. In fact, although most surgeons certainly used anaesthesia, large numbers of operations continued to employ no pain-killing agent. While the 'Anti-Chloroformers' constituted a vocal minority many operating surgeons entertained reservations over anaesthesia and adopted it hesitatingly or tardily. An Aberdeen friend informed Simpson in February 1848 that anaesthesia was 'not used nearly as much as it might'. Although using it in an excision of a shoulder joint, surgeons declined to use it for a lithotomy performed on a former soldier whom they thought possessed 'courage sufficiently to carry him through'. The surgeons supposed wrongly: 'I don't think I ever heard a patient bellow so lustily' Simpson's correspondent observed.[94] The introduction of ether coincided with Edward Cree's time at Edinburgh where, although an experienced naval surgeon, a veteran of the first Opium war and fights with pirates in Borneo, he had returned to enter the Royal College of Surgeons of Edinburgh. Cree watched operations under ether with interest which he regarded as a 'great blessing'. His surgery teacher James Syme, however, he found 'rather opposes it' because of the delay and the uncertainty in obtaining insensibility. Cree optimistically concluded that 'the matter is still in its infancy'.[95] Thomas Cunningham, a Belfast student at Edinburgh, reported to his brother in March 1847 that Syme remained suspicious of ether. He had had difficulty in procuring unconsciousness and had given up in impatience. He thought that 'it will not do at least for capital operations'.[96] Many surgeons trained in the period of painful surgery – who remained active and influential for decades – did not believe anaesthesia to be necessary: George Macilwain even in 1854 entertained 'the greatest doubt' of chloroform.[97] Many used it only to assist in the initial shocking incision. Others reckoned whether its use was justified on a 'calculus of suffering' expertly delineated and analysed by Martin Pernick. In 1848 an ophthalmologist decided not to administer chloroform to a woman because he felt her older and 'staid' to stand the stress while Robert Druitt decided not to use chloroform for a hernia operation because the patient was epileptic.[98] It was possible a decade or more after 1846 to contemplate operations for hare-lip or to remove a child's finger without it. James Paget recalled the case of a boy who was to lose part of a finger but who refused to allow the operation to proceed without chloroform. It was, for some unexplained reason, 'not convenient' to the surgeon to administer anaesthesia (perhaps because the risk of death might have contributed to the case against anaesthesia). The surgeon had a dresser give the boy a damp sponge to sniff. The boy apparently believed himself insensible and 'the operation swiftly done was not felt'.[99]

Medical texts make clear not only that their use was optional but that for some anaesthesia was not expected. William Mackenzie published his ophthalmic text *Cure of Strabismus* in 1851. He recommended that the best position for the operation was for adults to 'rest' on the breast of an assistant – where they could be secured in the old style. For children more than two assistants might be required but Mackenzie advised swaddling the child in a sheet so that arms and legs might be kept at rest while the assistants concentrated on restraining the patient's head.[100] Medical journals provide ample evidence of even major operations proceeding without anaesthesia. In 1852 J.M. Carnochan described the excision of the entire lower jaw of a man who could not be given ether or chloroform for fear of asphyxia, an operation which lasted 55 minutes.[101] James Miller, a passionate advocate for chloroform, accepted that painful operations must proceed despite the impossibility of administering anaesthesia. Obliged to remove 'a large amount of vascular tissue' from a man with cancer of the nose, Miller found that the gurgling of blood in the throat precluded the use of the inhaler and decided that he must proceed with a 'bloody and painful, but safe operation'.[102] Habits of mind acquired during their long acquaintance with surgery persisted. Charles Clay who specialised in ovariotomies is said to have asserted that if a patient could 'make up her mind to submit to so formidable [an] operation' without anaesthesia, he believed that 'her chance would be better without the chloroform or ether'.[103]

The culture of indifference or stoicism lingered. One of Syme's students recorded that he excised a testicular growth using a pair of scissors but no chloroform in 1861.[104] Other surgeons continued to express reservations but used anaesthesia because patients asked for it. A Charles Bleeck of Warminster wrote to the *Lancet* to describe how he had amputated a scirrhous breast using chloroform at the patient's request. She collapsed and was revived by artificial respiration. Bleeck continued without renewing the chloroform.[105] In 1856 surgeons at the Melbourne Hospital 'thought it to be inexpedient' to administer chloroform in amputating the leg of a man who had received a compound fracture falling off a horse when drunk.[106] In 1868 a woman about to undergo an operation for anal fistula at the same hospital was asked if she wanted chloroform.[107] Robert Jones, a pioneering orthopaedic surgeon in Liverpool in the 1880s who had trained under surgeons trained before 1850, 'occasionally shocked' younger colleagues by refusing to use anaesthetic.[108] Jones was not alone. A chaplain at the London Hospital recalled that the 'prejudice against anaesthetics was general and lasted some time'. He particularly remembered an older surgeon remark that he 'liked a good honest scream'.[109] Even major operations continued without anaesthesia, mostly at the insistence of surgeons, although sometimes in accordance with patients' wishes. John Bland-Sutton saw a senior at the Middlesex Hospital cut dead bone from a sailor's heel without anaesthesia in 1879 and his own first operation a few years later was to excise a tumour from the leg of a woman who had refused chloroform.[110] The continuation of painful surgery explains why the board of the Norfolk and Norwich Hospital resolved to consider 'the best method for stopping sound from the operation room' in 1849: the possibility of painless surgery emphasised the horror of the painful procedures that continued.[111]

This lukewarm acceptance explains how debate over the necessity, desirability or safety of anaesthesia continued for years. Persistent concerns over the safety of chloroform eventually resulted in the Royal Medical and ChirurgicalSociety appointing a committee in 1862 to consider the effects of its use which resulted in 'Rules' issued in 1864 although it did not diminish the use of anaesthetics.[112] As late as 1855, eleven years after the introduction of ether, Colonel E. Elers Napier felt constrained to defend the safety of chloroform. He pointed out that in 'many thousands' of operations under chloroform at Edinburgh only one death attributable to the anaesthetic could be traced while the 'comparatively few' operations without anaesthesia had cost the lives of four or five patients. Napier listed the statistics of operations without anaesthesia collected at hospitals in Britain and France which totalled over 2,500 operations performed 'several years' before the mid-1850s. The advantages of chloroform were as clear to Colonel Napier as they are to us: only those brought up to see patients suffer pain believed otherwise and they remained in a substantial, albeit diminishing, minority.[113]

Some of the practitioners most reluctant to endorse anaesthesia were military surgeons, who viewed anaesthesia somewhat differently to their hospital counterparts. Surgeon James who had served at

Waterloo remained convinced to the end that pain was 'advantageous in a physical and moral sense ... one of the greatest boons'.[114] In September 1854, as the British army entered action on the Alma in the Crimea, the *Illustrated London News* published Dr Hall's recommendation that the surgeons with the Army of the East should dispense with anaesthesia. 'However barbarous it may appear,' Hall wrote, 'the shock of the knife is a powerful stimulant'. He believed that it was better to hear a man 'bawl lustily' from pain than 'sink silently into the grave' from receiving chloroform.[115] Hall echoed an aphorism of the oft-quoted John Abernethy who had said to his students – presumably more than once – that 'there is no hartshorn like the cut of a knife'.[116] Hall's view, although harsh, was not simply barbarous. Rather, it reflected the experience of surgeons who had had to revive sinking patients on the table and to whom pain was a lesser evil than death. Unlike civil surgeons most of the military surgeon's work, in battle at least, concerned traumatic injury. Even those who deprecated primary amputation still confronted patients who had been recently wounded and who very likely suffered the accompanying symptoms of loss of blood and shock. Perhaps because of Hall's advice, however, the surgeons of one of the five British divisions to serve in the Crimea commonly did not use chloroform.[117]

'This blessed boon' : anaesthesia triumphant

The efforts of advocates such as Miller and Simpson and the self-evident benefits of painless surgery eventually persuaded opponents and sceptics of the value of anaesthesia. James Syme, although dubious of anaesthesia in the late 1840s, had become a supporter by the mid-1850s. He wrote to *The Times* to contest John Hall's view, arguing that not only did the use of chloroform not increase the danger of operating but that pain itself 'most injuriously exhausts the nervous energy of a weak patient'.[118] Even William Gull was recorded as administering chloroform for a hernia operation.[119] Despite the diminishing opposition of older or more conservative surgeons, by the end of the first full decade in which anaesthesia was available most opposition had declined to the fringe of medical opinion. Chloroform, wrote Henry Smith (Surgeon to the Westminster General Dispensary) in his survey of *The Improvements in Modern Surgery*, had been 'the great discovery of late years'.[120] With its assistance surgery accelerated the onward march which all living surgeons believed to be its destiny. Indeed the availability of chloroform allowed surgeons to continue and accelerate the innovation of the previous half-century. The headline 'New Surgical

Operation' began to appear more frequently in the press. *The Times* reported in December 1847 that thirty spectators watched Thomas Wakley (the journalist's son) dissect out the bones of a patient's foot under chloroform at the Royal Free Hospital. The patient felt nothing. That the operation took only six minutes, however, suggests how established styles persisted.[121]

While largely abolishing acute surgical pain in the operating room the acceptance of anaesthesia did not solve other problems. It did not alleviate chronic pain and post-operative remedies remained as ineffective as before. Anaesthesia did not remove the fear of the knife or many of the complications or difficulties of wielding it: even among surgeons the Caesarean remained 'a rare and fearful operation'.[122] It did nothing to solve intractable post-operative infection and indeed, in that it encouraged more operations, may have worsened it. Even the possibility of painless surgery did not immediately alter the public's residual and deeply-rooted fear of surgeons. As Henry Bigelow acknowledged, 'years .. must elapse before the surgeon will cease ... to be identified with pain'.[123]

Nor did chemical anaesthesia entirely supplant mesmerism. The triumph of ether and chloroform removed the urgency for many of its advocates and it was soon relegated to the margins. Eccentric mesmeric partisans continued to damage their cause: John Mill, for example, relied on a 'clairvoyante' to assist his diagnosis.[124] Small wonder that when the Royal Medical and Chirurgical Society's librarian accepted the gift of two books on the subject he denied the donors 'the usual courtesy' of acknowledging or announcing the gift.[125] Mesmeric surgery continued nevertheless. In 1854 Mr Tubbs of Upwell in Cambridgeshire operated upon a Mrs Flowerday at his Mesmeric Infirmary. Tubbs excised her breast in an operation of 'unusual slowness'. Mrs Flowerday sat in 'complete repose ... still, silent and relaxed'. At its conclusion she walked up some steps and back to her room in a trance.[126]

The availability of anaesthesia, however, did relieve the great dread at the heart of surgical practice for both patients and operators. Henry Smith again made clear that because of chloroform, operators could embark upon 'the most terrible operations without doing violence to those feelings which will always animate the really good surgeon'. No longer need surgeons affect an 'apparent insensibility'. No longer, because of 'this blessed boon' need operators feel that firmness of purpose would war with 'the most generous and most gentle sympathy'.[127]

The accepted version of the introduction of aneasthesia is

universally presented as the story of the introduction of chemical anaesthesia. Henry Bigelow was prescient when he quoted a British journal's prediction that 'we shall hear no more of mesmerism and its absurdities'.[128] Mesmerism remains consigned to the fringe of history as well as medicine: John Elliotson's advocacy is presented in terms of the *Lancet's* strictures and Robert Liston's derision. A history commemorating the 150th anniversary of anaesthesia accorded one sentence to mesmerism perpetuating the fallacy that 'generous doses of alcohol' was one of the 'mainstays of analgesia' before 1846.[129] Whatever mesmerism's imperfections, it is still true that in the early 1840s hundreds of patients were spared the pain of surgery by its use. Sadly, that fact was denied at the time and has been ignored ever since.

Notes.

1. J. Wilde, *The Hospital, a Poem in Three Books, Written in the Devon and Exeter Hospital,* (Norwich: Stevenson, Matchett & Stevenson, 1809), 48.

2. Copy of undated letter by William Roots in the papers of J.F. South, Add. Ms 342& 343, RCSEng.

3. Charles Bell, *The Anatomy and Philosophy of Expression* [1806] (London: J. Murray, 1844), 156.

4. Anthony Carlisle, Lecture XV, 'Conclusion and moral conduct of operations', 42.f.28, RCSEng.

5. *Lancet,* 1832–33, Vol. I, 744–47.

6. James Moore, *A Method of Preventing or Diminishing Pain in Several Operations of Surgery* (London: T. Cadell, 1784), 13.

7. Barry Milligan, *Pleasures and Pains: Opium and the Orient in Nineteenth Century British Culture* (Charlottesville: University Press of Virginia, 1995), 22.

8. Dorothy Porter & Roy Porter, *Patient's Progress: Doctors and Doctoring in Eighteenth Century England* (Cambridge: Polity, 1989), 220.

9. John Pearson, *The Life of William Hey, Esq.* (London: Hurst, Robinson & Co., 1822), 7.

10. Thomas Chevalier, *A Treatise on Gun-Shot Wounds* (London: Samuel Bagster, 1806), 119.

11. Astley Cooper & Frederick Tyrrell, *The Lectures of Sir Astley Cooper, Bart. ...* (London: Thomas Tegg, 1824), 169 .

12. J.W. Chelius, (trans. and ed. J.F. South), *A System of Surgery,* 2 vols (London: Henry Renshaw, 1847), Vol. II, 854n .

13. H.B. Gibson, *Pain and its Conquest* (London: Peter Owen, 1982),

33.

14. Samuel Wilks & G.T. Bettany, *A Biographical History of Guy's Hospital* (London: Ward & Lock, London, 1892), 340.

15. *The Times*, 28 September 1801, 3b.

16. *Lancet*, 1850, 504.

17. 'On the Inhalation of Sulphuric Ether Vapour', *Edinburgh Medical & Surgical Journal*, Vol. 67, 1847, 504–19.

18. Gibson, *op. cit.* (note 13), 38-40.

19. 'Dr Quadri on the Medical Use of Morphia', *Edinburgh Medical & Surgical Journal*, Vol. 26, 1826, 190–94.

20. 'Dr Robertson on the Salts of Morphia', *Edinburgh Medical & Surgical Journal*, Vol. 37, 1832, 278.

21. George Pickering, *Creative Malady: Illness in the Lives and Minds of Charles Darwin, Florence Nightingale ... [and] Elizabeth Barrett Browning* (London: Allen & Unwin, 1974), 261–63.

22. 'An Invalid' [Harriet Martineau], *Life in the Sick Room* (London: Edward Moxon, 1844), 7; 109.

23. *London Medical Gazette*, 23 June 1843.

24. Anon, *Motives and Encouragements to Bear Afflictions Patiently ...* (London: Society for Promoting Christian Knowledge, 1811), 18.

25. J. Allison, *Mesmerism: Its Pretensions as a Science Physiologically Considered* (London: Whittacker & Co., 1844), 16.

26. 'Clericus', *Remarks on Dr Maitland's Superstition and Science* (London: James Ridgway, 1856), np.

27. *Lancet*, 1843–44, Vol. I, 500.

28. H. Hale Bellot, *University College London 1826–1926* (London: University of London Press, 1929), 162-64.

29. Elliotson to UCH Medical Committee, 4 July 1838, UCHOFF/MIN/1/1.

30. W.P. Alison, *History of Medicine* (London: Blackwood, 1833), 52.

31. Ross Leitch, *Mesmerism in 1845* (Edinburgh, 1845), 39.

32 . [William Lang], *Mesmerism: its History, Phenomena, and Practice* (Edinburgh: Fraser & Co., 1843), Chapter IV.

33. *Medical Times*, 5 August 1848.

34. Leitch, *op. cit.* (note 31), 38.

35. W. Topham & W. Squire Ward, *Account of a Case of Successful Amputation of the Thigh During the Mesmeric State* (London: H. Ballière, 1842), 12–15.

36. John Elliotson, *Numerous Cases of Surgical Operations Without Pain* (London: H. Ballière, 1843), 8–65.

37. R.M. Thomson and others, *Record of Cases Treated in the Mesmeric*

Hospital ... (Calcutta: W. Risdale, 1847).

38. James Esdaile, *Mesmerism in India and its Practical Application in Surgery and Medicine* (London: Longman, Brown, Green & Longmans, 1846); *Natural and Mesmeric Clairvoyance* (London: Hipployte Ballière, 1852); *The Introduction of Mesmerism ... into the Public Hospitals of London* (Perth: Dewar & Son, 1856).
39. *London Medical Gazette*, 26 February 1847.
40. Esdaile, *The Introduction of Mesmerism into the Public Hospitals of London*, 8–9.
41. Esdaile, *Mesmerism in India*, xviii.
42. [Lang], *op. cit.* (note 32), 64.
43. Cock, 'Anecdota Listoniensia', *University College Hospital Magazine*, 1911, 60.
44. Liston to Miller, 22 February 1839, MS 6095, WIHM.
45. 'On the Powers of Life to Sustain Surgical Operations', Charles Bell, *Practical Essays* (Edinburgh: Maclachlan, Stewart & Co., 1841), 1.
46. Eve Blantyre Simpson, *Sir James Y. Simpson* (Edinburgh: Oliphant, Anderson & Ferrier, 1896), 51.
47. *The Times*, 28 December 1846, 3e.
48. Thomas Baillie, *From Boston to Dumfries: the First Surgical Use of Ether in the Old World* (Dumfries: Dinwiddie, 1966), 9.
49. Alison Winter, *Mesmerized: Powers of Mind in Victorian Britain* (Chicago: University of Chicago Press, 1998), 180.
50. James Miller, *Surgical Experience of Chloroform* (Edinburgh: Sutherland & Knox, 1848), 7.
51. *Illustrated London News*, 30 January 1847.
52. Miller, *op. cit.* (note 50), 8.
53. *The Times*, 13 January 1847, 5a.
54. *London Medical Gazette*, 8 January 1847.
55. *The Times*, 27 March 1847, 7c.
56. Gwen Wilson, *One Grand Chain: The History of Anaesthesia in Australia 1846–1962*, Vol. I, 1846–1934 (Melbourne: Australian and New Zealand College of Anaesthetists, 1995), 41–46, 95.
57. *The Times*, 16 January 1847, 5b.
58. 'L.R.C. P. Edin', *Medical Musings, Grave and Gay* (London: William Stevens, 1907), 13 .
59. *Medical Times*, 9 January 1847.
60. *The Times*, 15 January 1847, 3b.
61. J.Y. Simpson, *Account of a New Anaesthetic Agent* (Edinburgh: Sutherland & Knox, 1848), 8.
62. *The Times*, 12 January 1847, 5f.
63. *The Times*, 29 January 1847, 6f.

64. Minutes of Council, January 1849, A4g, RCSEng.

65. *The Times,* 29 November 1847, 5f.

66. *Lancet,* 20 November 1847.

67. George Keith, *Fads of an Old Physician* (London: A. & C. Black, 1897), 100–101.

68. *The Times,* 24 March 1847, 8f.

69. *The Times,* 3 February 1848, 8c; *London Medical Gazette,* 11 February 1848.

70. *Australian Medical Journal,* June-September 1847.

71. J. Duns, *Memoir of Sir James Y. Simpson, Bart.* (Edinburgh: Edmonston & Douglas, 1873), 271.

72. Simpson, *op. cit.* (note 61), 12; Simpson, *Remarks on the Superinduction of Anaesthesia in Natural and Morbid Parturition ...* (Edinburgh: Sutherland & Knox, 1848), 15n.

73. Miller, *op. cit.* (note 50), p. 7.

74. 'On the Effects of Ether on the Different Classes of Animals', Theodore Acland (ed.), *A Collection of the Published Writings of William Withey Gull* (London: 1856), 571–75.

75. *Medical Times,* 18 August 1849.

76. Miller, *op. cit.* (note 50), 35.

77. Anon, *Remarks on a Treatise on the Rectum* (Edinburgh: Stevenson, [1852]), 1.

78. 'Dr Pickford on Aether Inhalation', *Edinburgh Medical & Surgical Journal,* Vol. 68, 1847, 256–58.

79. Frank Hastings Hamilton, *A Treatise on Military Surgery and Hygiene* (New York: Ballière Brothers, 1865); Simpson, *op. cit.* (note 72), 14.

80. Skey, *Operative Surgery* (London: John Churchill, 1850), 16.

81. J.Y. Simpson, *Anaesthetic Midwifery: Report on its Early History and Progress* (Edinburgh: Sutherland & Knox, 1848), 45.

82. Annotation on letter 'Turner' to Dr Black, 23 November 1872, JYS 47, RCSEd.

83. Simpson, *op. cit.* (note 81), 43.

84. Duns, *op. cit.* (note 71), 271. He was doubtless alerted by a French case in which two sisters alleged that a dentist had molested them under the influence of ether. The dentist was sentenced to six years hard labour in the prison hulks.

85. Archibald Cockburn to Simpson, 30 January 1849, JYS 143, RCSEd.

86. Simpson, *op. cit.* (note 79), 6

87. Simpson, *Anaesthesia in surgery: Does it Increase or Decrease Mortality?* (Edinburgh: Sutherland & Knox, 1848), 14–15.

88. Skey, *op. cit.* (note 80), 17.

89. F.G. William Mullar, *Remarks on the Operation of the Perineal Section* (Edinburgh: Robert Seton, 1850), 9.

90. John Erichsen, *On the Study of Surgery* (London: Taylor, Walton & Maberly, 1850), 29.

91. George Guthrie, *Commentaries on the Surgery of the War in Portugal, Spain, France, and the Netherlands* (London: Renshaw, 1853), 54 .

92. George Ballingall, *Outlines of Military Surgery* (Edinburgh: A.&C. Black, 1844, 1846), 298.

93. Miller, *op. cit.* (note 50), 14.

94. William Williams to Simpson, 14 February 1848, JYS 128, RCSEd.

95. Michael Levien, (ed.), *The Cree Journals: the Voyages of Edward H. Cree, Surgeon R.N. ...* (Exeter: Webb & Bower, 1981), 185.

96. Thomas Cunningham to John Cunningham, 18 March 1847, DK 7.46/55, EUA.

97. George Macilwain, *Memoirs of John Abernethy*, 2 vols (London: Hurst & Blackett, 1854), Vol. II, 225.

98. Norman Moore, & Stephen Paget, *The Royal Medical and Chirurgical Society of London, 1805-1905* (Aberdeen: Aberdeen University Press, 1905), 93.

99. James Paget, *Studies of Old Case Books* (London: Longmans & Co., 1891), 158.

100. William Mackenzie, *The Cure of Strabismus by Surgical Operation* (London: Longmans, Orme, Brown, Green & Longmans, 1851), 13.

101. John Carnochan, *Amputation of the Entire Lower Jaw* (New York: Van Norden & Amerman, 1852), 7, 10.

102. Miller, *op. cit.* (note 50), 42.

103. Hamilton, *op. cit.* (note 79), 617.

104. Myrtle Simpson, *Simpson the Obstetrician: A Biography* (London: Gollancz, 1972), 181–82.

105. *Lancet*, 1850, 283.

106. *Australian Medical Journal*, Vol. I, 1856, 191–93.

107. Wilson, *op. cit.* (note 56), Vol. I, 1846, 137–38.

108. Frederick Watson, *The Life of Sir Robert Jones* (London: Hodder & Stoughton, 1934), 66.

109. E.W. Morris, *A History of the London Hospital* (London: Edward Arnold, 1910), 169.

110. John Bland-Sutton, *The Story of a Surgeon* (London: Methuen, 1930), 72; 74.

111. Peter Eade, *The Norfolk and Norwich Hospital 1770–1900* (London: Jarrold & Sons, 1900), 88.

112. Moore & Paget, *op. cit.* (note 98), 103; 122.

113. *The Times*, 5 February 1855, 8f.

114. J.H. James, *Chloroform vesus Pain and Paracentesis of the Bladder* (London: Churchill, 1870), 7; 9.

115. *Illustrated London News*, 23 September 1854.

116. *The Times*, 11 October 1824, 3b. Hartshorn, a solution of ammonia, was used to revive patients in syncope.

117. Hamilton, *op. cit.* (note 79), 614.

118. *The Times*, 12 October 1854, 9a.

119. Moore & Paget, *op. cit.* (note 98), 93.

120. Henry Smith, *The Improvements in Modern Surgery* (London: John Churchill, 1854), 21.

121. *The Times*, 30 December 1847, 6b.

122. *The Times*, 11 December 1860, 5e.

123. Henry Jacob Bigelow, *An Introductory Lecture delivered at Massachusetts Medical College* (Boston: David Clapp, 1850), 13.

124. John Mill, *The Use of Clairvoyance in Medicine* (London: 1858), 40.

125. Moore & Paget, *op. cit.* (note 98), 98.

126. *The Times*, 2 May 1854, 12d.

127. Smith, *op. cit.* (note 120), 21–22.

128. Bigelow, *op. cit.* (note 123), 33.

129. G.B. Rushman, N.J.H. Davies & R.S. Atkinson, *A Short History of Anaesthesia: the First 150 Years* (Oxford: Butterworth-Heinemann, 1996), 1.

Epilogue
'Long fixed in the memory':
The Legacy of Painful Surgery

Over the course of twenty years the naval surgeon Stephen Hammick performed amputations on 287 patients (only 16 of whom died) and witnessed a further 400 amputations.[1] He must have performed or watched countless other procedures. What did the memory of that experience mean for Hammick and his patients? Like his colleagues, his students and his patients, those who had performed, witnessed or endured surgery before anaesthesia lived with the memory of it for ever after.

'A cause of disquiet': patients' memories of surgery

George Wilson, whose foot James Syme had amputated in 1841, wrote seven years later how memories of the operation 'haunted' him for 'a long time ... and even now they are easily remembered'. Writing to James Simpson in support of his crusade in favour of chloroform, George Wilson fervently wished that he could drink 'some Lethean draught' to erase the memory. Such memories, he reflected, 'occasion a suffering of their own ... a cause of disquiet which favours neither mental or bodily health'.[2] Wilson conceded that he may have possessed a 'more active and roving fancy' but believed that he was not unique in the way the experience remained with him.

It is true that other patients disclaimed any notable distress. In 1911 students at University College spoke for an hour to an old man who as a twelve-year-old, just before the introduction of chemical anaesthesia, had lost a leg at the hands of Robert Liston.[3] He had suffered from white swelling of the knee and Liston advised him to submit to amputation. He recalled how Liston had come to him on a Friday and asked when he would have the operation. 'Will it hurt?' he had asked. 'No more than having a tooth out' Liston replied. 'Oh', the man recalled the boy replying, 'I'll have it done tomorrow ... then I shall be all right on Sunday'. 'Very well,' Liston had replied gravely. The man could not recall Liston's face but after more than sixty years he could remember his voice as 'extraordinarily pleasant'. The following day he was blindfolded and taken to the theatre, laid on a table and held firmly. 'Was the operation very painful?' the students asked. 'No,' he replied, but added, 'although I was bellowing all the time'. He recalled counting the strokes of the saw – six. When told that the limb had been removed he answered 'That's a lie'. That evening, in accordance with the prevailing doctrine of granulation, Liston adjusted the flaps and tied the stump. This, the man said, was 'the most painful part of the whole business'. The interview offers a fragmentary insight into one of the last amputations Liston performed before he adopted ether.

Liston's case books disclose that the boy's name was Henry Pace.[4] 'A great sufferer', he had been admitted late on 23 September 1846. He had been afflicted with the tubercular swelling of the right knee joint since having scarlet fever at six. Now, the withered lower leg was contracted and bent at a right angle to the thigh, chronically painful. Two days after admission, Liston operated. Although he was still in hospital three weeks later his notes, kept by a student dresser, are sketchy and do not disclose when he was discharged. Henry Pace's was the second-last public capital operation that Liston undertook before using ether for the first time in December. Given the trauma of painful surgery, Henry Pace is unlikely to have either truly forgotten the experience: but nor may he have been inclined to reveal it to casual enquirers.

Even as Henry Bigelow celebrated how the advent of anaesthesia had 'shaken ... the balance of surgical right ... to its centre', he recognised that surgeons would long be indentified with the infliction of pain. As we have seen, painful surgery was an experience of such profundity that merely witnessing it, not to speak of performing or enduring it, remained with all those involved. In his autobiography Charles Darwin acknowledged that the 'cases' he saw in the Edinburgh Royal Infirmary left 'vivid pictures' which he still saw in his mind's eye. His memories of the two operations he saw proved even more traumatic: he confessed that they 'fairly haunted me for many a long year'.[5] Medical educators before 1850 exposed their students to surgery so that they could see beyond it and comprehend and grasp the lessons they taught. 'By the sufferings of the patient', a contributor to the *Lancet* wrote, 'the observer becomes sympathetically interested in his welfare, and impressions painfully produced are long fixed in the memory'.[6]

The methods of the era of painful surgery lived on. Those who had developed their style before 1846 naturally continued to operate rapidly. In that their juniors tended to imitation even men such as Henry Smith (who qualified in 1846) adopted William Fergusson's

Figure 12.1

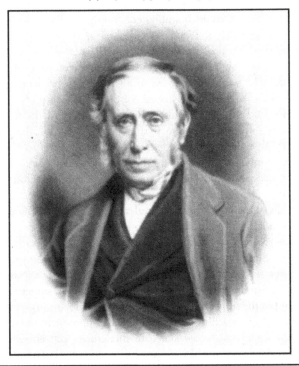

*A photograph of James Syme (1799-1870)
at the age of 65, at the end of his long career. His eyes, with which he
had witnessed twenty-five years of painful surgery, compel attention.*

style of extreme celerity. It is certain that Frederick Treves (even if he did not see painful surgery) did encounter some of its legacies in the brusquerie of the address of his surgical teachers.

'Well do I remember ...': surgeons' recollections

The effort of observing or performing surgery took its toll. James Paget, who had counselled students to control the will to bear watching pain, also conceded that ultimately the suppressed trauma would emerge. He reflected that memory of pain 'expected, watched for, long thought of, or talked of, will come ...'.[7] We can only speculate on the impact of the burden of disturbed nights and guilty feelings especially in retrospect as the full horror of painful surgery became apparent in relief, as it were, after 1846.

Surgery was – and remains – an unavoidably physical experience. Surgeons working without gloves and gowns confronted the corporeal reality of surgery directly. They held mortifying limbs, stopped bleeding by seizing bleeding arteries with their fingers, felt tumours and growths in the body and applied force in reducing fractures. Fergusson devoted a page of his text to the importance of 'touch'.[8] Many entertained ambivalent feelings at best toward their chosen calling. Plarr's *Lives of the Fellows of the Royal College of Surgeons* drew on the obituary of Samuel Barnes of Exeter (1776-1858). Barnes, Surgeon to the Devon and Exeter Hospital from 1813, it reads, 'was a good operator, for he knew what he meant to do and did it. Yet he did not dislike nor did he love his profession. It was', it adds significantly, 'his business.'[9] Others did dislike their profession. Fifteen of the 38 medical men who arrived in the colony of South Australia in the decade after 1836 decided not to practise; perhaps as much to evade the pressures of their calling as to settle a land of opportunity.[10] The enlistment registers of the East India Company's Bengal Army disclose that in the 1840s alone at least twenty-six surgeons or medical students chose to enlist as private soldiers in its small European force in preference to remaining in the profession.[11]

James Simpson, who had done as much as anyone to urge his colleagues to accept anaesthesia, reflected on the transformation which its introduction brought, not to the practice of surgery but to the mind of the surgeon. Pondering on the cruelties of surgery which Ambrose Paré's teachings had supplanted, Simpson observed that surgeons would not be awakened to the 'cruelty and enormity' of established practices until a change had occurred. Having seen the blessing which ether and chloroform brought, he wrote how he and his colleagues were at last able to see how 'sufferings and inhumanities' had become 'utterly unnecessary ... utterly uncalled for'.[12] After the mid-1840s surgeons were able to regard painful surgery with the horror with which it has since been indelibly associated. In the meantime, however, even as surgeons accepted anaesthesia and adopted practices that would break the nexus between surgery and pain, they lived with the legacies of the era which they had seen end.

Hints of the effects on those who trained or practised before 1846 can be found in surgeons' memoirs and recollections. In 1887, as the Australian colonies began to regard themselves as belonging to one continent if not yet a nation, medical practitioners gathered in Adelaide for the inaugural Intercolonial Medical Congress. T.

Naughton FitzGerald of the Melbourne Hospital spoke at the 'Section on Surgery', reviewing 'The Progress of Surgery'.[13] FitzGerald congratulated his fellows on the fiftieth anniversary of both Queen Victoria's accession and of the formation of the British Medical Association. (The BMA, the lineal descendant of the Provincial Medical Association, represented the triumph of the despised provincial practitioner over the exclusive royal colleges.) Speaking in the florid style of late-Victorian public oratory FitzGerald recalled the great figures of surgical history, still a memory: Lawrence and Skey at Bart's, Hawkins and Brodie at St George's, Guthrie at Westminster and Fergusson, newly arrived in London. He acknowledged the continental figures Lisfranc and Civiale, Dieffenbach and Langenbeek. Naturally he noted the limitations of surgery fifty years before and contrasted the progress made in ensuing decades. Only when recalling his own memories of that time did FitzGerald hint at the trauma that his formal, oratorical, positive recollection concealed. 'Some of us,' he continued, 'can well remember the operating theatre of old, ensanguined like a slaughter-yard, the air rent with the shrieks of the unhappy victims quivering under the knife ...'.

How such memories came and when – in the night; in old age when memories emerge unbidden with clarity – we do not know. Many, like FitzGerald, must surely have been tormented by the recollection of scenes they had witnessed even if they declined to commit them to paper. In a memoir of her husband Marion Bell remembered how 'nobody suffered more than he from a disturbed night'.[14] In 1841, the year before his death, Charles Bell described the sight of a patient on the table. He recalled 'the limbs stiffened though agonizing pain; the face turgid, and the eyes prominent and suffused ...'.[15] He had seen the sight hundreds of times for half a century and it retained its horror. One of James Syme's oldest friends recalled how he became 'at times moody', suggesting perhaps disquiet with the operations he had performed over thirty years of operating without anaesthesia.[16] Addressing the annual meeting of the British Medical Association in 1865, he spoke on the changes he had witnessed – and to a large extent fostered– in the fifty years since he began practising. 'Well do I remember', he said, 'the shrieks of unfortunate patients ...'. Even the 'Napoleon of Surgery' it seems, entertained recriminations and regrets over what he had had to do as a surgeon. The trauma of performing, undergoing or even hearing painful surgery surely did not simply evaporate with the introduction of chloroform. For generations after 1846 the fears and foreboding surely remained to colour the dreams and fuel the fears of those who had lived through that time. We, like they, have understandably chosen not to consider it but we need to acknowledge that for unknown numbers of those born before, say, 1835 – the people who so avidly read John Brown's 'Rab and his Friends' – secretly carried the burden of anguish, the fear of pain.

'The skill of the competent butcher': the history of surgery

Late in 1896, fifty years after the first surgical operation to be conducted under chemical anaesthesia, the British journal *The Hospital* observed the anniversary, reflecting on the changes that the innovation had brought. Before operations became painless, its editor mused, surgeons contemplated operating only because they could preserve limb or life. Because of anaesthesia they had been able to treat a vast range of injuries and conditions. *The Hospital's* celebration was, of course, entirely justified. The acceptance of anaesthesia relieved patients from pain and enabled surgeons to continue to develop operations bringing immense changes to the practice of medicine and to the alleviation of suffering. But *The Hospital's* editor also expressed what had already become the conventional view of the era of painful surgery, and especially its surgeons. Anaesthesia, he wrote, had enabled 'a class of men' to practise surgery who 'would not have been willing – would not, indeed, have been able – to practise surgery at all' before 1846. Protesting, unconvincingly, that he meant no disparagement he described the surgeon of the era of painful surgery as, at best, 'a cultured man, with the skill of the competent butcher'. In contrast the surgeon of the painless present was 'an "artist"'. Within living memory of its end the era of painful surgery was being presented as crude and barbaric.[17]

The Hospital's view of painful surgery has never been challenged since. Indeed it has become an orthodoxy. The *Oxford Companion to Medicine*, for example, portrays the surgeons of the period before 1846 as 'largely inattentive to the sufferings wreaked by surgery'.[18] We are commonly told that surgeons were able to perform a 'small number' of procedures, that operations were usually over in minutes, that surgeons were indifferent to the shrieks of their patients. This book seeks to challenge these conventional views, suggesting that there is much in received knowledge that is incorrect, unsubstantiated, requires revision or which is open to question and demands further research.

Epilogue

'Dreams of the dreadful knife': a memoir

I can capture the place exactly; the time less precisely. In the library of Scott Street Primary School some time in 1967 I read Addison Whipple's children's biography, *All About Nelson*. I remember his description of the amputation of Nelson's right arm by Thomas Eshelby on the orlop deck of HMS *Theseus* after the disastrous storming of Tenerife in July 1797.

> There was nothing to kill the pain of the operation, for anesthetics had not yet been discovered. While the surgeon cut through the flesh and what was left of the bone, Nelson could only close his eyes and grit his teeth ...

The setting was incongruous. I sat in the air-conditioned library of a brand new school, built on the edge of Whyalla, a raw South Australian steel town. Glancing up, I could have looked out over the saltbush plain which would shortly be filled with more Housing Trust houses like the one I lived in, a few dirt-pavemented, freshly-surfaced streets away. There, as a ten year old, within a year of arriving in this remote desert town half a world away from the British city of Liverpool in which I had grown up, I encountered a scene which has remained a part of my mental life. It recurred at random in my waking hours and, for a time, came to me unbidden in dreams. For nearly thirty years the vision of that amputation exerted an appalled fascination and became the subject of a surreptitious interest.

Like Tennyson's nurse 'my sleep was broken with dreams of the dreadful knife'. For a time I had nightmares in which I saw a hospital in which soldiers during the Napoleonic wars underwent shockingly crude operations. I awoke from these nightmares with profound relief but in a state of greater disorientation and alarm than any other dream I have ever had. Thereafter, scenes and description accumulated in memory. Shortly after reading the biography of Nelson I saw the film of *Gone with the Wind* for the first time. I saw the scene in a hospital in besieged Atlanta in which Scarlett O'Hara rushes in distress from the operating room – the horror conveyed almost exclusively on Vivien Leigh's face. Few such scenes depicted what I imagined graphically. Indeed, until this book was almost finished I had not actually witnessed an actual surgical operation. But the horror was by now embedded in my imagination, and it never really left it until in 1995 I began to think seriously about this book.

This book began as an attempt to exorcise this preoccupation,

319

musing on what it meant for me and what it can mean for us all. Looking back on it with a sort of reflective maturity as a professional historian, I am ready both to explore publicly what the fascination might mean and find in it a significance, a higher purpose, perhaps. In a sense, I want to share this journey with you because I have come to feel that it has served a purpose, not just for me, but for us all. This isn't simply a cathartic confession; a tour of some of the darker recesses of a mind; a reflection on the febrile creativity of an adolescent imagination. It is a reflection which will enable us to confront what humans have done to each other, and how they've lived with it. Although they may have similar effects the scenes which periodically tormented me are not like, say, the mindless terrors of the adolescent horror movie – a genre to which, interestingly, I was never drawn. Staying with me this far has been much more unpleasant for you than it has been for me. Nightmares came to me only occasionally over thirty years but you've encountered it in one dose, as it were, and the experience may well have been an ordeal. I'm sorry: but I'm glad that you haven't looked away. In the end, I hope, it will have been worthwhile.

The choice I made until 1995 was to accept that this was a part of my life, that from time to time a passage in a book or a scene in a film would recall the incident in the cockpit of HMS *Theseus*. Then I became bolder and made another choice. Instead of trying to forget the scene, I entered into it, to the cockpits of Nelson's ships, the barns and churches around Waterloo and the operating rooms of a dozen hospitals. I learned about what happened there and what it looked like; I know what a retractor is, what happens when a tourniquet breaks and what should and shouldn't happen during a lithotomy. And in the end, thirty odd years on, as I sat in the Public Record Office in Kew and read the surgeon's journal of HMS *Theseus*, I found that painful surgery had lost his power to scare. Knowledge, I discovered, is indeed power.

•

What is the point of such a study such as this? Joseph Wilde, the 'comedian' who, lying ill in the Devon and Exeter Hospital, pondered his intent in writing his mock epic *The Hospital*. He wanted, he wrote

T' Explore the depth of human misery
And trace th' extremes poor mortals may endure.

My purpose in examining the experience of painful surgery and the relationships between those who shared its burden in the hope of relief is similar. I hope that it may offer insights into what humanity had encompassed and endured; an awareness of the immense range of human qualities: courage, compassion and nobility, as well as unthinking cruelty, ambition and indifference. Those who entered the operating rooms of early-Victorian Britain were not so different from us. We may see in them ourselves. How might we have responded to the challenges imposed by contemporary surgery, whether as surgeons, students or subjects?

The people with whom this book deals looked and sounded like ourselves but they shared an experience which is almost totally foreign to anything we are likely to encounter. There is in this respect something useful in this enquiry even for those for whom medical history is unfamiliar or uncongenial. Much of recent historical scholarship exhibits a tendency to enquire into the lives of individuals or groups with whom historians of our time find some affinity. Attempting to understand how surgeons could repeatedly bring themselves to inflict pain, even in the cause of healing, demands the exercise of a salutary historical imagination. This is an important corrective. Large numbers of western historians believe that it is impossible to recapture the reality of the past and focus instead on an analysis – albeit often creative, stimulating and valuable – of the evidence and writing about it as if to deny or abandon that reality. This book deals with pain as a reality. People felt and witnessed real pain: we must accept and confront that reality.

Finally then, there is the phenomenon of pain. Drawing upon Martin Pernick's pioneering work *A Calculus of Suffering* we must consider the philosophy and psychology of medicine, particularly in relation to pain, its infliction and endurance. On a more abstract level we must grapple with the culture of pain: the ways in which it has been variously experienced and described, even though nerves and brains before 1846 must structurally be identical to our own. At bottom just as we can witness but never actually share another's pain, it is possible that at the end of an arduous journey we may not in fact be any closer to understanding one of the great facts of the human condition. The experience of pain may prove to be as elusive in scholarship as it was unavoidable in reality. Even so, the attempt is worthwhile and should not be avoided for fear of pain.

Notes

1. [Review of] Hammick's *Practical Remarks on Amputation, Edinburgh Medical & Surgical Journal,* Vol. 34, 1830, 185.

2. J. Duns, *Memoir of Sir James Y. Simpson, Bart.* (Edinburgh: Edmonston & Douglas, 1873), 266.

3. Cock, 'Anecdota Listoniensa', *University College Hospital Magazine,* 1911, 55.

4. Liston case book, December 1845-February 1847, UCH/MR/1/61, UCL.

5. Charles Darwin, (Nora Barlow, ed.), *The Autobiography of Charles Darwin 1809–1882* (London: Collins, 1958), 47–48.

6. *Lancet,* 1830–31, Vol. I, 2.

7. James Paget, *Studies of Old Case Books* (London: Longmans & Co., 1891), 160.

8. William Fergusson, *A System of Practical Surgery* (London: John Churchill, 1846), 31.

9. Victor Plarr, *Lives of the Fellows of the Royal College of Surgeons,* 2 vols (London: Simpkin, Marshall Ltd, 1930), Vol. I, 62.

10. J.B. Cleland, 'Pioneer Medical Men in South Australia', PRG 1384/1, MLSA.

11. Peter Stanley, *White Mutiny: British Military Culture in India, 1825-1875* (London: Christopher Hurst & Co., 1998), 15.

12. Duns, *op. cit.* (note 2), 251.

13. *Transactions of the Intercolonial Medical Congress of Australiasia* (Adelaide, 1887), 122–23.

14. Marion Bell's memoir of her late husband, in George Jospeh Bell, (ed.), *Letters of Sir George Bell* (London: John Murray, 1870), 410.

15. Charles Bell, *Practical Essays* (Edinburgh: Maclachlan, Stewart & Co., 1841), 7.

16. Alexander Peddie, *Recollections of John Brown* (London: Percival & Co., 1893), 14.

17. *The Hospital,* quoted in *The Times,* 16 October 1896, 7f.

18. John Walton, Paul Beeson & Ronald Bodley Scott (eds), *The Oxford Companion to Medicine,* 2 vols, (Oxford: Oxford University Press 1986), Vol. I, 44.

Image Credits

The author and publishers would gratefully like to acknowledge the sources for the following figures included in this book:

I.1   Sir Astley Cooper (1768-1841). Courtesy: *Wellcome Library,* London.

I.2   Robert Liston (1794-1847). Courtesy: *Royal College of Surgeons of England.*

2.1   Joshua Reynolds's portrait of John Hunter (1728-93). Courtesy: *Royal College of Surgeons of England.*

3.1   Charles Bell's depiction of the stages in the amputation of the arm. Courtesy: *Royal Australasian College of Physicians.*

3.3   Amputation and the use of the tourniquet.... Courtesy: *Royal Australasian College of Physicians.*

4.1   The cramped and dark state of a warship's cockpit in battle. Courtesy: *National Maritime Museum.*

4.2   George James Guthrie (1785-1856). Courtesy: *Wellcome Library.*

4.3   The field of Waterloo. Courtesy: *Anne S.K. Brown Military Collection, Brown University Library.*

4.4   Charles Bell's watercolour of Private James Ellard. Courtesy: *Wellcome Library.*

5.2   1808 depiction of a ward in the Middlesex Hospital. Courtesy: *Wellcome Library.*

5.3   The Women's Operating Theatre of Old St Thomas's Hospital. Courtesy: *The Old Operating Theatre, Museum and Herb Garret, 9A St. Thomas Street, London, SE1 9RY, UK.*

5.4   Engraving of Rahere Ward, St Bartholomew's Hospital, 1832. Courtesy: *Wellcome Library.*

6.1   A London medical student in 1840. Courtesy: *Wellcome Library*.

6.2   Thomas Rowlandson's 'The Dissecting Room'. Courtesy: *Wellcome Library*.

6.3   Caricature of James Syme. Courtesy: *Wellcome Library*.

6.4   The Examination of a Young Surgeon. Courtesy: *National Library of Medicine, Bethesda*.

7.1   John Abernethy (1764-1831). Courtesy: *Wellcome Library*.

7.2   Watercolour depicting surgeons performing an operation on an 'R. Power'. Courtesy: *Wellcome Library*.

7.3   Joseph Henry Green (1791-1863). Courtesy: *Wellcome Library*.

8.1   A surgeon with four assistants about to amputate an arm at the shoulder. Courtesy: *Royal Australasian College of Physicians*.

8.3   A caricature lampooning the reaction of Bransby Cooper. Courtesy: *Wellcome Library*.

9.1   'The Danger of the Streets' from *Profitable Amusement for Children*. Courtesy: *British Library*.

11.1 Sir Anthony Carlisle (1768-1840). Courtesy: *Wellcome Library*.

11.2 Charles Bell (1774-1842). Courtesy: *Royal College of Surgeons of England*.

12.1 A photograph of James Syme (1799-1870). Courtesy: *Wellcome Library*.

Bibliography

Archival sources

ALEXANDER TURNBULL LIBRARY, WELLINGTON, NEW ZEALAND
9 MS Papers MAN 1300 Gideon Mantell Papers
 Medical and Surgical papers, 1819–32
 Notes on Medical Cases, 1815–21
MS Papers 4203 Clifford Hughes Papers, 1841–42
MS Papers 0647 Scott Papers, 1825

BRITISH LIBRARY, LONDON
Add. Ms 34928 Nelson Papers
Add. Ms 49172Anonymous account of Fuentes D'Onore
Liverpool Papers Add. Ms 40305; Add. Ms 40371 2
Peel Papers Add. Ms 40344 2

THE HUNTINGTON LIBRARY, SANTA MONICA
Dickens Papers

*LOTHIAN HEALTH SERVICES ARCHIVES, UNIVERSITY OF
 EDINBURGH*
LHB1/ Records of the Edinburgh Royal Infirmary

MITCHELL LIBRARY, STATE LIBRARY OF NEW SOUTH WALES
A3970 William Getty Papers
A4245 Macarthur Papers (Dr John Bowman)
MSS 594/1 Elyard Papers
MSS 846/1 John Gold Papers
MSS 1816 Charles Nathan, 'Charles and Harriet, or The Singing Surgeon'
ML 5-391C James McIntyre Papers

MORTLOCK LIBRARY OF SOUTH AUSTRALIANA, ADELAIDE
PRG V 1008, Testimonials etc. of Dr G.F. Moreton, 1833–46
PRG 502, Journal of Dr John Woodforde, 1836–37
PRG D6912, Certificate of Thomas Hawker
PRG 1384/1, J.B. Cleland, 'Pioneer medical men in South Australia', nd

NATIONAL ARCHIVES OF SCOTLAND, EDINBURGH
Melville Papers, GD51/2/1087

NATIONAL ARMY MUSEUM, LONDON
NAM 9109-86 William Jones Papers
NAM 8202-17 J. McGrigor Papers
NAM 8010-16 John Denny Papers
NAM 7008-11 William Dent Papers
NAM 6807-262-1 Arthur Pine Papers
NAM 6403-17 George Williams Papers
NAM 8807-52 Thomas Maynard Papers

NATIONAL LIBRARY OF SCOTLAND, EDINBURGH
Acc. 3897 Casebook of a Scottish doctor, 1826–27
Acc. 5811 IIa Commonplace book of Andrew and John Johnston, 1797–1817
Acc. 6289/23 Correspondence of Dr John Brown
Acc. 6684; 6690; 8931; 11019 Malcolm Papers
Acc. 9266 Correspondence of Thomas Goldie Scott, 1842–45
Acc. 10000/305 Thomas Buchanan, 'An Essay on the Mode of Inspecting the Human Ear'
Ms 13 Letters on Scottish Affairs, 1810–30
Ms 2778 'Memoranda relating to a visit to London', Charles Anderson, 1793
Ms 3004 'A Correct statement of Mr Robert Todd's education'
Ms 3117 Correspondence of Dr Robert Douglas
Ms 5006 Miscellaneous political manuscripts
Ms 8922 Case book of David Maule, Royal Glasgow Infirmary, 1799–1801
Ms 9236 Correspondence of John Thompson, 1815
Ms 9756 Lady Clementina Malcolm Papers
Ms 9818 Correspondence of Leonard Horner, 1817
Ms 16428 Correspondence of Thomas Graham, Baron Lyndoch
Ms 20311 Letters of Mungo Park [junior], 1819–20
Ms 23118 Correspondence of Sir Walter Scott
Ms 24504 Correspondence of Lord Monboddo, 1787

NATIONAL MARITIME MUSEUM, GREENWICH
NMM ADL/Q/35, John Neill Papers

NATIONAL WAR MUSEUM OF SCOTLAND, EDINBURGH
M.1996.11 George Guthrie Papers

ORIENTAL AND INDIA OFFICE COLLECTIONS, BRITISH LIBRARY
L/MIL/9/372 Assistant Surgeons' Papers, 1820
L/MIL/9/377 Assistant Surgeons' Papers, 1825

L/MIL/9/382 Assistant Surgeons' Papers, 1830–31
MSS.Eur.F 133/1 James Anderson Papers
MSS.Eur.F 133/10 John Boyce Papers
MSS.Eur.E.382 John Colvin Papers
MSS.Eur.F 133/53 Joseph Fitzpatrick Papers
MSS.Eur.D.758 Frederick Loinsworth Papers
MSS.Eur.F 133/99 John Macdonnell Papers
MSS. Eur.D.1036 Reginald Orton Papers
MSS.Eur.D.909 George Spilsbury Papers
Photo.Eur 308 Henry Spry Papers
MSS.Eur.F.133/168 J. Walls Papers

PUBLIC RECORD OFFICE, LONDON

Papers of the Commissioners for Inquiry into Charities
CHAR2/385 Guy's Hospital
CHAR2/386 St Bartholomew's Hospital
CHAR2/387 St Thomas's Hospital

Admiralty records
ADM 13/103 Courts Martial 1803–56
ADM 101/118/1 'Physical and Surgical Journal, HMS Russel, 1797–98
ADM 101/102/8 Surgeon Leonard Gillespie's private diary HMS
    Racehorse
ADM 101/123/2 Journal of His Majesty's Ship Theseus, 1797
ADM 101/120/3 Journal of His Majesty's Frigate Shannon, 1812–13
ADM 101/85/7 Journal of His Majesty's Ship Ardent, 1797–98
ADM 101/125/1 Surgeon's Journal, Victory 1805

Probate records
PROB 12/229 Determinations, Middlesex, 1831
PROB 6/207 Wills, 1831

War Office records
WO71/216-19 Army, Courts Martial, 1808
WO71/182-85 Army, Courts Martial, 1799

ROYAL AUSTRALASIAN COLLEGE OF SURGEONS, MELBOURNE
Journal of Surgical Wards Nos 2, 5 and 6, Edinburgh Surgical Hospital,
    1844
Ms notes of 'Mr Abernethy's Lectures', c. 1809

ROYAL COLLEGE OF SURGEONS OF EDINBURGH
James Duncan Papers
James Simpson Papers
John Robert Hume Papers

ROYAL COLLEGE OF SURGEONS OF ENGLAND, LONDON
NC 1f No. 334 Sir Everard Home's lectures, c. 1811
42.b.13-16 John Abernethy's Lectures on Surgery
42.b.12 Mr Abernethy's Surgical Lectures, 1806
Ms Add. 155 Rowland Fawcett case book, 1823–27
Ms Add 150 Rowland Fawcett Commonplace book, c. 1822
Ms Add 370 Benjamin Brodie receipt books, 1806–28
Ms Add 388 Letters of William Dent, 1808–24
67.b.9 Astley Cooper Papers
42.f.28 Anthony Carlisle lectures, 1818
Box 1(46) 'Pain'
Ms 342-343 J.F. South correspondence, 1801–66
Ms Add 287 George Guthrie Papers
Ms Add 84 W. Fergusson, Statement to the Mangers of the Royal
    Infirmary, 1834
275.g.41-42 Royal College of Surgeons of England, Visitors" book,
    1823–26; 1830–32
Glass Case 333 Benjamin Travers Papers
A4g Minutes of Council, Vol. VIII, 1843–49
Cabinet VI(1) Astley Cooper Papers
330 (16) James Paget, 'Medical students at St Bartholomew's'
330 (33) James Paget, 'Notes on Shock and Reaction'
Ms Add FER 87 & 88 Fergusson *Practical Surgery*, interleaved

ROYAL NAVAL MUSEUM, PORTSMOUTH
RNM Document 1986/537 Wounds and Hurts certificates, 1797–1815
RNM Document 118 Orders and Regulations, HMS *Egmont*, 1794–97
RNM Document 116 Muster List and Order Book, HMS *Active*, 1805
RNM Document 1988/417(2), Orders and Letters of Sir William Beattie
    [sic]
RNM Document 242 Reports of the Medical Commissioner, Physician
    General and Director General, 1822–54

UNIVERSITY COLLEGE HOSPITAL, LONDON, D.M.S WATSON
    LIBRARY
UCH/MR/1 Case books of Robert Liston, 1839–47
UCHOFF/MIN/1/1 Minutes of Medical Committee, 1834–48
University College correspondence
Brougham Papers

UNIVERSITY OF EDINBURGH ARCHIVES
Dc.2.52 Notes on lectures on military surgery
Dc.3.20 Notes from lectures on military surgery, 1846–47
DK.4.23 Notes from the Surgical lectures of Robert Liston
DK.7.46 Cunningham Papers
DK.7.58 'Twenty four hours of my pupilage'

Gen 585 Essay on the excision of the head of the femur, c. 1836
Gen 594 J. Thomson & W. Somerville, Sketches of the wounded at
    Waterloo

WELLCOME INSTITUTE FOR THE HISTORY OF MEDICINE
MS 5817 Journal of H.V Carter
MS 6061 Notebook of R. Jones
MS 6084-95 Liston–Miller correspondence
MS 7147 Diary of an English student
RAMC 394-396 Isaac James Papers
RAMC 484/1-2; RAMC 336 James Elkington Papers
RAMC 630/1-2 Papers of Sir Charles Bell
RAMC 96 'Description of a series of watercolour drawings'
RAMC 95 Bell Waterloo watercolours

Parliamentary Papers

Army Medical Department, PP 1810, Vol. XIV
Report from the Select Committee on Anatomy, PP 1828, Vol. VII, Part 1
Royal Navy Surgeons, PP 1830, Vol. XVIII
Royal College of Surgeons, PP 1833, Vol. XXXIV
Select Committee on Medical Education, House of Commons Papers, PP
    1834, Vol. XIII
32nd Report of the Charity Commissioners, PP 1840, Vol. XIX
Royal Colleges of Physicians and Surgeons, PP 1846, Vol. XXXIII
Report on the Hospitals of the United Kingdom, PP 1864 XXVIII

Contemporary books

John Abernethy, *Introductory Lectures Exhibiting Some of Mr Hunter's
    Opinions Respecting Life Diseases* (London: Longman, Hurst, Rees,
    Orme & Brown, 1819) (RACS)
_____, *Lectures on Anatomy, Surgery and Pathology* (London: James
    Bullock, 1828) (SLNSW)
_____, *Physiological Lectures Exhibiting a General View of Mr
    Hunter's Physiology* (London: Longman, Hurst, Rees, Orme & Brown,
    1822) (RACS)
_____, *The Surgical Works*, 3 vols (London: Longman, 1811)
    (RACS)
Theodore Acland (ed.), *A Collection of the Published Writings of William
    Withey Gull* (London: 1856) (RCPE)
'Dr Aiken & Mrs Barbauld', *Evenings at Home; or, the Juvenile Budget
    Opened* (London: William Milner, 1844) (NLS)
John Aitkin, *A Probationary Essay on Stone in the Bladder and Lithotomy*
    (Edinburgh: 1816) (RACS)

Thomas Alcock, 'An Essay on the Education and Duties of the General
Practitioner in Medicine and Surgery' in *Transactions of the Associated
Apothecaries and Surgeon Apothecaries of England and Wales* (London:
the Society, 1823) (BL)

Rutherford Alcock, *A Summary of the Results Recorded in a Series of Lectures
... on Amputation ...* (London: the Lancet, 1841) (WIHM)

_____, *Notes on the Medical History and Statistics of the British
Legion of Spain* (London: John Churchill, 1838) (WIHM)

W.P. Alison, *History of Medicine* (London: Blackwood, 1833) (RACS)

J. Allison, *Mesmerism: Its Pretensions as a Science Physiologically Considered*
(London: Whittacker & Co., 1844) (NLS)

'An Officer', [David Roberts], *The Military Adventures of Johnny Newcome*
[1816] (London: Methuen & Co., 1904)

Anon, *Motives and Encouragements to Bear Afflictions Patiently ...* (London:
Society for Promoting Christian Knowledge, 1811) (NLS)

____, *Profitable Amusement for Children; or Puerile Tales Uniting Instruction
with Entertainment* (London: Verno & Hood; J.Harris, 1802) (BL)

____, [Mary Stanley], *Hospitals and Sisterhoods* (London: 1854) (BL)

____, *Remarks on a Treatise on the Rectum* (Edinburgh: Stevenson, [1852])
(RACS)

____, *Stories of Waterloo* (London: 1847) (MLG)

James Arnott, *On Neuralgic, Rheumatic, and Other Painful Afflictions*
(London: 1851) (RCSEng)

_____, *The Question Considered; is it Justifiable to Administer
Chloroform ...?* (London: John Churchill, 1854) (RCSEng)

_____, *The Hunterian Oration,* (London: J. Scott, 1843) (WIHM)

John Ashburner, *Facts in Clairvoyance* (London: 1848) (RCSEng)

James Blake Bailey, *The Diary of a Resurrectionist 1811–1812* (London:
Swan Sonnenschein & Co., 1896) (NLS)

William Bainbrigge, *Remarks on Chloroform in Alleviating Human Suffering*
(London: S. Highley, 1848) (RCSEng)

George Ballingall, *A Clinical Lecture delivered to the Students of Surgery in
the Royal Infirmary of Edinburgh* (Edinburgh: A. Balfour, 1827)
(WIHM)

_____, *Case of the High Operation of Lithotomy , in which
Unusual Difficulty was experienced in the Extraction of the Stone*
(Edinburgh: Medico-Chirurgical Society of Edinburgh, 1826)
(WIHM)

_____, *Introductory Lecture to a Course of Military Surgery*
(Edinburgh: Hugh Paton, [1846?]) (WIHM)

_____, *Outlines of Military Surgery* (Edinburgh: A.&C. Black,
1844, 1846) (WIHM/ NLS)

William Mitchell Banks, *The Gentle Doctor* (Liverpool: Lee & Nightingale,
1893) (WIHM)

Benjamin Bell, *A System of Surgery*, 3 vols (Edinburgh: Bell & Bradfute,
1801) (WIHM; RACS)

_____, *The Life, Character and Writings of Benjamin Bell*
(Edinburgh: Edmonston & Douglas, 1868) (RCSEd)

Charles Bell, *The Anatomy and Philosophy of Expression* [1806] (London: J.
Murray, 1844) (NLA)

_____, *A System of Operative Surgery* (London: Longman, Hurst,
Rees, Orme & Brown, 1814) (BLUM)

_____, *Illustrations of the Great Operations of Surgery* (London:
Longman, 1821) (RACP)

_____, *Institutes of Surgery*, 2 vols (Edinburgh: Longmans & Co.,
1838) (ECL)

_____, *Observations on Injuries of the Spine and of the Thigh Bone*
(London: Thomas Tegg, 1824) (BL)

_____, *Practical Essays* (Edinburgh: Maclachlan, Stewart & Co.,
1841) (ECL)

_____, *Surgical Observations* (London: Longmans & Co. 1816)
(RCSEd)

George Jospeh Bell, (ed.), *Letters of Sir George Bell* (London: John Murray,
1870) (BLUM)

John Bell, *The Principles of Surgery*, 2 vols (Edinburgh: T. Cadell & W.
Davies, 1801) (BLUM; RACS)

_____, *Letters on Professional Character and Manners* (Edinburgh: J.
Moir, 1810) (BL)

_____, *Memorial Concerning the Present State of Military and Naval
Surgery* (Edinburgh: Mundell & Son, 1800) (NLS)

Henry Jacob Bigelow, *An Introductory Lecture delivered at Massachusetts
Medical College* (Boston: David Clapp, 1850) (WIHM)

_____, *Surgical Anaesthesia: Addresses and Other Papers*
(Boston: Little, Brown & Co., 1900) (RCSEd)

H. Home Blackadder, *Observations in Phagendaena Gangrenosa* (Edinburgh:
Balfour & Clarke, 1818) (RCSEng)

John Bland-Sutton, *The Story of a Surgeon* (London: Methuen, 1930)
(NLS)

Anthony Brett-James, (ed.), *Edward Costello: The Peninsular and Waterloo
Campaigns* (London: Longmans, 1967)

Benjamin Brodie, (C. Hawking, ed.), *Autobiography*, (London: Longmans
& Co., 1865) (RACP)

_____, *An Introductory Discourse on the Duties and Conduct of
Medical Students and Practitioners* (London: Longman & Co., 1843)
(BL)

_____, *Clinical Lectures on Surgery* (Philadelphia: Lea &
Blanchard, 1846) (WIHM)

John Brown, *Horae Subsecivae* (London: Edmonston & Douglas, 1907)
(ANU)

_____, *Letters of John Brown* (London: A.& C. Black, 1907) (ANU)

_____, *Rab and His Friends & Other Papers & Essays* (London: Dent,
1911) (ANU)

William Burney, *A New Universal Dictionary of the Marine* (London: T. Cadell & W. Davies, 1815) (BL)

J. Burton-Sanderson & J.W. Hulke, *The Collected papers of Sir W. Bowman*, 2 vols (London: Harrison & Sons, 1892) (WIHM)

John Carnochan, *Amputation of the Entire Lower Jaw* (New York: Van Norden & Amerman, 1852) (WIHM)

J.C. Carpue, *An Account of Two Successful Operations for Restoring a Lost Nose* ... (London: Longman & Co., 1816) (BL)

Thomas Castle (ed.), *A Manual of Modern Surgery* ... (London: E. Cox & Son, 1828) (BL)

William Chamberlain, *Tirocinium Medicum, or a Dissertation on the Duties of Youth Apprenticed to the Medical Profession* (London: William Chamberlain, 1812) (WIHM)

Robert Chambers, *A Biographical Dictionary of Eminent Scotsmen*, 2 vols (Edinburgh: Blackie & Son, 1875) (UE)

J.W. Chelius, (trans. and ed. J.F. South), *A System of Surgery*, 2 vols (London: Henry Renshaw, 1847) (WIHM)

Thomas Chevalier, *A Treatise on Gun-Shot Wounds* (London: Samuel Bagster, 1806) (NAM)

Lydia Child, *The Mother's Book* (Glasgow: T.T. & J. Tegg, 1834) (MLG)

J.F. Clarke, *Autobiographical Recollections* (London: J. & A. Churchill, 1874) (ANU)

John Clarke, *Commentaries on Some of the Most Important Diseases of Children* (London: Longman, Hurst, Rees, Orme & Brown, 1815) (RCSEd)

'Clericus', *Remarks on Dr Maitland's Superstition and Science* (London: James Ridgway, 1856) (ECL)

J.C. Colquhoun, *Isis Revelata: An Inquiry into the Origin, Progress and Present State of Animal Magnetism*, 2 vols (Edinburgh: Maclachlan & Stewart, 1836) (MLG)

Andrew Combe, *The Management of Infancy ... Intended Chiefly for the Use of Parents* (Edinburgh: Machlachlan & Stewart, [1840], 1890) (ECL)

George Combe (ed.), *The Life and Correspondence of Andrew Combe, MD* (Edinburgh: Machlachlan & Stewart, 1850) (ANU)

Astley Cooper, *Lectures on the Principles and Practice of Surgery* (London: Edward Portwine, John Thomas Cox, 1824–7; 1835; 1837) (RACS)

_____ & Frederick Tyrrell, *The Lectures of Sir Astley Cooper, Bart.* ... (London: Thomas Tegg, 1824) (RACS)

_____ & Benjamin Travers, *Surgical Essays* (London: Cox & Son, 1818) (RACP)

_____, *The Anatomy and Surgical Treatment of Abdominal Hernia* (London: Longman, Hurst, Rees, Orme & Brown, 1827) (BL)

Bransby Cooper, *The Life of Sir Astley Cooper, Bart.*, 2 vols (London: John Parker, 1843) (RACS)

_____, *Surgical Essays: the Result of Clinical Observations* (London: Longman, Hurst, Rees, Orme & Brown, 1833) (MLG)

Bibliography

Samuel Cooper, *A Dictionary of Practical Surgery* (London: Longman, Hurst, Rees, Orme & Brown, 1829) (RACP)
_____, *The First Lines of the Practice of Surgery* (London: Longman, Hurst, Rees, Orme & Brown, 1840) (RACP); (RACS, 1813)
_____, *Introductory Address to the Students of University College* (London: Longman, Brown, Green & Longman, 1844) (NLS)
George Corfe, *Mesmerism Tried by the Touchstone of Truth* (London: Hatchard & Son, 1848) (NLS)
J. Coster, *Manual of Surgical Operations* (Philadelphia: H.C. Carey & I Lea, 1825) (LC)
Edward Cotton, *A Voice from Waterloo* (London: B.L. Green, 1849) (NAM)
William Sands Cox, *A Memoir on Amputation of the Thigh, at the Hip-Joint* (London: Reeve & J. Churchill, 1845) (WIHM)
_____, *Maingault's Illustrations of the Different Amputations Performed on the Human Body* (London: Barlow, 1831) (WIHM)
George Crabbe, *The Borough* (London: J. Hatchard, 1810) (ANU)
Philip Crampton, *Cases of the Excision of Carious Joints* (Dublin: Hodges & McArthur, 1827) (RCSEng)
James Crichton-Browne, *Victorian Jottings from an Old Commonplace Book* (London: Etchells & Macdonald, 1926) (ECL)
John Green Crosse, *An Inaugural Address, Delivered at the Opening of the Norfolk and Norwich Hospital Museum* (Norwich: Bacon & Co., 1845) (NLS)
C. Cecil Curwen, (ed.), *The Journal of Gideon Mantell: Surgeon and Geologist* (Oxford: Etchells & Macdonald, OUP, 1940) (NLS)
Charles Darwin, (Nora Barlow, ed.), *The Autobiography of Charles Darwin 1809–1882* (London: Collins, 1958) (SLSA)
'Jonathan Dawplucker', *Remarks upon the First Volume of Mr Bejamin Bell's System of Surgery* (London: Robinson, 1799 [?]) (NLS)
William Dewees, *Treatise on the Physical and Medical Treatment of Children* (London: John Miller, 1826) (RCSEng)
Charles Dickens, *The Pickwick Papers* (London: Chapman & Hall, 1857)
_____, *Sketches by Boz: Illustrative of Every-Day Life & Every-Day People*, 'The Hospital Patient' (London: John Macrone, 1836) (BL)
[Samuel Dickson?], *Sir Benjamin Brodie's Doings in Diseases of the Joints and Spine* (London: John Oliver, 1852) (WIHM)
Sydney Doane, *Surgery Illustrated Compiled from the Works of Cutler, Hind, Velpeau, and Blasius* (New York: Harper & Brothers, 1837) (BL)
William Dodd, *The Factory System Illustrated*, [1842] (London: Frank Cass, 1968)
John Syng Dorsey, *Elements of Surgery* (Philadelphia: 1823) (WIHM)
Robert Druitt, *The Surgeon's Vade Mecum* (London: Henry Renshaw, John Churchill, 1851) (BL)
_____, *The Principles and Practice of Modern Surgery* (Philadelphia: Lea & Blanchard, 1842) (RACS)

J. Duns, *Memoir of Sir James Y. Simpson, Bart.* (Edinburgh: Edmonston & Douglas, 1873) (SLSA)

[Charlotte Eaton], *Narrative of a Residence in Belgium During the Campaign of 1815* (London: John Murray, 1817) (NLS)

'L.R.C. P. Edin', *Medical Musings, Grave and Gay* (London: William Stevens, 1907) (ECL)

Edinburgh Eye Infirmary, *Annual Reports,* 1834–45 (ECL)

John Elliotson, *Address Delivered at the Opening of the Medical Session in the University of London* (London: 1832) (NLS)

——————, *Human Physiology* (London: Longman & Co., 1840) (UE)

——————, *Numerous Cases of Surgical Operations Without Pain* (London: H. Ballière, 1843) (NLS)

Ellen Epps (ed.), *Diary of the Late John Epps, MD* (London: Kent & Co., [1875]) (NLS)

John Erichsen, *The Science and Art of Surgery* (London: Walton & Maberly, 1853) (BL)

——————, *Observations on Aneurism* (London: Sydenham Society, 1844) (RCSEd)

——————, *On the Study of Surgery* (London: Taylor, Walton & Maberly, 1850) (NLS)

James Esdaile, *Mesmerism in India and its Practical Application in Surgery and Medicine* (London: Longman, Brown, Green & Longmans, 1846) (ECL)

——————, *Natural and Mesmeric Clairvoyance* (London: Hipployte Ballière, 1852) (NLS)

——————, *The Introduction of Mesmerism ... into the Public Hospitals of London* (Perth: Dewar & Son, 1856) (ECL)

William Falconer, *A Dissertation on the Influence of the Passions on the Disorders of the Body* (London: C. Dilly, 1791) (NLS)

Arthur Farre, *On Some of the Circumstances which have Retarded the Progress of Medicine* (London: John Churchill, 1849) (NLS)

James Fergusson, (ed.), *Notes and Recollections of a Professional Life* (London: Longman, Brown, Green & Longmans, 1846) (NWMS)

William Ferguson, *A System of Practical Surgery* (London: John Churchill, 1846) (RACS)

John Forbes, *Mesmerism True – Mesmerism False ...* (London: 1845) (RCSEng)

John Ford (ed.), *A Medical Student at St Thomas's Hospital, 1801–1802 The Weekes Family Letters* (London: Wellcome Institute for the History of Medicine, 1987)

J. Cooper Forster, *The Surgical Diseases of Children* (London: J.W. Parker, 1860) (RCSEng)

W.E. Frye, *After Waterloo: Reminiscences of European Travel 1815–1819* (London: William Heinemann, 1908) (NAM)

Henry Willam Fuller, *Advice to Medical Students* (London: John Churchill, 1857) (WIHM)

Bibliography

Elizabeth Gaskell, *The Life of Charlotte Brontë* (London: J.M. Dent, 1946)

W.T. Gairdner, *Medical Education, Character, and Conduct* (Glasgow: Maclehose & Sons, 1883) (WIHM)

R.D. Gibney, (ed.), *Eighty Years Ago, or the Recollections of an Old Army Doctor* (London: Bellairs & Co., 1896) (NLS)

William Gibson, *Institutes and Practice of Surgery* (Philadelphia: J. Kay, Jnr & Brother, 1841) (BL)

Mary Gilmore, *Old Days: Old Ways A Book of Recollections* (Sydney: Angus & Robertson, 1934)

William Glover, *Exposure of the Unfounded Statements and Insinuations of a Paragraph in the Caledonian Mercury ...* (Edinburgh: A. Balfour, 1828) (ECL)

Benjamin Golding, *The Origin, Plan, and Operations of the Charing Cross Hospital* (London: W.H. Allen, 1867) (BL)

William Grattan, *Adventures with the Connaught Rangers, 1809–1814* (London: Edward Arnold, 1902)

J.H. Green, *A Letter to Sir Astley Cooper, Bart ...* (London: Sherwood, 1825) (WIHM)

Joseph Green, *Spiritual Philosophy: Founded on the Teaching of the Late Samuel Taylor Coleridge*, 2 vols (London: Macmillan, 1865) (BL)

James Gregory, *Additional Memorial to the Managers of the Royal Infirmary* (Edinburgh: Murray & Cochrane, 1803) (NLS)

_____, *Censorian Letter to the President and Fellows of the Royal College of Surgeons of Edinburgh* (Edinburgh: Murray & Cochrane, 1805) (ECL)

_____, *Memorial to the Managers of the Royal Infirmary* (Edinburgh: W. Creech, 1800) (NLS)

_____, *On the Duties and Qualifications of a Physician* (London: W. Creech, 1805) (WIHM)

William Gregory, *Letters to a Candid Enquirer on Animal Magnetism* (London: Taylor, Walton & Maberly, 1851) (MLG)

H.J.C. Grierson, (ed.) *The Letters of Sir Walter Scott 1815–1817* (London: Constable, 1933)

William Griffin, *An Essay on the Nature of Pain* (Edinburgh: J. Moir, 1826) (RCSEng)

Rees Gronow, *The Reminiscences and Recollections of Captain Gronow*, 2 vols (London: J.C. Nimmo, 1900) (NWMS)

George Guthrie, *Commentaries on the Surgery of the War in Portugal, Spain, France, and the Netherlands* (London: Renshaw, 1853) (NLS)

_____, *On Gunshot Wounds of the Extremities* (London: Longman, Hurst, Rees, Orme & Brown, 1815) (ECL)

_____, *On the ... Operation for the Extraction of a Cataract* (London: W. Sams, 1834) (UE)

_____, *On Wounds and Injuries of the Abdomen and the Pelvis* (London: J. Churchill, 1847) (NLS)

William Augustus Guy, *On Medical Education* (London: Henry Renshaw, 1846) (WIHM)

James Hamilton, *Hints for the Treatment of the Principal Diseases of Infancy and Childhood adapted to the Use of Parents* (Edinburgh: Peter Hill, 1824) (ECL)

Frank Hastings Hamilton, *A Treatise on Military Surgery and Hygiene* (New York: Ballière Brothers, 1865) (NMM)

William Hammond, *Military Medical and Surgical Essays* (Philadelphia: J.B. Lippincott, 1864) (RCSEng)

William Hay, (ed. S.C.I. Wood), *Reminiscences 1808–1815 Under Wellington* (London: Simpkin, Marshall & Co., 1901) (NWMS)

Pat Hayward, (ed.), *Surgeon Henry's Trifles* (London: Chatto & Windus, 1970)

Joyce Hemlow, (ed.), *The Journals and Letters of Fanny Burney (Madame D'Arblay)* Vol. VI, (Oxford: OUP, 1975)

William Ernest Henley, *A Book of Verses* (London: David Nutt, 1888) (NLS)

John Hennen, *Principles of Military Surgery* (London: John Wilson, 1829) (WIHM)

Mitchell Henry, *The Address delivered at the Opening of the Middlesex Hospital Medical College* (London: Mitchell & Son, 1859) (WIHM)

W. Hetling, *Introductory Lectures to the Principles and Practice of Surgery* (Bristol: Bristol Infirmary, 1832) (UE)

William Hey, *Practical Observations in Surgery* (London: T. Cadell Jnr & W. Davies, [1803; 1814]) (BL; RACS)

William Hey (jun), *The Retrospective Address in Surgery* (Worcester: Deighton, 1843) (WIHM)

Christopher Hibbert, (ed.), *The Wheatley Diary: A Journal and Sketch-book kept during the Peninsular War and the Waterloo Campaign* (London: Longman, 1964)

Thomas Hood, *Hood's Own: or, Laughter from Year to Year* (London: A.H. Baily & Co., 1839) (NLA)

_____, *The Poetical Works of Thomas Hood* (London: E. Moxon, 1890) (ANU)

M. House & G. Storey (eds), *The Letters of Charles Dickens* 7 vols, (Oxford: Clarendon Press, 1965-99)

Alexander Hutchison, *Some Farther Observations on the Subject of the Proper Period for Amputating in Gunshot Wounds* (London: J. Callow, 1817) (WIHM)

_____, *Practical Observations in Surgery*, (London: 1816) (WIHM)

Basil Jackson, *Notes and Reminscences of a Staff Officer* (London: John Murray, 1903) (NWMS)

George Jackson, *The Perilous Adventures and Vicissitudes of a Naval Officer 1801–1812* (Edinburgh: Blackwood & Sons, 1927) (NWMS)

J.H. James, *Chloroform versus Pain and Paracentesis of the Bladder* (London: Churchill, 1870) (NLS)

_____, *On the Causes of Mortality after Amputation of the Limbs* (Worcester: Deighton, 1850) (RCSEng)

William James, *A Full and Correct Account of the Chief Naval Occurrences of the Late War between Great Britain and the United States of America* (London: Black, Kingsbury, Parbury & Allen, 1817) (NWMS)

George Jones, *The Battle of Waterloo*, 3 vols (London: John Booth, T. Edgerton, 1817) (NWMS)

G.M. Jones, *On Excision of the Knee Joint* (London: J.E. Adlard, 1854) (WIHM)

George Keith, *Fads of an Old Physician* (London: A. & C. Black, 1897) (RCSEd)

James Kennedey, *Instructions to Mothers and Nurses on the Management of Children* ... (Glasgow: R. Griffin, 1825) (RCSEng)

Robert Masters Kerrison, *Inquiry into the Present State of the Medical Profession in England* (London: Longman, Hurst, Rees, Orme & Brown, 1814) (RACS)

Charles Kingsley, *The Water Babies: A Fairy Tale for a Land-Baby* (London: Macmillan, 1863) (NLS)

[William Lang], *Mesmerism: its History, Phenomena, and Practice* (Edinburgh: Fraser & Co., 1843) (MLG)

James Latta, *A Practical System of Surgery*, 3 vols (Edinburgh: G. Mudie, A. Guthrie & J. Fairbairn, 1795) (WIHM)

Christopher Lawrence & others, (eds), *"Take Time by the Forelock": the Letters of Anthony Fothergill to James Woodforde, 1789–1813* (London: Wellcome Institute for the History of Medicine, 1997)

William Lawrence, *The Hunterian Oration* (London: J. Churchill, 1834) (UE)

Ross Leitch, *Mesmerism in 1845* (Edinburgh, 1845) (RCSEng)

Michael Levien, (ed.), *The Cree Journals: the Voyages of Edward H. Cree, Surgeon R.N.* ... (Exeter: Webb & Bower, 1981)

B.H. Liddell Hart, (ed.), *The Letters of Private Wheeler 1809–1828* (London: Michael Joseph, 1951)

Robert Liston, *Elements of Surgery* (London: Longman, Orme, Brown, Green & Longmans, 1840) (SLV)

_____, *Lectures on the Operations of Surgery* (Philadeliphia: Lea & Blanchard, 1846) (LC)

_____, *Letter to the Honourable the Managers of the Royal Infirmary* ... (Edinburgh: J. Robertson, 1822) (ECL)

_____, *Letter to the Ladies and Gentlemen Contributors to the Royal Infirmary of Edinburgh* (Edinburgh: Balfour & Clarke, 1821) (ECL)

_____, *Letter to the Right Hon. The Lord Provost* ... (Edinburgh: John Robertson, 1822) (ECL)

_____, *Practical Surgery* (London: John Churchill, 1846) (SLV)

John Lizars, *Observations on Extraction of Diseased Ovaria* (Edinburgh: Daniel Lizars, 1825) (WIHM)

_____, *A System of Practical Surgery* (Edinburgh: W.H. Lizars, 1838) (RACS)

_____, *Cases Illustrating the Failure of the Operation of Perineal Section* ([Edinburgh]: 1850 (RCSEd)

_____, *John Lizars ... against James Syme,* July 1852 (Edinburgh: W.H. Lizars, 1852) (WIHM)

_____, *On Fracture of the Neck of the Thigh Bone* (Edinburgh: 1850) (RCSEd)

_____, *Operation for the Cure of Clubfoot* (Edinburgh: W.H. Lizars, 1842) (WIHM)

William Logan, (ed.), *Words of Comfort for Bereaved Parents* (London: Religious Tract Society, 1877) (MLG)

John Macfarlane, *Clinical Reports of the Surgical Practice of the Royal Infirmary* (Glasgow: D. Roberston, 1832) (MLG)

George Macilwain, *Memoirs of John Abernethy,* 2 vols (London: Hurst & Blackett, 1854) (RACS)

_____, *Surgical Observations on the More Important Diseases of the Mucous Canals of the Body* (London: Longman, Rees, Orme, Brown & Longmans, 1830) (NLS)

William Mackenzie, *The Cure of Strabismus by Surgical Operation* (London: Longmans, Orme, Brown, Green & Longmans, 1851) (WIHM)

George Macleod, *Notes on the Surgery of the War in the Crimea* (London: John Churchill, 1858) (WIHM)

John Mann, *Recollections of My Early and Professional Life* (London: W. Rider & Sons, 1887) (ANU)

Thomas Marryat, *Therapeutics or the Art of Healing* (Bristol: W. Sheppard, 1806) (RACS)

'An Invalid' [Harriet Martineau], *Life in the Sick Room* (London: Edward Moxon, 1844) (NLS)

Henry Mayhew, *London Characters* (London: Chatto & Windus, 1881) (ANU)

James M'Grigor, *The Autobiography and Services of James McGrigor* (London: Longman, Green, Longmans & Roberts, 1861) (NWMS)

James M'Queen, *A Narrative of the Political and Military Events of 1815* (Glasgow: [1816?]) (NWMS)

John Mill, *The Use of Clairvoyance in Medicine* (London: 1858) (ECL)

James Miller, *The Principles of Surgery* (Edinburgh: Adam & Charles Black, 1844) (BL)

_____, *A Probationary Essay on the Dressing of Wounds* (Edinburgh: 1840) (RCSEd)

_____, *Supplementary Statement* ([Edinburgh: 1852]) (RCSEd)

_____, *Surgical Experience of Chloroform* (Edinburgh: Sutherland & Knox, 1848) (RACS)

John Millingen, *The Army Medical Officer's Manual Upon Active Service* (London: Burgess & Hill, 1819) (NWMS)

_____, *Curiosities of Medical Experience* (London: Richard Bentley, 1839) (RACS)

Silas Wear Mitchell, *Doctor and Patient* (Philadelphia: J.B. Lippincott, 1888) (BL)

James Moore, *A Method of Preventing or Diminishing Pain in Several Operations of Surgery* (London: T. Cadell, 1784) (RCSEng)

F.G. William Mullar, *Remarks on the Operation of the Perineal Section* (Edinburgh: Robert Seton, 1850) (RCSEd)

W.C.E. Napier, (ed.), *The Early Military Life of General Sir George Napier* (London: John Murray, 1886) (BL)

Florence Nightingale, *Notes on Hospitals* (London: John Parker & Sons, 1863) (MLG)

Drewry Ottley, *The Life of John Hunter, FRS* (London: Longman, Rees, Orme, Brown, Green & Longmans, 1835) (RACS)

James Paget, *Studies of Old Case Books* (London: Longmans & Co., 1891) (BL)

Stephen Paget (ed.), *Memoirs and Letters of Sir James Paget* (London: Longmans & Co., 1902) (RACS)

Joseph Pancoast, *A Treatise on Operative Surgery* (Philadelphia: Carey & Hart, 1852) (LC)

Robert Paterson, *Memorials of the Life of James Syme* (Edinburgh: Edmonston & Douglas, 1874) (SLSA)

John Pearson, *The Life of William Hey, Esq.* (London: Hurst, Robinson & Co., 1822) (NLS)

Alexander Peddie, *Recollections of John Brown* (London: Percival & Co., 1893) (UM)

Thomas Percival, *Medical Ethics, or A Code of Institutes and Precepts ...* (Oxford: J.H. Parker, 1849) (RACS)

Thomas Pettigrew, *Biographical Memoirs of the Most Celebrated Physicians, Surgeons, etc., etc.*, 3 vols (London: Fisher, Son & Co., 1839–40) (RACS)

_____, *On Superstitions Connected With the History and Practice of Medicine and Surgery* (London: J. Churchill, 1844) (RACS)

Amédée Pichot, *The Life and Labours of Sir Charles Bell* (London: R. Bentley, 1860) (SLSA)

Royal College of Surgeons of Edinburgh, *Regulations to be Observed by Candidates ...* (Edinburgh: 1832; 1845) (ECL)

_____, *Plan for the Better Regulation of the Surgical Department of the Royal Infirmary* (Edinburgh: 1800) (ECL)

Royal Infirmary of Edinburgh, *Regulations of the Royal Infirmary* (Edinburgh: 1816) (ECL)

_____, *Regulations respecting Clerks* (Edinburgh: 1816) (ECL)

_____, *Regulations respecting Dressers* (Edinburgh: 1816; 1831) (ECL)

_____, *Regulations respecting Nurses* (Edinburgh: 1816) (ECL)

_____, *Regulations respecting Students* (Edinburgh: 1816) (ECL)

William Robinson, (ed.), *Jack Nastyface: Memoirs of a Seaman* (London: Wayland, 1973)

Edward Sabine, (ed.), *Letters of Colonel Sir Augustus Simon Frazer* (London: 1859) (NLS)

John Scott, *Paris Revisited in 1815* (London: Longman & Co., 1817) (NLS)

J.Y. Simpson, *Account of a New Anaesthetic Agent* (Edinburgh: Sutherland & Knox, 1848) (RACS)

_____, *Anaesthesia in Surgery: Does it Increase or Decrease Mortality?* (Edinburgh: Sutherland & Knox, 1848) (RACS)

_____, *Anaesthetic Midwifery: Report on its Early History and Progress* (Edinburgh: Sutherland & Knox, 1848) (RACS)

_____, *Answer to the Religious Objections Advanced Against the Employment of Anaesthetic Agents* (Edinburgh: Sutherland & Knox, 1847) (RACS)

_____, *Ovariaotomy Is It – or Is It Not – an Operation Justifiable upon the Common Principles of Surgery?* (Edinburgh: Sutherland & Knox, 1846) (RACS)

_____,*Remarks on the Superinduction of Anaesthesia in Natural and Morbid Parturition ...* (Edinburgh: Sutherland & Knox, 1848) (RACS)

Frederic Skey, *Operative Surgery* (London: John Churchill, 1850) (RACS)

_____, *On a New Operation for the Cure of Lateral Curvature of the Spine* (London: Longman, Orme, Brown, Green & Longmans, 1841) (WIHM)

G.C. Moore Smith (ed.), *The Autobiography of Lieutenant General Sir Harry Smith* (London: Constable, 1903) (NWMS)

Henry Smith, *The Improvements in Modern Surgery* (London: John Churchill, 1854) (WIHM)

Nathan Smith, *Medical and Surgical Memoirs* (Baltimore: William A. Francis, 1831) (BL)

Nowell Smith, (ed.), *The Letters of Sydney Smith* (Oxford: OUP, 1953)

John Snow, *On Chloroform and Other Anaesthetics* (London: John Churchill, 1858) (RCSEng)

John Flint South, *Memorials of John Flint South* (Fontwell: Centaur Press, 1970)

Alexander Stewart, *Medical Discipline, or Rules and Regulations for the More Effectual Preservation of Health ...* (London: Murray & Highley, 1798) (RACS)

F. Campbell Stewart, *The Hospitals and Surgeons of Paris* (Philadelphia: Langley, 1843) (BL)

Brian Stuart, (ed.), *Soldier's Glory, being, Rough Notes of an Old Soldier by Sir George Bell* (London: G. Bell & Sons, 1956)

James Syme, *Principles of Surgery* (Edinburgh: Sutherland & Knox, 1842) (RACS)

_____, *Observations in Clinical Surgery* (Edinburgh: Edmonston & Douglas, 1861) (RACS)

John & Dorothea Teague, (eds), *Where Duty Calls Me: The Experiences of William Green of Lutterworth in the Napoleonic Wars* (West Wickham: 1975)

John Thomson, *Report on Observations made in the British Military Hospitals in Belgium after the Battle of Waterloo* (Edinburgh: William Blackwood, 1816) (NLS)

R.M. Thomson and others, *Record of Cases Treated in the Mesmeric Hospital … * (Calcutta: W. Risdale, 1847) (RCSEng)

W. Topham & W. Squire Ward, *Account of a Case of Successful Amputation of the Thigh During the Mesmeric State* (London: H. Ballière, 1842) (NLS)

Transactions of the Intercolonial Medical Congress of Australiasia (Adelaide, 1887) (SLNSW)

Thomas Trotter, *Medicina Nautica: An Essay on the Diseases of Seamen* (London: Longman, Hurst, Rees & Orme, 1804) (NMM)

William Turnbull, *The Naval Surgeon, Comprising the Entire Duties of Professional Men at Sea* (London: R. Phillips, 1806) (NMM)

Jane Vansittart, (ed.), *Surgeon James's Journal* (London: Cassell, 1964)

James Veitch, *A Fasiculus; including Observations on the Ligation of Arteries* (London, 1851) (RCSEng)

_____, *Observations on the Ligature of the Arteries* (London, 1824) (RCSEng)

B.R. Ward, (ed.), *A Week at Waterloo: Lady De Lancey's Narrative* (London: John Murray, 1906) (UE)

James Wardrop, *Aneurism, and its Cure by a New Operation* (London: Longman, 1828) (RCSEd)

Samuel Warren, *Passages from the Diary of a Late Physician*, 2 vols (Edinburgh: William Blackwood, 1834) (NLS)

Patrick Herron Watson, *Introductory Address Delivered at Surgeons' Hall, Edinburgh* (Edinburgh: Edinburgh Medical Journal, 1867) (WIHM)

Charles West, *Lectures on the Diseases of Infancy and Childhood* (London: Longman, Brown, Green & Longmans, 1852) (MLG)

_____, *The Profession of Medicine* (London: Longman, 1850) (WIHM)

J. Wilde, *The Hospital, a Poem in Three Books, Written in the Devon and Exeter Hospital,* (Norwich: Stevenson, Matchett & Stevenson, 1809) (BL)

Arthur Wilson & Muriel Kent (eds), *A Diary of St Helena: the Journal of Lady Malcolm* (London: Allen & Unwin, 1929) (NLS)

Jessie Aitken Wilson, *Memoir of George Wilson*, (Edinburgh: Edmonston & Douglas, 1860) (ECL)

Forbes Winslow, *Physic and Physicians: A Medical Sketch Book*, 2 vols (London: Longman, Orme, Brown, 1839) (UA)

Contemporary articles

'An eye witness', Waterloo, the day after the battle', *United Service Journal*, 1829, Pt 1, 84–92

Joseph Bell, 'The Surgical Side of the Royal Infirmary, 1854–92', *Edinburgh Hospital Reports*, Vol. 1, 1893

F. William Cock, 'Anecdota Listoniensia', *University College Hospital Magazine*, Vol. II, 1911, No. 2

_____, 'Anecdota Listoniensia No. 2', *University College Hospital Magazine*, Vol. II, 1912, No. 3

W.W. Francis, (ed.), 'Repair of Cleft Palate by Philibert Roux in 1819', *Journal of the History of Medicine and Allied Sciences*, 1963, Vol. XVIII, No. 3

W.B. Hodge, 'On the Mortality arising from Military Operations', *Journal of the Statistical Society of London*, Sep 1856

J. Paget, 'What becomes of Medical Students?', *St Bartholomew's Hospital Reports*, Vol. 5, 1869

Contemporary serials

A List of the Officers of the Army, 1793 (NWMS)

A List of the Officers of the Army, 1798 (NWMS)

A List of All the Officers of the Army and Royal Marines, 1815 (NWMS)

Army List of the East India Company's Troops on the Bengal Establishment, 1837, (NAM)

Australian Medical Journal (RACS)

Bengal and Agra Directory, 1850 (NAM)

Bengal and East India Calendar, 1793 (NAM)

Blackwood's Magazine (NLS)

Cornhill Magazine (NLS)

Edinburgh Hospital Reports (ECL)

Edinburgh Medical and Surgical Journal (NLS; WIHM)

Edinburgh Medical Journal (WIHM)

Gentleman's Magazine (NLS)

Glasgow Medical Journal, 1831–33 (MLG)

Guy's Hospital Reports, (RACS)

Illustrated London News (NLS)

Lancet (1823–1900) (ANU; RACS, WIMH)

London Medical Gazette (WIMH)

London Medical and Surgical Journal (WIHM)

Medical Directory (RCSEng)

Medical Times (WIMH)
Original Calcutta Annual Directory, 1816 (NAM)
Punch 1841–50 (ANU)
Reports of the Royal Infirmary of Edinburgh (NLS; ECL)
The Royal Military Panorama (NWMS)
St Bartholemew's Hospital Reports (RACS)
The Scotsman (NLS)
Steel's Original and Correct List of the Royal Navy, London, 1806, 1810
   (RNM;NWMS)
The Times, 1790–1875 (NLA)

Secondary books

James Johnston Abraham, *Lettsom: His Life, Times, Friends and Descendants*
   (London: William Heinemann, 1933)
D. Arnold & A.D. Harvey, *Collision of Empires: Britain in Three World Wars*
   (London: Phoenix, 1994)
Thomas Baillie, *From Boston to Dumfries: the First Surgical Use of Ether in
   the Old World* (Dumfries: Dinwiddie, 1966)
Michael Barfoot, *To Ask the Suffrages of the Patrons: Thomas Laycock and the
   Edinburgh Chair of Medicine, 1855* (London: Wellcome Institute for
   the History of Medicine, 1995)
H. Hale Bellot, *University College London 1826–1926* (London: University
   of London Press, 1929)
G.T. Bettany, *Eminent Doctors: Their Lives and Works* (London: John Hogg,
   1885)
Richard Blanco, *Wellington's Surgeon General: Sir James McGrigor* (Durham:
   Duke University Press, 1974)
J. Blomfield, *St George's 1733–1933* (London: Medici Society, 1933)
Anthony Bowlby, *The Hunterian Oration on British Military Surgery in the
   Time of Hunter and in the Great War* (London: Arnold & Sons, 1919)
J.G. Brighton, *Sir P.B.V. Broke Bart ...* (London: Sampson Lowe & Co.,
   1866)
R.C. Brock, *The Life and Work of Astley Cooper* (Edinburgh: E. & S.
   Livingstone, 1952)
J.M. Bulloch, *Gordon Highlanders Wounded at Waterloo* (Aberdeen: 1916)
Roger Buckley, *The British Army in the West Indies: Society and the Military
   in the Revolutionary Age* (Gainesville: University Press of Florida, 1998)
W.F. Bynum & Roy Porter, (eds), *William Hunter and the Eighteenth-
   Century Medical World* (Cambridge: CUP, 1985)
_____, *Companion Encyclopedia of the History of
   Medicine and Science*, 2 vols (London: Routledge, 1993)
W.F. Bynum, *Science and the Practice of Medicine in the Nineteenth Century*
   (Cambridge: CUP, 1991)
H.G. Cameron, *Mr Guy's Hospital 1726–1948* (London: Longman, Green
   & Co., 1954)

Neil Cantlie, *A History of the Army Medical Department*, 2 vols (Edinburgh: Churchill Livingstone, 1974)

Frederick F. Cartwright, *The Development of Modern Surgery* (London: Arthur Barker, 1967)

A.E. Clark-Kennedy, *The London: A Study in the Voluntary Hospital System Vol. I The First Hundred Years 1740–1840* (London: Pitman Medical Publishing, 1962)

_____, *London Pride: the Story of a Voluntary Hospital* (London: Hutchinson, 1979)

Hubert Cole, *Things for the Surgeon: A History of the Resurrection Men* (London: Heinemann, 1964)

Clarendon Creswell, *The Royal College of Surgeons of Edinburgh Historical Notes from 1505 to 1905* (Edinburgh: Oliver & Boyd, 1926)

Adrian Desmond, *The Politics of Evolution: Morphology, Medicine, and Reform in Radical London* (Chicago: University of Chicago Press, 1989)

_____, *Huxley: From Devil's Disciple to Evolution's High Priest* (London: Michael Joseph, 1997)

Adrian Desmond & James Moore, *Darwin* (Harmondsworth: Penguin, 1992)

Jesse Dobson, *John Hunter* (Edinburgh: E. & S. Livingstone, 1969)

Peter Eade, *The Norfolk and Norwich Hospital 1770–1900* (London: Jarrold & Sons, 1900)

John Elting, *Swords Around a Throne: Napoleon's Grande Armée* (New York: Free Press, 1988)

Mary English, *Victorian Values: The Life and Times of Dr Edwin Lankester* (Bristol: Biopress, 1990)

H.B. Gibson, *Pain and its Conquest* (London: Peter Owen, 1982)

Gordon Gordon-Taylor & E.W. Walls, *Sir Charles Bell: His Life and Times* (Edinburgh: E. & S. Livingstone, 1958)

David Hamilton, *The Healers: a History of Medicine in Scotland* (Edinburgh: Canongate, 1981)

Negley Harte & John North, *The World of UCL 1828–1990* (London: University College London, 1991)

James Henderson, *Sloops and Brigs* (London: Coles, 1972)

J.G. Humble & Peter Hansell, *Westminster Hospital 1716–1966* (London: Pitman Medical, 1966)

Edgar Johnson, *Sir Walter Scott: the Great Unknown*, 2 vols (London: Hamilton, 1970)

Royston Lambert, *Sir John Simon 1816–1904 and English Social Administration* (London: Macgibbon & Kee, 1963)

Harold D. Langley, *A History of Medicine in the Early US Navy* (Baltimore: Johns Hopkins, University Press, 1995)

Christopher Lawrence, *Medical Theory: Surgical Practice – Studies in the History of Surgery* (London: Routledge, 1992)

_____, *Medicine in the Making of Modern Britain, 1700–1920* (London: Routledge, 1994)

Bibliography

_____ & Steven Shapin, *Science Incarnate: Historical Embodiments of Natural Knowledge* (Chicago: University of Chicago Press, 1998)

Susan Lawrence, *Charitable Knowledge: Hospital Pupils and Practitioners in Eighteenth-Century London* (Cambridge: CUP, 1996)

Stuart Legg, (ed.), *Trafalgar: An Eye-Witness Account of a Great Battle* (London: Hart Davis, 1966)

Michael Lewis, *A Social History of the Navy* (London: George Allen & Unwin, 1960)

Christopher Lloyd, *The British Seaman 1200–1860: A Social Survey* (London: Paladin, 1970)

_____ & Jack Coulter, *Medicine and the Navy 1200–1900* (Edinburgh: E. & S. Livingstone, 1961)

Irvine Loudon, *Medical Care and the General Practitioner 1750–1850* (Oxford: Clarendon, 1986)

Leslie Marchand, *Byron: A Biography* (London: John Murray, 1957)

Roderick McGrew & Margaret McGrew (eds), *Encyclopaedia of Medical History* (New York: McGraw-Hill, 1985)

Margaret McNair, *Nursing in South Australia: First Hundred Years 1837–1937* (Adelaide: Nurses' Memorial Foundation of South Australia, 1938)

Victor Medvei & John Thornton, *The Royal Hospital of St Bartholemew (1123–1973* (London: St Bartholomew's Hospital Medical College, 1974)

Alexander Miles, *The Edinburgh School of Surgery Before Lister* (London: A. & C. Black, 1918)

Barry Milligan, *Pleasures and Pains: Opium and the Orient in Nineteenth Century British Culture* (Charlottesville: University Press of Virginia, 1995)

Norman Moore, & Stephen Paget, *The Royal Medical and Chirurgical Society of London, 1805-1905* (Aberdeen: Aberdeen University Press, 1905)

E.W. Morris, *A History of the London Hospital* (London: Edward Arnold, 1910)

A. L. T. Mullen, *The Military General Service Roll* (London: London Stamp Exchange, 1990)

James Mumford, *Surgical Memoirs, and other essays* (New York: Moffat, Yard & Co., 1908)

Charles Newman, *The Evolution of Medical Education in the Nineteenth Century* (London: OUP, 1957)

C. Northcote Parkinson, *Britannia Rules: the Classic Age of Naval History, 1793–1815* (London: Weidenfield & Nicolson, 1977)

Noel Parry & José Parry *The Rise of the Medical Profession: A Study of Collective Mobility* (London: Croom Helm, 1976)

F.G. Parsons, *The History of St Thomas's Hospital, Vol. III, from 1800 to 1900* (London: Methuen, 1936)

Martin S. Pernick, *A Calculus of Suffering: Pain, Professionalism and Anesthesia in Nineteenth Century America* (New York: Columbia University Press, 1985)

M. Jéanne Peterson, *The Medical Profession in Mid-Victorian London* (Berkeley: University of California Press, 1978)

George Pickering, *Creative Malady: Illness in the Lives and Minds of Charles Darwin, Florence Nightingale … [and] Elizabeth Barrett Browning* (London: Allen & Unwin, 1974)

Victor Plarr, *Lives of the Fellows of the Royal College of Surgeons*, 2 vols (London: Simpkin, Marshall Ltd, 1930)

Dorothy Porter & Roy Porter, *Patient's Progress: Doctors and Doctoring in Eightenth Century England* (Cambridge: Polity, 1989)

William Porter, *The Medical School in Sheffield, 1828–1928* (Sheffield: Northend, 1928)

D'Arcy Power & H.J. Waring, *A Short History of St Bartholomew's Hospital 1123–1923* (London: C. Whittingham & Griggs, 1923)

F.N.L. Poynter, *The Evolution of Medical Education in Britain* (London: Pitman Medical, 1966)

———————, (ed.), *The Evolution of Hospitals in Britain* (London: Pitman Medical, 1964)

George Qvist, *John Hunter 1728-1793* (London: W. Heinemann, 1981)

Isobel Rae, *Knox: the Anatomist* (Edinburgh: Oliver & Boyd, 1964)

W.J. Reader, *Professional Men: The Rise of the Professional Classes in Nineteenth Century England* (London: Weidenfield & Nicolson, 1966)

Guenter Risse, *Hospital Life in Enlightenment Scotland: Care and Teaching at the Royal Infirmary of Edinburgh* (Cambridge: CUP, 1986)

———————, *Mending Bodies, Saving Souls: A History of Hospitals* (New York: OUP, 1999)

Ella Hill Burton Rodger, *Aberdeen Doctors at Home and Abroad* (Edinburgh: W. Blackwood, 1893)

Lisa Rosner, *Medical Education in the Age of Improvement: Edinburgh Students and Apprentices 1760–1826* (Edinburgh: Edinburgh University Press, 1991)

G.B. Rushman, N.J.H. Davies & R.S. Atkinson, *A Short History of Anaesthesia: the First 150 Years* (Oxford: Butterworth-Heinemann, 1996)

Elaine Scarry, *The Body in Pain: the Making and Unmaking of the World* (New York: OUP, 1985)

John Shepherd, *Spencer Wells: the Life and Work of a Victorian Surgeon* (Edinburgh: E. & S. Livingstone, 1965)

Eve Blantyre Simpson, *Sir James Y. Simpson* (Edinburgh: Oliphant, Anderson & Ferrier, 1896)

Myrtle Simpson, *Simpson the Obstetrician A Biography* (London: Gollancz, 1972)

F.B. Smith, *The People's Health 1830–1910* (London: Croom Helm, 1979)

Bibliography

S. Squire Sprigge, *The Life and Times of Thomas Wakley* (London: Longmans, 1899)

W.C. Spencer, *Westminster Hospital - An Outline of its History* (London: H.J. Glaisher, 1924)

Peter Stanley, *White Mutiny: British Military Culture in India, 1825-1875* (London: Christopher Hurst & Co., 1998)

Violet Tansey & D.E.C. Meikie, *The Museum of the Royal College of Surgeons of Edinburgh* (Edinburgh: Royal College of Surgeons of Edinburgh, 1982)

H. Campbell Thomson, *The Story of the Middlesex Hospital Medical School* (London: John Murray, 1935)

John Walton, Paul Beeson & Ronald Bodley Scott (eds), *The Oxford Companion to Medicine*, 2 vols, (Oxford: Oxford University Press 1986)

James Walvin, *A Child's World: A Social History of English Childhood, 1800-1914* (Harmondsworth: Penguin, 1984)

S.G.P. Ward, *Wellington's Headquarters: A Study in the Administrative Problems in the Peninsula, 1809-1814* (Oxford: OUP, 1957)

Frederick Watson, *The Life of Sir Robert Jones* (London: Hodder & Stoughton, 1934)

J. Frederick Watson, *The History of Sydney Hospital from 1811 to 1911* (Sydney: W.A. Gullick, 1911)

William White, *Great Doctors of the Nineteenth Century* (London: Edwin Arnold, 1935)

Samuel Wilks & G.T. Bettany, *A Biographical History of Guy's Hospital* (London: Ward & Lock, London, 1892)

Gwen Wilson, *One Grand Chain: The History of Anaesthesia in Australia 1846-1962*, Vol. I, 1846-1934 (Melbourne: Australian and New Zealand College of Anaesthetists, 1995)

T.G. Wilson, *Victorian Doctor, Being the Life of Sir William Wilde* (London: Methuen, 1942)

Alison Winter, *Mesmerized: Powers of Mind in Victorian Britain* (Chicago: University of Chicago Press, 1998)

Geoffrey Yeo, *Nursing at Bart's: A History of Nursing Service and Nurse Education at St Bartholomew's Hospital, London* (London: St Bartholomew's and Princess Alexandra and Newham College of Nursing, 1995)

Agatha Young, *Scalpel: Men who made Surgery* (London: Robert Hale, 1957)

A.J. Youngson, *The Scientific Revolution in Victorian Medicine* (New York: Croom Helm, 1979)

Secondary articles and chapters

S.T. Anning, 'The Practice of Surgery in Leeds 1823-1824', *Medical History*, 1979, 23: 59-95

Anon, 'A Medical Man after Waterloo', *Journal of the Society of Army Historical Research*, Vol. 46, 1968, 124

Myron F. Brightfield, 'The Medical Profession in early Victorian England, as depicted in the novels of the period (1840–1870)', *Bulletin of the History of Medicine*, Vol. XXXV, 1961, 240–53

John Bruce, 'The Footprints of Scottish Paediatric Surgery', *Journal of the Royal College of Surgeons of Edinburgh*, 1976

J.C. Goddard, 'An insight into the life of Royal Naval surgeons during the Napoleonic War', Part 2, *Journal of the Royal Naval Medical Service*, Vol. 78, Spring 1992, 27–36

Lindsay Granshaw, '"Fame and fortune by means of bricks and mortar": the medical profession and specialist hospitals in Britain, 1800–1948', in Lindsay Granshaw & Roy Porter, *The Hospital in History* (London: Routledge, 1989), 199–220

M.R. Howard, 'British medical services at the battle of Waterloo', *British Medical Journal*, Vol. 297, 24–31 December 1988, 1653–56

W.B. Howie, 'Complaints and Complaint Procedures in the Eighteenth- and Early Nineteenth Century Provincial Hospitals in England', *Medical History*, 1981, 25, 345–62

Alastair Johnson, 'The Diary of Thomas Giordani Wright: Apprentice Doctor in Newcastle upon Tyne, 1824–29', *Medical History*, 1999, 43, 468–84

Irvine Loudon, 'A Doctor's Cash Book: The Economy of General Practice in the 1830s', *Medical History*, 1983, 27, 249–68

_____, 'The Nature of Provincial Medical Practice in Eighteenth-Century England', *Medical History*, 1985, 29, 1–32

A.M. McIntosh, 'Surgery in Sydney in the 1830's', *Medical Journal of Australia*, June 1956, 998–1001

F.H. Robarts, 'The Origins of Paediatric Surgery in Edinburgh', *Journal of the Royal College of Surgeons of Edinburgh*, Vol. 14, Nov 1969, 299–315

E.M. Sigsworth, 'Gateways to death?: Medicine, Hospitals and Mortality, 1700–1850', in Peter Mathias (ed.), *Science and Society 1600–1900* (Cambridge: CUP, 1972)

E.M. Sigsworth & P. Swan, 'An Eighteenth-Century Surgeon and Apothecary: William Elmhurst (1721–1773)', *Medical History*, 1982, 26, 191–98

Grainger Stewart, 'Sketch of the History of the Royal Infirmary and the Development of Clinical Teaching', *Edinburgh Hospital Reports*, Vol. 1, 1893

John Harley Warner, 'Therapeutic Explanation and the Edinburgh Bloodletting Controversy: Two Perspectives on the Medical Meaning of Science in the Mid-Nineteenth Century', *Medical History*, 1980: 24, 241–58

John B. Wilson, 'A Surgeon's Private Practice in the Nineteenth Century', *Medical History*, 1987, 31, 349–53

Index

Printed in the United States
by Baker & Taylor Publisher Services